PHYSICAL AC
AND MENTAL HEALTH

The Series in Health Psychology and Behavioral Medicine

Charles D. Spielberger, *Editor-in-Chief*

Byrne, Rosenman   Anxiety and the Heart

Chesney, Rosenman   Anger and Hostility in Cardiovascular and Behavioral Disorders

Crandall, Perrewe   Occupational Stress: A Handbook

Elias, Marshall   Cardiovascular Disease and Behavior

Forgays, Sosnowski, Wrzesniewski   Anxiety: Recent Developments in Cognitive, Psychophysiological, and Health Research

Gilbert   Smoking, Personality, and Emotion

Hackfort, Spielberger   Anxiety in Sports: An International Perspective

Hobfoll   The Ecology of Stress

Johnson, Gentry, Julius   Personality, Elevated Blood Pressure, and Essential Hypertension

Lamal   Behavioral Analysis of Societies and Cultural Practices

Lonetto, Templer   Death Anxiety

Morgan, Goldston   Exercise and Mental Health

Morgan, William   Physical Activity and Mental Health

Pancheri, Zichella   Biorhythms and Stress in the Physiopathology of Reproduction

Sartorius et al.   Anxiety: Psychobiological and Clinical Perspectives

Seligson, Peterson   AIDS Prevention and Treatment: Hope, Humor, and Healing

PHYSICAL ACTIVITY AND MENTAL HEALTH

Edited by

William P. Morgan
Department of Kinesiology
University of Wisconsin-Madison
Madison, Wisconsin

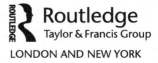

LONDON AND NEW YORK

First published 1997 by Taylor & Francis

2 Park Square, Milton Park, Abingdon, Oxon OX14 4RN
711 Third Avenue, New York, NY 10017, USA

Routledge is an imprint of the Taylor & Francis Group, an informa business

First issued in paperback 2016

PHYSICAL ACTIVITY AND MENTAL HEALTH

This book was set in Times Roman by Brushwood Graphics, Inc. The editors were Christine Williams and Maureen McNally. Cover design by Michelle Fleitz.

A CIP catalog record for this book is available from the British Library.

Library of Congress Cataloging-in-Publication Data
Physical activity and mental health / edited by William P. Morgan.
    p. cm. — (Series in health psychology and behavioral medicine, ISSN 8756-467X)
    Includes bibliographical references

    1. Exercise therapy. 2. Mental illness—Prevention. 3. Exercise—Psychological
aspects. 4. Depression, Mental—Exercise therapy. 5. Anxiety—Exercise therapy.
6. Mental health promotion. I. Series.
RC489.E9P48   1996
616.89′05—dc20   96-20373
                                                                            CIP

ISBN 978-1-56032-365-5 (hbk)
ISBN 978-1-138-99492-8 (pbk)
ISSN 8756-467X

To
Stephen E. Goldston
Former Director of the Office of Prevention
at the National Institute of Mental Health
in recognition of his insights, vision, and
support in connection with the physical activity
and mental health movement.

Contents

PART II PSYCHOLOGICAL RESPONSES
TO PHYSICAL ACTIVITY

Contributors

STEVEN N. BLAIR, P.E.D.
The Cooper Institute for Aerobics Research
Division of Epidemiology and Clinical
  Applications
12330 Preston Road
Dallas, TX 75230

JANET BUCKWORTH, Ph.D.
Sport and Exercise Science Program
Ohio State University
344 Larkins Hall
337 West 17th Avenue
Columbus OH 43210

FRANCIS CHAOULOFF, Ph.D.
INSERM CGF 94-05
Génétique du Stress
Université Bordeaux II
B.P. 10
146 rue Léo Saignat
33076 Bordeaux Cédex
France

ROD K. DISHMAN, Ph.D.
Exercise Psychology Laboratory
Department of Exercise Science
University of Georgia
Athens, GA 30602

ANDREA L. DUNN, Ph.D.
The Cooper Institute for Aerobics
  Research
Division of Epidemiology and Clinical
Applications
12330 Preston Road
Dallas, TX 75230

PAVEL HOFFMANN, Ph.D.
Department of Physiology
University of Göteborg
Medicinaregatan 11
S-413 90 Göteborg
Sweden

DANIEL S. KIRSCHENBAUM, Ph.D.
Center for Behavioral Medicine
Northwestern University Medical School
676 North S. Clair, Suite 1790
Chicago, IL 60611

KELLI F. KOLTYN, Ph.D.
Department of Exercise and Sport Sciences
University of Florida
P.O. Box 118205
Gainesville, FL 32611-8205

EGIL W. MARTINSEN, M.D.
Department of Psychiatry
Central Hospital of Sogn og Fjordane
N-6800 Førde
Norway

WILLIAM P. MORGAN, Ed.D.
Department of Kinesiology
University of Wisconsin-Madison
2000 Observatory Drive
Madison, WI 53706-1189

PATRICK J. O'CONNOR, Ph.D.
Department of Exercise Science
University of Georgia
115 L Ramsey Center
300 River Road
Athens, GA 30602

JOHN S. RAGLIN, Ph.D.
Associate Professor
Department of Kinesiology
Indiana University
Bloomington, IN 47405-4801

ROBERT J. SONSTROEM, Ph.D.
Department of Physical Education,
    Health, and Recreation
Tootell Physical Education Center
University of Rhode Island
Kingston, RI 02881-0810

JOHAN KVALVIK STANGHELLE, M.D.
Sunnaas Rehabilitation Hospital
N-1450 Nesoddtangen
Norway

Preface

Physical activity has been advocated by health scientists and physicians for many years as a means of preventing health problems such as obesity and hypertension, and its therapeutic efficacy has also been extolled following various cardiovascular, musculoskeletal, and hormonal disturbances. It has also been recognized that physical activity has an influence on mental health, and the famous Harvard University psychologist William James stated that "it is pretty well understood now that the result of physical training is to train the nervous centres more than the muscles" (1899, p. 220). While there continues to be an absence of compelling causal evidence corroborating these views, there is strong correlational data in support of a lifestyle that incorporates regular physical activity. In addition to the association between regular physical activity and more desirable health status, a good case can be made for regular exercise on theoretical grounds alone. During the past two decades these views have been extended to include the belief that regular physical activity can also prevent the onset of emotional problems, and there is now limited evidence suggesting that physical activity can be an effective treatment for mental health problems. Survey data have revealed, for example, that many primary care physicians routinely prescribe physical activity for the treatment of anxiety and depression.

Given the pandemic nature of such mental health problems as anxiety and depression—together with the cost and time associated with traditional psychotherapy as well as the cost and potential side effects or after effects of various drugs used in the treatment of these problems—it is important to quantify the psychotherapeutic efficacy of physical activity. It has been reported that 4.5% to 9.3% of women and 2.3% to 3.2% of men in the United States meet the criteria established for major depression at any given point in time (Depression Guideline Panel, 1993), and it has also been noted that the majority of cases go unrecognized and untreated. Furthermore, it has recently been pointed out by Muñoz, Holon, McGrath, Rehm, and VandenBos (1994) that, "most of the major advances in public health have come as a consequence of breakthroughs in the area of prevention rather than treatment" (p. 54). If physical activity were shown to be effective in the primary and secondary prevention of mental health problems, and if there were no significant after effects or side effects, physical activity could become the treatment of choice. There have been attempts to consolidate existing knowledge on this topic, but these efforts have not been comprehensive nor have they attempted to elucidate the potential mechanisms underlying affective improvement.

Because our earlier volume titled *Exercise and Mental Health* (Morgan & Goldston, 1987) was a critical and commercial success, we had considered updating it. Due to developments in the field as a whole, however, it was felt that a new book would be more appropriate. Chapter 2, which deals with the prevention of sedentary patterns of physical activity, has undergone minor revisions because there has not been a great deal of research on this subject since the earlier volume appeared. The chapters dealing with adherence to physical activity (chapter 4) and drug therapy and physical activity (chapter 5) also appeared in the earlier volume, and these chapters have been revised, updated, and expanded. The rest of the material has been written expressly for this publication. The first section of the book deals with general principles involving prevention, prescription, adherence, drug therapy, and various methodological issues that must be taken into consideration when evaluating the efficacy of physical activity. The second section provides a state-of-the-art summary of our knowledge about the effect of physical activity on anxiety, depression, and self-esteem. Chapter 9 in this section deals with the influence of overtraining on mental health, because it is now recognized that physical activity can actually produce some of the very problems it is intended to prevent. This particular paradox, while well recognized in exercise science, has been largely ignored in most contemporary reviews dealing with physical activity and mental health. The final section of the book considers potential or hypothesized mechanisms for the affective beneficence that is noted to follow both acute and chronic physical activity. The endorphin, norepinephrine, serotonin, and thermogenic hypotheses are addressed in this section. These hypotheses are not intended to be exhaustive, but they do seem to be the most compelling and tenable at this point in time. Finally, while these hypotheses are treated independently, it is recognized that psychoneuroendocrinological interaction and redundancy exist.

It is hoped that this book will be valuable to psychologists, physicians, exercise scientists, physical educators, and exercise leaders concerned with the preservation and restoration of health in their students, clients, and patients. This book has been conceptualized and organized in such a way that it will prove useful in courses in which the principal focus involves the influence of physical activity on mental health. Furthermore, it is hoped that this book will serve as a desk reference for health professionals interested in using physical activity in primary and secondary prevention efforts. It should also prove useful to scientists and funding agencies in the development of research ideas and agendas because a number of questions remain unanswered.

Problems of the type addressed in this book are most likely to be solved if approached from a multidisciplinary perspective. All of the contributors have published considerable research on the focus of their respective chapters in refereed journals. This research has been supported by numerous agencies and organizations, and the contributors have acknowledged support where appropriate. Finally, it is our belief that prevention—not treatment—offers the best solution to the pandemic mental health problems that characterize modern society. This book attempts to demonstrate the extent to which physical activity, a nonpharmacological strategy, can be effective in this regard.

Appreciation is expressed to Wendy Dickinson for her expert technical assistance in the preparation of this book, as well as to my doctoral students, Ann Wertz Garvin, Sarah Moss, and Malani R. Trine, for providing thorough support and proofreading.

William P. Morgan, Ed.D., F.A.C.S.M.
University of Wisconsin-Madison

Part One

General Principles

Chapter 1

Methodological Considerations

William P. Morgan

The link between physical activity and mental health is an interesting one that deserves further exploration. However, the efficacy of physical activity in the prevention of mental health problems, as well as in the treatment of psychological problems once they occur, has historically been based on a number of hypotheses that have yet to be confirmed. This book attempts to present an overview of our existing knowledge about physcial activity and mental health, as well as to create a research agenda for the future. Some of the existing research has led to the conclusion that physical activity does not possess affective beneficence, and this has been due in part to the inadequacy of research designs and assessment procedures. Conversely, additional research has been equally problematic, and this work has led to the conclusion that physical activity is not only beneficial, but is a panacea for many emotional ills. It is apparent that much of the existing literature in this area has suffered from a number of methodological shortcomings, and there is a need for experimentation dealing with the conditions under which physical activity will have a positive impact on mental health. It is imperative that future inquiry in this area be approached with rigorous research designs, appropriate and powerful statistical models, and state-of-the-art psychometric methods. There has been a tendency for workers in this field to argue that one model or method is better than another, but it will become apparent as this book proceeds that such debates merely reflect pseudoarguments. In short, the best or preferred method is usually governed by the question being asked. It is also important to recognize that basic, fundamental design principles must be taken into account in order to eliminate or minimize behavioral artifacts, regardless of the method being employed.

It has been emphasized in most earlier reviews that research in this area has been characterized by a number of methodological problems (Folkins & Sime, 1981; Hughes, 1984; Morgan, 1969a, 1970a, 1974, 1984, 1985a; Morgan &

O'Connor, 1988; Morgan, O'Connor, & Koltyn, 1990). As a matter of fact, Hughes (1984) concluded that only 12 of 1,100 published articles involving the influence of physical activity on mental health were acceptable on the basis of selected methodological criteria. According to Hughes the published research in this field is characterized by the absence of randomization, small sample size, inadequate psychological measures, and experimenter expectancy effects, among other flaws. While the rejection of 99% of the published literature in this field probably reflects an extreme position, there have clearly been numerous methodological problems in this area of inquiry. Each of the chapters in this book deals with clinical and research topics that rely on unique investigative paradigms, and each has its own unique methodological issues and problems. The authors deal with those methodological concerns that are unique or specific to the research areas covered in their respective chapters. There are additional methodological issues of a general nature, which are reviewed in this chapter in order to eliminate the need to discuss these general considerations at length in subsequent chapters.

It has been recognized for many years that a number of behavioral artifacts are known to have a direct impact on studies involving psychological outcomes (Rosenthal, 1966; Rosenthal & Rosnow, 1969) and physical performance (Morgan, 1972). In this connection the area of physical activity and mental health is approximately at the same stage of development as the field of psychotherapy was in the early 1950s when Eysenck (1952) published his seminal paper dealing with the efficacy of psychoanalysis versus psychotherapy. While both interventions were found to result in psychological improvement (44% vs. 64%, respectively), it was also noted that "untreated controls" improved in 72% of the cases. Needless to say, this paper raised serious concerns about the efficacy of both psychoanalysis and psychotherapy. A parallel observation was made by Levitt (1971) in an equally instructive paper involving the influence of psychotherapy on children. His review revealed that emotionally disturbed children who received psychotherapy, and those who elected not to receive psychotherapy, had comparable improvement rates.

Eysenck's 1952 paper has been criticized widely because of various methodological problems, but the fact remains that there was simply an absence of compelling scientific evidence in support of these traditional interventions at the time his paper was published. It is probably unreasonable to judge a study that was published more than four decades ago by current methodological standards, and whether or not one finds the results acceptable, Eysenck's paper had the desirable effect of provoking a great deal of needed research. The subsequent four decades of research have improved our understanding of the extent to which psychotherapy can be expected to work, as well as the conditions under which it can be maximized. While the parallel is perhaps not identical, there are several striking similarities with regard to the influence of physical activity on mental health. It is time to move beyond simplistic and unproven arguments of causality and to recognize that much of what passes as fact in this area is, in reality, speculation based on a series of yet-to-be-confirmed hypotheses. There is a need to distinguish between fact and fancy, and this book represents an effort to "set the record straight" to the extent possible. This chapter deals with the methodological principles one must entertain when evaluating existing research, and provides a modest prescription for what needs to be done in conducting future research in the area of physical activity and mental health.

ETHICAL CONSIDERATIONS

Guidelines

The study of psychological outcomes associated with physical activity must be conducted within the guidelines and principles established by professional organizations such as the American Psychological Association (APA), the American Physiological Society (APS), and the American College of Sports Medicine (ACSM). These and related ethical codes are revised periodically, and it is the investigator's responsibility to ensure that all experimental procedures are in compliance with current guidelines. A brief overview of selected guidelines follows.

A number of years ago Beecher (1958) proposed that a prerequisite for experimentation on other humans be the willingness on the part of investigators to first test themselves on the planned intervention. However, self-experimentation may be impractical, and it could be misleading. Beecher (1958) cites the famous medical experiment by Hunter, who inoculated himself in 1767, with gonorrheal pus in order to demonstrate that the disease could be transmitted in this fashion. Unfortunately, he contracted not only gonorrhea, but syphilis as well, and this led to the erroneous conclusion "that gonorrhea and syphilis were merely manifestations of the same disease" (p. 7). At any rate, demonstration that one is willing to undergo an experimental treatment should be thought of as *necessary* rather than *sufficient* evidence that the procedure is safe.

The judgements made by the Nuremberg Military Tribunal regarding experimentation with humans served as the basis for many of the guidelines currently employed, and the 10 points presented in the Nuremberg Code have been discussed by Beecher (1958). Additional guidelines with regard to the rights of human participants were published in the 1964 Declaration of Helsinki, and since 1966 the U.S. Department of Health, Education, and Welfare and the U.S. Department of Health and Human Services (DHHS) have required peer-group approval of all human experimentation funded by the federal government. Institutions receiving federal funding in the United States must also demonstrate that research funded by other sources as well as unfunded research undergo peer review by an institutional review board (IRB) if human participants or animals are involved. In addition, ethical codes pertaining to experimentation with humans and animals have been developed by professional and scientific organizations such as the APA and APS. While this section focuses on issues surrounding experimentation with humans, it is important to recognize that equally rigorous guidelines exist with regard to the use of animals for experimental purposes. It is noteworthy from a general perspective, as well as for this book in particular, that in the 1985 amendments to the Animal Welfare Act, the U.S. Congress ordered the Agriculture Department to "write rules to require, among other things, that universities provide exercise for dogs and improve the psychological well-being of non-human primates" (Burd, 1993, p. 30). One might argue that the U.S. Congress should also order that school districts receiving federal funds be required to provide exercise for the children enrolled in their schools! While it is sometimes difficult to make ethical judgments of proposed experiments, the experience of most IRBs suggests that it is possible, and it is imperative that investigations concerned with the study of physical activity and mental health comply with published ethical standards.

Informed Consent

Informed consent is a rather straightforward matter in many experiments, but the issue can be problematic in certain types of investigations. Several principles should serve as guides to investigators when designing a study. It should be understood that investigators employ informed consent procedures that comply with guidelines published by relevant groups (e.g., IRB, DHHS, APA, APS). There are three basic considerations to be made when requesting informed consent from a potential participant, and this applies to both verbal and written statements. First, the potential participant should be informed of what will be done in the experiment, including the actual procedures and time requirements. It may be necessary to illustrate the actual intervention (i.e., model) in some cases. Second, it should be emphasized that the individual should feel free to discontinue his or her involvement in the study at any point. Third, if there are known side effects or after effects of the planned procedure, these should be made clear when requesting informed consent. Muscle soreness, fatigue, and injuries are certainly possibilities in most exercise studies. A number of overtraining studies have been conducted in recent years, and it is known that overtraining sometimes leads to depression of clinical significance (Morgan, Brown, Raglin, O'Connor, & Ellickson, 1987). Volunteers for experiments involving an overtraining stimulus should be informed of this possibility, and it would seem prudent for investigators to provide treatment should any undesired effects occur. It was once thought that if anxiety neurotics exercised they would experience anxiety and panic attacks because of excess lactate production (Pitts & McClure, 1967). While this view is no longer regarded as valid for all patients suffering from anxiety disorders (see chapter 7), it would still seem appropriate to caution patients with panic disorder about this possible side effect. Stein et al. (1992), for example, reported that 1 of 16 patients with panic disorder experienced panic following submaximal exercise on a bicycle ergometer. Hence, while the likelihood of panic in this patient group is low, the possibility does exist, and it would be appropriate to inform such patients of this potential outcome.

It is possible that a given treatment might result in after effects or side effects that the investigator may not be aware of at the outset of an experiment. While this can make obtaining a true informed consent problematic, there are some safeguards that can be employed. Volunteers for an experiment can be informed that no negative effects are anticipated, nor have any been reported for the planned treatment, but that the investigators will terminate the experiment if any negative effects occur. A study may also need to be terminated because the positive effects (e.g., survival rate) of a given treatment (e.g., aspirin) might exceed those noted for an untreated (e.g., placebo) sample. This actually occurred in the multicenter aspirin trial conducted by the National Institute of Health, and there are numerous other examples of this type in the medical literature.

There are times when it is difficult to obtain valid informed consent from individuals who represent special populations. Individuals who cannot read or who speak a different language, young children, and patients from various diagnostic subgroups (e.g., Alzheimer's disease, depression, schizophrenia, mental retardation) might not understand a verbal or written informed consent statement. It is important that investigators who anticipate conducting research with special populations become familiar with the unique guidelines in place for the population they plan to study.

It is recognized that numerous behavioral artifacts are known to influence investigations dealing with psychological outcomes. Because factors such as demand characteristics, pretest sensitization, experimenter expectancy effects, and the Hawthorne effect (discussed later in this chapter) can have a significant impact on individuals participating in experiments (Morgan, 1972), it is sometimes necessary to deceive the participant regarding the true purpose of a study. However, deception paradigms run the risk of violating certain ethical and legal principles, and it is important that the use of deception be carried out in accordance with established guidelines. This will usually include a debriefing session following completion of the study in which participants are informed of the true purpose of the study and provided with a summary of the findings if desired.

While it is imperative that volunteers for a study be informed of its general purpose, it is not necessary that they be informed of the investigator's actual working hypothesis. Indeed, there is compelling evidence that compliant volunteers will respond to an intervention on the basis of what Orne (1962) has labeled "demand characteristics." This phenomenon, along with other behavioral artifacts, are reviewed in the next section.

RESEARCH STRATEGIES

Acute and Chronic Physical Activity

It is important for several reasons that attempts to describe, predict, or explain the psychological outcomes of physical activity make a clear distinction as to whether or not the nature of a given intervention involves an acute or chronic stimulus. First, psychological benefits that result from a single episode (acute) may not be demonstrable across time (e.g., 10 weeks or longer; chronic). That is, the sense of well-being and enhanced mood experienced following a single bout of physical activity may be episodic, and this transitory affective state may return to baseline levels within hours. Hence, a given level of baseline mood state may remain the same following chronic physical activity over several months. Conversely, it is possible that acute physical activity has little or no influence on a specific psychological construct (e.g., self-esteem), but this same variable may improve following chronic physical activity.

Throughout this book *acute physical activity* is regarded as those interventions ranging in time from 10 to 15 min through several hours. Psychological changes in such cases will typically involve those taking place during a single bout of physical activity as well as those occurring in the minutes and hours following a single episode. *Chronic physical activity* is viewed as acute episodes repeated at least several times per week for months or years.

State-Trait Measures

It has been shown that psychological constructs such as anxiety are best conceptualized as states (situational) or traits (enduring dispositions). The most frequently employed anxiety model (Spielberger, 1983) in use today, for example, is based on this conceptual distinction (see chapter 7). Conversely, some psychological constructs such as extroversion-introversion and neuroticism-stability are viewed as stable dimensions of personality (Eysenck & Eysenck, 1975). It has been shown, for example, that these *traits* change very little in marathon runners tested over a 25-year period (Morgan & Costill, 1996). One would not expect traits to change following acute physical activity, and it is even unlikely that substantial changes would occur commonly following most chronic interventions. Theoretically therefore, it would be more productive to use traits as predictor variables. Trait anxiety, for example, has been found to be a good predictor of state anxiety responses when employed in research paradigms designed to provoke state anxiety (Morgan & Raven, 1985; Spielberger, 1983). Another commonly employed trait in exercise and sport psychology is self-motivation, which is effective in predicting exercise adherence (Dishman, Ickes, & Morgan, 1980). Spielberger's model of anxiety predicts that state anxiety will increase following various physical and mental stressors, and this has been shown to occur in a variety of settings (Spielberger, 1972, 1983, 1989; Morgan & Ellickson, 1989; Raglin, 1992). Finally, while state anxiety has been shown to decrease predictably following physical activity, trait anxiety is not influenced following single bouts of exercise (Morgan, 1973c; see chapter 7). It is important that investigators employ psychological states and traits within the theoretical framework in which these constructs have been conceptualized and developed.

Prescription of Physical Activity

The prescription of physical activity is addressed in chapter 3, as well as in guidelines published by the ACSM and in those jointly published by the Centers for Disease Control (CDC) and ACSM by Pate et al. (1995). Factors to be considered in developing an exercise prescription for clinical or research purposes consist of the *mode* (e.g., walking vs. running), *duration* (e.g., minutes or hours), *frequency* (e.g., times per day or week), and *intensity* (e.g., metabolic demand). The issue of intensity represents the element in any physical activity equation that is currently the most debated. Pate et al. (1995) pointed out that one must first decide the objective before establishing the intensity, and this point is reinforced by Dunn and Blair (chapter 3). That is, health benefits have been shown to occur with habitual physical activity performed at low to moderate metabolic demands, whereas performance must be at a higher intensity if improvement in physical fitness is desired.

There has been a gradual move away from the use of rigid formulae based on a percentage of an individual's VO_2max or heart rate reserve. However, this literature has been based in large part on physiological markers, and there is not a great deal known about psychological outcomes associated with physical activity performed at lower metabolic levels. However, there is limited evidence that gains in physical performance can be greater when exercise intensity is based on "perceived" exertion (Borg, 1973; Morgan & Borg, 1976) as opposed to heart rate (Koltyn & Morgan, 1992b). It has also been shown that the "preferred" intensity (i.e., 75% of VO_2max) of experienced distance runners (Morgan, 1994a) may differ from the intensities often employed (e.g., 60% or 80% of VO_2max) in exercise studies. There are also several reports indicating that preferred exercise intensity is higher in extroverts compared with introverts (Morgan, 1973a, 1994a), and this observation is congruent with Eysenckian theory (Eysenck & Eysenck, 1975). At any rate, the related issues of perceived and preferred exertion need to be considered in future research. It is quite probable that investigators who ask participants in research studies to exercise at their *customary* or *preferred* level of intensity would be more likely to observe positive psychological outcomes than would investigators who require all individuals to exercise at the same relative intensity (e.g., 70% of VO_2max), because the latter (i.e., nonpreferred) might be perceived as aversive. That is, a given relative intensity might be too low for some individuals and too high for others, and rigid prescriptions of this nature theoretically would not facilitate exercise adherence (see chapter 4).

One additional matter that has not received adequate attention in the past relates to the possible role of circadian rhythms during exercise states. There is some evidence of an interaction between exercise intensity and the time of day at which exercise is performed. It has been reported by Hill, Cureton, and Collins (1989) that exercise performed at intensities below the ventilatory threshold was characterized by similar ratings of perceived exertion in the morning and afternoon. However, exercise performed at intensities above the ventilatory threshold was perceived as lower in the morning. Furthermore, these investigators reported that 20% of the differences in effort sense was due to lower ventilatory demands in the morning. These results have implications for the prescription of exercise because perceived exertion is known to be correlated with variables such as anxiety, depression, neuroticism, and extroversion (Morgan, 1994a).

Threshold Effects

It has been shown that physical activity can have undesirable psychological effects when performed to excess (Morgan et al., 1987; Morgan, Costill, Flynn, Raglin, & O'Connor, 1988). This problem is referred to as *overtraining*, and the resulting syndrome has been termed *staleness* in the field of sports medicine. Excessive training and its undesired psychological consequences are discussed in detail in chapter 9.

There is also reason to believe that some individuals become dependent on or addicted to physical activity (Morgan, 1979a). This particular problem has also been described as *obsessive-compulsive behavior* by Polivy (1994). However, there is an absence of epidemiological research involving this dark side of physical activity, and the nature of this apparent self-imposed abuse is not well understood. It is not surprising, however, that physical activity might become counterproductive when pursued to extremes.

Nature of the Individual

It is well established in the field of psychology that behavior and psychological outcomes following interventions are governed to a large degree by individual differences. This same principle is also recognized in the field of exercise science, but clinical and research applications are often made without taking this into account. It has been customary, for example, to administer tests of maximal aerobic power to groups of individuals and then require these individuals to perform physical activity at a relative intensity such as 70% of VO_2max. The problem with this approach is that these individuals differ widely on psychological variables such as anxiety, depression, extroversion, and neuroticism, and it is known that perceived exertion, preferred exertion, and pain perception are all correlated with these psychometric variables (Morgan, 1973a, 1994a; Morgan & Horstman, 1978). Furthermore, individuals also differ on a wide variety of physiological variables such as muscle fiber types in exercising muscle, lactate threshold, percent body fat, and so on. In other words, there has been a tendency in exercise science research to match participants in experiments on a single metabolic variable (i.e., relative percent of VO_2max) and to permit a host of equally relevant psychological and physiological variables to remain uncontrolled. This practice, of course, can only be defended on the grounds that such an approach is the most convenient, and the time has come to consider the adoption of alternative clinical and research paradigms. The "lifestyle" approach discussed in chapter 3 offers one such alternative.

Future research should take both the individual's psychological and physiological profiles into account, and while it may be possible to defend a single exercise prescription for all individuals (e.g., 70% of VO_2max), it would make more sense to anchor prescriptions of physical activity on the *hedonic* side of the hedonia-anhedonia continuum. In other words, it does not make sense to employ aversive physical activity, and then conclude that physical activity per se does not lead to positive psychological outcomes. Also, because this is, in fact, commonly practiced in many exercise programs, it is not surprising that many individuals drop out of exercise programs.

There is some research in this area that has failed to demonstrate that physical activity leads to positive psychological outcomes. One of the obvious reasons for such a finding has been that participants in many of these studies have scored in the normal range on various psychological measures such as anxiety and depression. Actually, it would be remarkable to find that an individual who scored in the normal range at the outset of a physical activity program were to experience a reduction in anxiety and depression. Hence, it is not surprising that investigators have failed to observe anxiolytic or antidepressant effects, or both, with such samples. Conversely, investigations carried out with clinically depressed individuals, for example, have shown consistently that an antidepressant effect occurs following a program of physical activity (see chapter 6). There is also limited evidence that a single exercise session can lead to improved mood and reduced depression in college students who are classified as depressed, and exercise intensities of 40%, 60%, and 80% of maximum were found to be equally effective (Nelson & Morgan, 1994). However, this effect has not been noted for individuals who score in the normal range on measures of anxiety and depression (Morgan, Roberts, & Feinerman, 1971). These findings lead to the conclusion that outcomes are dependent in part on the psychological nature of the individual being studied.

Control Comparisons

It is important that investigations concerned with the psychological outcomes of physical activity include a control condition or control group for comparative purposes. It has also been emphasized by Isaac and Michael (1995) that individuals who serve as members of a control group "should experience *all things* in common with the treatment group *except* the critical factor, per se" (p. 93). This particular design feature is often overlooked in research dealing with the influence of physical activity on psychological outcomes. McGowan, Pierce, and Jordan (1991) reported, for example, that a single bout of physical activity resulted in improved mood whereas no change in mood state was observed in a control group. However, the control group attended a lecture and took a quiz while the other subjects took part in physical activity. It is possible that the lecture or the quiz provoked state anxiety (Spielberger, 1983) or suppressed the usual reduction in anxiety known to accompany "no treatment" control conditions (see chapter 7).

There are many other examples of inadequate control groups in this area of inquiry, and it almost appears as though investigators sometimes employ "straw-person" designs that have been developed in such a way that physical activity interventions are assured of being superior to control treatments. Rather than randomly selecting or assigning participants to control groups, there has been a tendency to use intact, readily available, "convenience" samples in much of this work. Likewise, it is not only common for the control period to differ in critical ways such as time of exposure, but control groups have sometimes been administered treatments that conceivably could have anxiolytic effects. Subjects in control groups have been instructed to employ imagery (e.g., imagine that you are running), and imagery of exercise can actually result in metabolic and perceptual effects (Wang & Morgan, 1992).

The use of a control group should be viewed as a *necessary* rather than a *sufficient* design requirement, and it is often preferable to include a traditional treatment such as psychotherapy, biofeedback, or hypnotherapy for the purpose of drawing comparisons. Use of a comparison treatment has the advantage of overcoming the problem of "any" versus "no" treatment. In other words, the question of whether or not physical activity results in psychological improvement should be expanded to include the question of "compared to what"? An example of such an approach is the study by Greist et al. (1979), who compared running therapy with two forms of traditional psychotherapy, and found the running intervention to be equivalent to one form of psychotherapy and superior to the other. While a strict control group is often inadequate for quantifying the efficacy of a given intervention, the use of traditional treatments for comparison purposes can be problematic. Nevertheless, it is important to ask the question, "compared to what," when evaluating the efficacy of physical activity. This is one of the reasons why placebo groups have been employed in drug (Boshes, 1960) and surgical (Cobb, Thomas, Dillard, Merendino, & Bruce, 1959) studies for many years. Indeed, there have been cases in which both experimental drugs and surgical procedures (Cobb et al., 1959) have been found to be no more effective than a placebo.

The importance of employing placebo treatments where possible is explored in a subsequent section. Unfortunately, it is sometimes difficult to create an adequate placebo treatment, and some investigators have elected to employ control treatments and groups in which the participants are either passive or relatively inactive from a physical standpoint. Bahrke and Morgan (1978), for example, randomly assigned 75 adult men to 20 min of aerobic exercise (treadmill walking), noncultic meditation (Benson, 1975), or a no-treatment control group in which participants rested quietly in a sound-dampened chamber (8 dB). Since the no-treatment control group was monitored physiologically, and in a sense received "special attention," this can be regarded as a placebo treatment. Each group experienced a significant reduction in state anxiety that was comparable among the three groups. This finding resulted in formulation of the "distraction hypothesis," which suggests that reduced anxiety following acute physical activity may be due in part to distraction from the cares and worries of the day that is afforded by exercise. While some authors have interpreted or classified this observation as a psychological effect, it has also been shown that comparable periods of quiet rest also lead to a significant reduction in plasma epinephrine and norepinephrine levels (Michaels, Huber & McCann, 1976).

A similar placebo group has been used in exercise research reported by Raglin and Morgan (1987), who replicated and extended the earlier observations by Bahrke and Morgan (1978). The anxiolytic effect was comparable following exercise and quiet rest, but the effect persisted for a longer period of time following exercise. Another approach consists of using a minimal exertion group (e.g., horseshoes, shuffleboard) in addition to a control group for comparison purposes (Morgan & Pollock, 1978). This type of treatment probably comes closer to a true placebo. It is important that investigators consider the influence of treatments that result in distraction, as well as the special attention (i.e., Hawthorne) effect when evaluating the efficacy of physical activity. Some form of comparison exceeding that of an untreated control is needed, and this issue is explored further in the section dealing with the Hawthorne effect.

Summary

Although it seems reasonably clear that physical activity is *associated* with positive psychological outcomes, it is equally clear that much of the published literature in this field has been characterized by various methodological problems. Furthermore, while it is often implied, and sometimes stated explicitly, that this *association* reflects a *causal* link, there is an absence of scientific evidence in support of casualty. The nature of causal explanation in psychology has been addressed effectively by Moore (1984). This book has been structured in such a way that causal attributes might be elucidated in future research. There are a number of research strategies that have been employed by investigators in this field, and it is apparent that psychological outcomes are dependent in part on factors such as (a) the use of acute and chronic physical activity paradigms, (b) the use of state and trait measures, (c) the prescription of physical activity, (d) threshold effects, (e) the nature of the individual being studied, and (f) the type of control group or condition employed. All of these factors must be taken into account in both evaluating existing research and planning future investigations and clinical interventions. There are also a number of additional methodological issues dealing with research design that must be considered in conducting research involving the psychological outcomes of physical activity, and these are reviewed next.

BEHAVIORAL ARTIFACTS

Volunteerism

It has been recognized for many years that the phenomenon known as "volunteerism" can be a significant problem in behavioral research (Rosenthal & Rosnow, 1975). It can also be equally problematic in biological research, but this problem has been largely ignored in exercise and sport science. This is somewhat surprising because exercise scientists often rely on small samples of 5 to 6 individuals who are often unique in a number of ways. At any rate, by virtue of the fact that investigators should employ an informed consent procedure, potential participants are free to accept (i.e., volunteer) or reject (i.e., nonvolunteer) a researcher's invitation to take part in a study. Furthermore, it is known that a subset of those who volunteer to take part in studies never report to the test site (i.e., pseudovolunteer). The usual criticism of investigations that are biased because volunteers were studied fails to address the difficulty associated with the alternative approach: An investigator would certainly be criticized for using *nonvolunteers*! In other words, for most of the research that is conducted in the area of physical activity and mental health, one must rely on the use of volunteers.

A good example of the problem that can arise from volunteerism was presented by Rohles, Nevins, and Springer (1967), who hypothesized that thermal stress tolerance is governed in part by the individual's level of trait anxiety. These investigators administered the Taylor Manifest Anxiety Scale to a large number of volunteers, and identified those individuals with the lowest ($N = 35$) and highest ($N = 35$) levels of trait anxiety. They next invited all of these individuals to volunteer for a study involving thermal stress in order to quantify the response patterns of groups differing in trait anxiety. These investigators were unable to test their anxiety hypothesis because *all* of the low-anxiety individuals, but *none* of the high-anxiety individuals, volunteered to be in the study. It is possible that much of the literature involving heat stress physiology can only be generalized to the low-anxiety end of the continuum, and it is also possible that little or nothing can be said about the response patterns of individuals with high trait anxiety—the group most likely to have stress responses when exposed to heat or other stressors.

The main question should be whether or not the sample of volunteers employed in a given study is representative of the target population about whom one hopes to generalize. If it can be shown, for example, that the volunteers for a given study are representative of the target population on the parameter or parameters of interest, the study can be said to possess generalizability or external validity. This principle may seem so obvious that it does not warrant attention, but the published literature demonstrates that this point is often ignored. It should be apparent that physical activity research carried out with depressed patients cannot be generalized to other patient groups or to normal individuals, and the converse generalization should not be made either. Furthermore, research findings derived from inpatient populations do not necessarily apply to outpatient groups and vice versa.

It is also possible for a given experiment to lack what has come to be known as "ecological validity." Orne (1962) has defined ecological validity as "appropriate generalization from the laboratory to nonexperimental situations" (p. 776). This is an important issue because many behavioral scientists believe that variables always change when they are studied in the laboratory. In other words, a study might possess good "internal validity" but lack generalizability from the laboratory to the field setting where application of results is often desired.

Summary   There is considerable evidence that volunteers for experiments differ psychologically from nonvolunteers and pseudovolunteers (Morgan, 1972; Rosenthal & Rosnow, 1975). It has also been reported that volunteers may be more responsive to demand characteristics than nonvolunteers. In addition, it is also known that perception of effort and physical performance are correlated with selected psychological states and traits (Morgan, 1973a, 1973b, 1985c, 1994a). For these reasons, it is very important that the generalizability of results in selected experiments dealing with the psychological outcomes of interventions such as exercise be restricted to the population from which the sample was drawn.

Experimenter Expectancy Effects

There are three types of experimenter expectancy effects, and while their results are comparable, they differ in unique ways. The experimenter effect that is most widely recognized is known as the *halo effect*, which was first described by Thorndike (1920). The halo effect involves the tendency of a rater to ascribe positive or negative attributes to the ratee on the basis of his or her knowledge about the participant's role (e.g., experimental or control group) in a given study. In other words, the experimenter rates a given outcome as higher or lower than it actually is because of the positive or negative "halo." A related problem involves what has come to be known as the *Rosenthal effect* (Rosenthal, 1966), which results from the participant actually scoring higher or lower because of the experimenter's expectancy. The third problem is due to what Orne (1962) has labeled *demand characteristics*. A brief summary of each of these artifacts follows.

Halo Effect   It has been recognized for many years that raters have a tendency to ascribe certain qualities to the ratee on the basis of other known characteristics of that person. In other words, it is difficult for even the most objective rater to evaluate an individual on one quality independent of his or knowledge about other qualities possessed by the person being rated. This constant error can be substantial, and it was first described by Thorndike (1920), who labeled it the "halo" effect. The error can be either negative or positive, depending on the ratee's status, and therefore, the rater should be unaware (i.e., blinded) of the individual's other qualities when performing assessments. This principle should be applied not only when projective psychological measures such as the Rorschach test or objective measures such as the Minnesota Multiphasic Personality Inventory (MMPI) are employed, but also where objective physiological measures are concerned. Investigators and technicians who record and analyze the electroencephalogram (EEG) of human test subjects or the brain tissue of animals, for example, should not be aware of group affiliation. In other words, the principle of blinding applies to collection and analysis of both "hard" and "soft" data.

Application of this principle is particularly important in studies in which investigators are evaluating the psychological or physiological outcomes, or both, of an exercise program. In other words, the evaluator should not be aware of the individual's diagnostic status (e.g., depressed, anxious, normal), nor should he or she be aware of the individual's group affiliation (e.g., experimental, control, placebo). If the rater is aware of the individual's diagnostic or treatment status, it is quite possible for a negative or positive halo to influence the assessment in an intentional or unintentional way. The magnitude of this error usually increases as one proceeds from objective to subjective measures. Hence, investigations should be designed in such a way that the rater(s) responsible for measuring the dependent variable(s) is unaware of the ratee's other attributes (e.g., treatment received). This principle is applied routinely when evaluating the efficacy of various drugs in the treatment of psychological disorders, and efforts are usually made in drug studies to ensure that neither the person providing the drug (e.g., investigator, physician, nurse) nor the individual receiving the drug (e.g., patient) is aware of the substance's (e.g., pill, capsule, injection) actual content (e.g., placebo, experimental drug, control drug). The necessity of employing double-blind paradigms will be explored in the discussion involving the Hawthorne effect.

Rosenthal Effect   The experimenter expectancy effect described by Rosenthal (1966) suggests that an individual or group of individuals can actually score higher or lower on a particular outcome measure because of the expectancies communicated to them by the clinician or experimenter. This can be thought of as a "self-fulfilling prophecy" in the sense that a teacher, for example, might expect children classified as possessing high, average, and low scores on a standard IQ test to perform at differential levels academically. Rosenthal (1966) presents numerous examples from educational, industrial, and clinical settings that confirm the impact of experimenter expectancy on various outcome measures. It is not always clear whether expectancies are communicated in an intended or unintended manner, but it would be reasonable to predict that antidepressant or anxiolytic effects, or both, would be more likely to occur following physical activity when the clinician or investigator expects such an effect to take place. This outcome, however, would be the result of the participant in such a study actually scoring lower on a measure of depression or anxiety, rather than the experimenter rating the person as being improved because of the halo effect.

Demand Characteristics   Not only do investigations dealing with experimenter effects demonstrate the possibility that experimenters communicate (intentionally or unintentionally) expectancies to the individual being tested, but such studies also reveal that participants are not passive receivers of stimuli. Orne (1962) has likened the participant's performance in a study to problem-solving behavior, in which the individual tries to determine the true purpose of the study, and he or she responds in accordance with the perceived hypothesis. The totality of cues responsible for communicating the experimental hypothesis to the participant are referred to as "demand characteristics" (Orne, 1962). Orne also pointed out that demand characteristics are more likely to have an impact when subtle as opposed to obvious cues are given. It almost seems as though obvious cues are not as believable to the test subject.

It would not be difficult to imagine that individuals participating in an exercise program for 30 min/day, 3 to 5 days per week for 20 weeks or longer would be influenced by demand characteristics. While the underlying hypothesis might not be stated explicitly to participants in such a study, it is quite likely that the administration of questionnaires designed to measure mood states before and after such an intervention would generate expectancies. Likewise, because most self-report questionnaires are quite transparent, it would be easy for participants to distort their responses. This is one reason why investigators must make an effort to determine whether or not baseline or posttest augmentation or suppression occurs. While debriefing during postexperimental interviews can sometimes serve to quantify the extent to which demand characteristics may have operated in a given experimental milieu, this is not always effective. Indeed, Levy (1967) conducted an experiment in which a confederate actually provided participants with the working hypothesis, but 75% of the individuals would not admit to prior knowledge during the debriefing that followed the experiment. It has been pointed out by Evans (1968) that postexperimental interviews are influence by the "pact of ignorance" that implicitly exists between the investigator and the participant in the experiment. Evans (1968) has suggested that participants in studies often deduce more information about the experimental hypothesis than they should, and investigators just as often prefer not to be aware of this. In other words, there is a tendency for both the investigator and participant to want the experiment to "work," or have a successful outcome.

It has been demonstrated by Desharnais, Jobin, Coté, Lévesque, and Godin (1993) that improvement in self-esteem occurs following an exercise program when the exercisers are led to believe that such an effect will occur. However, these investigators did not observe improved self-esteem in a control group that did not have an expectancy created regarding enhanced self-esteem, even though the control group performed the same type of exercise and experienced a significant gain in aerobic power. It is quite clear that investigators must make every attempt to minimize the influence of demand characteristics in studies designed to quantify the influence of physical activity on psychological states and traits.

The Hawthorne Effect

The behavioral artifact known as the Hawthorne effect is based on the tendency for participants in experiments to improve following the manipulation of a selected independent variable (e.g., drug, exercise, placebo) simply because of the "special attention" associated with the treatment. The Hawthorne effect can be thought of as the influence resulting from *any* versus *no* treatment. In other words, improved mood states following a given intervention such as exercise or psychotherapy might simply reflect an improvement resulting from the special attention afforded by the intervention. Furthermore, the observation that such a treatment exceeds the effects noted for an untreated control group is not very profound because this would merely suggest that the intervention is "better than nothing." Again, one can never be confident that psychological outcomes in such circumstances result from any treatment versus no treatment.

The experimental contaminant known as the Hawthorne effect is based on the famous experiment carried out at the Hawthorne Plant of the Western Electric Company in Chicago. The investigation was conducted by the Western Electric Company in connection with the National Research Council, and the initial concern related to evaluating the influence of illumination on worker efficiency (Roethlisberger & Dickson, 1939). In this investigation, which has been summarized in an earlier book (Morgan, 1972), the principal finding was that performance was either improved or maintained under stressful circumstances, regardless of the actual treatment. Furthermore, in one of the experiments the control group also improved, indicating that simply involving individuals in an experiment was sufficient to produce an effect. The results of this study emphasize that experimental treatments must be contrasted not only with those of an untreated control condition, but that a third group should receive a "sham" treatment (i.e., placebo) in order to quantify that portion of an observed effect due to any versus no treatment.

Even though the Hawthorne effect has been widely accepted by behavioral scientists for many years, its significance has been called into question by some authors. Snodgrass, Levy-Berger, and Haydon (1985), for example, have pointed out that several problems with the original research reported by Roethlisberger and Dixon (1939) raise questions about the generalizability of their findings. Snodgrass et al. (1985) pointed out that no statistical analyses were reported; some of the participants (i.e., plant workers) were replaced during the study; and, because the study was performed during the Great Depression, workers may have feared losing their jobs if they did not comply with expectations. Despite the fact that the original work did not conform with contemporary standards of research design, the principal findings have been replicated in numerous studies (Boshes, 1960; Cobb et al., 1959; Desharnais et al., 1993; Glick & Margolis, 1962; Greenberg, Bornstein, Zborowski, Fisher, & Greenberg, 1994; Kirsch, 1994; Morgan, 1972).

Placebo Paradigms   It was noted by Boshes (1960) a quarter of a century ago that all experiments involving placebo groups must be conducted in such a way that neither the patient nor the individual presenting the drug or placebo should be aware of the pill's actual contents. In one of the number of examples presented in support of this view, Boshes (1960) reports that morphine reduces intense pain in about 75% of cases, while placebo is about 35% effective in the same types of cases. In other words, placebo is about 50% as effective as one of our most powerful drugs. Furthermore, placebo is about 77% as effective as morphine in treating moderate pain, and any drug or a placebo is about 60% to 70% effective if the patient is anxious.

The position advanced by Boshes (1960) was supported in a paper by Glick and Margolis (1962), who evaluated the influence of experimental design on outcome in drug research. These investigators reviewed 34 published studies involving the drug chlorpromazine, and a comparison was made between single-blind and double-blind studies. Those studies that employed double-blind placebo treatments resulted in a mean improvement of 38%, which was significantly lower than the 60% noted for those investigations in which a single-blind design was used.

It is not always possible to employ a double-blind design in studies involving psychological outcomes. This can be particularly problematic in psychotherapy and exercise studies, and there may not be an acceptable placebo treatment for comparison purposes in some cases. A double-blind paradigm is preferred whenever possible, followed by a single-blind approach; and when neither of these can be used, some effort must be made to ensure that the members of the research team who are responsible for measuring psychological (e.g., scoring tests, conducting interviews) or physiological (e.g., biochemical assays, electrocardiogram [ECG], EEG) variables not be aware of the individual's group status (i.e., experimental, control, placebo, minimal treatment).

There is a substantial placebo response in depression, but little is known about the factors underlying this effect. In an effort to identify the predictors of placebo response, Brown, Johnson, and Chen (1992) studied 241 depressed patients who were administered placebo on a double-blind basis for 3 to 6 weeks. These patients were classified as responders ($\geq$50% improvement), extreme nonresponders (<25%), and partial responders (all others). Patients who improved with placebo were characterized by (a) a precipitating event, (b) a short illness, (c) depression of a moderate global severity, and (d) a good response to previous antidepressant treatment. This paper is instructive because it not only replicates the widely held belief that some individuals respond to placebo treatment while others do not (Luoto, 1964), but it also identifies some of the traits that characterize responders and nonresponders.

O'Leary and Borkovec (1978) have pointed out that investigators who study psychotherapy outcomes have recognized the need to control for expectancy effects and effects due to contact and attention by the therapist. These factors are usually thought to lead to problems involving the placebo effect, and while these factors must be controlled, this does not mean that a placebo group must necessarily be employed. As a matter of fact, O'Leary and Borkovec (1978) argue that a true psychotherapy placebo group "may be unethical, impractical, or methodologically unsound in psychotherapy research of moderate or greater length" (p. 821). These investigators propose several alternative comparison groups to replace placebo controls in psychotherapy research, and the necessity of "waitlist" control groups is emphasized. In a more recent paper, Kirsch (1994) has proposed that "hypnosis can be used therapeutically as a nondeceptive placebo" (p. 95). Kirsch (1994) points out that expectancy effects are usually seen as "less real" than other psychological mechanisms by most investigators, and hence something to be controlled or eliminated; but he goes on to ask, "But in what way is expectancy any less legitimate as a psychological factor?" (p. 97). The only problem with employing hypnosis as a placebo is that it does not conform with the usual connotation of an "inert" treatment. That is, hypnotic inductions not only alter response expectancies, but also can have significant physiological effects.

The use of a placebo group may not be ethical in certain situations, and it is also possible that blind paradigms cannot be used because of the side effects associated with various drugs. Greenberg et al. (1994) have proposed that the research methodology employed may be more important than the drug being studied. These investigators report that the advantage of antidepressant drugs over placebos becomes more modest as "the degree of blindness" increases. This supports the earlier finding of Glick and Margolis (1962), and it illustrates that a bias can occur due to side effects "unblinding" patients and clinicians. This finding is not restricted to drug studies, and investigators must take this into account when evaluating other interventions such as exercise because involvement in vigorous physical activity can have numerous side effects (both negative and positive) that can "unblind" raters.

It is clear that the use of placebo treatments can be problematic for several reasons, and Ojanen (1994) has argued that "the idea of a placebo group in exercise studies is, in practice, impossible" (p. 63). In a strict sense, one would hope that a placebo was inert if the purpose was merely to quantify the "special attention" effect. Conversely, Ojanen (1994) argues that a placebo should generate expectations, involvement, and subjective utility, and this treatment should "also offer something that is meaningful to the participants" (p. 63). Ojanen has also indicated that if the exercise employed in a placebo group is minimal, it will not activate placebo factors. However, it has been shown that minimal exercise (e.g., shuffleboard, horseshoes) used as a placebo not only results in an improved sense of well-being, but physiological changes may also occur. Morgan and Pollock (1978) reported, for example, that diversionary activity (i.e., placebo) is associated with a significant reduction in heart rate during treadmill exercise. This reduced sympathetic activity has been described by other investigators as well (Kavanagh, Shephard, Pandit, and Doney, 1970).

In the study by Kavanagh et al. (1970), the effectiveness of exercise and hypnotherapy was compared in the rehabilitation of patients with coronary heart disease (CHD). Following 1 year of physical exercise or autohypnosis it was found that both groups experienced an increase in confidence and sense of well-being. Even more surprising was the observation that both groups had an average improvement of 20% to 25% in estimated aerobic power along with a mean decrease of 5 bpm in resting pulse rate. In addition, both groups (on average) showed improvement in their ECG results over the year, and a number of the patients in both groups enjoyed dramatic symptomatic improvements. There are a number of plausible explanations for these findings, and Kavanagh et al. (1970) suggest that the changes may have been due to "the natural process of recovery following coronary occlusion," (p. 578) rather than to the exercise and hypnotherapy.

It is also possible that the improvements observed by Kavanagh et al. (1970) resulted from a change in sympathetic activity due to the effect of repeated testing. There is some evidence, for example, suggesting that participants in exercise experiments sometimes experience a reduction in physiological measures such as heart rate with repeated exposure to exercise tests designed to measure maximal capacity. Morgan and Pollock (1978) reported that heart rate measured at the 6th minute of a standard Bruce Treadmill Protocol decreased 15 bpm following 10 weeks of aerobic training, but nonexercising subjects who were assigned randomly to control and placebo groups experienced a decrease of 10 bpm in exercise heart rate. There is also evidence indicating that anticipation of exercise can lead to an elevation in heart rate and blood pressure. It has been speculated that these physiological changes are caused by anxiety, and this is important because a reduction in anxiety following exercise might result from a pseudobaseline due to the anticipation of exercise. Fortunately, this potential methodological problem was ruled out in a study by Purvis and Morgan (1978).

In the study reported by Purvis and Morgan (1978), 30 adult women completed maximal exercise tests on either a bicycle ergometer ($N = 15$) or treadmill ($N = 15$) on 3 separate days. State and trait anxiety (STAI), heart rate, and blood pressure were assessed at rest prior to each test. In other words, the volunteers in this investigation all completed a maximal exercise test on Day 1 of the study, and therefore had a basis for anticipating the exercise "stressor" on Days 2 and 3. The mean data for all variables fell within the normal range for college students under all conditions, and the statistical analysis of variance (ANOVA) revealed that no significant changes took place with repeated testing. These results suggest that anticipation of the "stress" associated with a maximal treadmill or bicycle ergometer test does not result in elevated heart rate, blood pressure, or state anxiety or trait anxiety (Purvis & Morgan, 1978). Hence, it is unlikely that the anxiolytic effect commonly reported following vigorous exercise is the result of baseline elevations due to anticipatory effects.

It is sometimes difficult to employ a true experimental design for ethical or practical reasons. In Kavanagh et al.'s study (1970), there was no control group employed for comparison purposes. However, in the case of patients with CHD being treated in a rehabilitation center, it might be impractical to include a group that receives no treatment. Also, because the autohypnosis had a significant effect, it can be concluded that hypnotherapy was meaningful to the patients. Ojanen (1994) maintains that such an activity cannot be viewed as a placebo because it is apparently meaningful and results in physiological and psychological changes. On the other hand, Kirsch (1994) has recently proposed that hypnosis can be used therapeutically as a nondeceptive placebo. Ojanen (1994) has actually proposed that "the real effects of exercise on mental health or psychological well-being cannot be studied" (p. 63), because these effects cannot be separated from placebo effects. His view does not represent the mainstream of contemporary thinking in this general area, and there is certainly evidence to the contrary presented throughout this book. Nevertheless, it is important to recognize that about two thirds of successful treatment outcomes represent nonspecific effects if the provider and patient both believe in the efficacy of a particular treatment (Roberts, Kewman, Mercier, & Hovell, 1993). In fact, certain surgical procedures are no longer employed because it has been shown that the outcomes of these interventions not only do not exceed those observed with a sham treatment, but at times these procedures have been shown to be harmful. An example of the former is the use of mammary artery ligation to treat angina (Cobb, et al., 1959). An example of the latter is the lobotomy procedure, which was once employed to treat various forms of mental illness (Valenstein, 1986).

Summary

It is clear that research involving psychological outcomes can be influenced directly or indirectly by the investigator(s), and these effects can be the result of both intentional and unintentional actions on the part of researchers. Investigators concerned with the use of physical activity as a method of preventing and treating psychological problems must make every effort possible to quantify those effects caused specifically by exercise as opposed to those resulting from various behavioral artifacts, e.g., the halo effect, Hawthorne effect, Rosenthal effect, volunteerism, demand characteristics, and pretest sensitization (Desharnais et al., 1993; Kavanagh et al., 1970; Morgan et al., 1990; Morgan & Pollock, 1978; Ojanen, 1994). Some of these effects can be eliminated or minimized by taking certain precautions such as "blinding" both participants and investigators when possible, as well as eliminating explicit or implicit cues regarding a study's true purpose or expected outcome. It is also important that attention be paid to possible undesired psychological effects such as exercise dependence (Baekeland, 1970), exercise addiction (Morgan, 1979a), compulsive behavior (Polivy, 1994), and panic attacks following exercise (Stein et al., 1992).

SAMPLE SIZE AND EXPERIMENTAL DESIGN

The decision of whether to employ a control group or to allow participants to serve as their own controls in a repeated measures design requires consideration of a number of factors. The extent to which repeated testing is known (or suspected) to influence the dependent measure(s) is a critical factor. The amount of interindividual variability for the dependent variable(s) is also quite important, and this in turn relates to the number of participants required to demonstrate a significant outcome if, in fact, there is one. It is known, for example, that any hypothesis can be proven or refuted simply by using an excessive or inadequate number of test subjects, respectively.

An investigator should first designate the target population of whom generalizations will be made, and then select participants randomly from this population. In the event that subjects cannot be selected randomly, the investigator should explain exactly how the participants were obtained, and it is preferable that individuals be assigned randomly to treatment conditions. Most investigations dealing with the influence of physical activity on psychological outcomes have violated each of these principles (Folkins & Sime, 1981; Hughes, 1984; Morgan, 1981, 1984; Morgan & O'Connor, 1988; Morgan et al., 1990), and the extant literature in this area is based on quasi-experimental designs (Campbell & Stanley, 1963). A number of authors have cited a report by Stern and Cleary (1982) as evidence that physical activity does not produce an antidepressant effect. The design employed by Stern and Cleary (1982) represents one of the few in which individuals were assigned randomly to control and exercise groups, and these investigators failed to observe an antidepressant effect following 24 months of exercise. However, this study was characterized by a number of methodological problems (Morgan, 1994b), and the participants in both the control and exercise groups were not depressed at the outset. It is unclear why the investigators, or authors who have subsequently reviewed the study, would be surprised that an antidepressant effect was not observed. There has been a tendency for workers in this area of inquiry to assume that research carried out with nondepressed samples of healthy volunteers can be generalized to depressed patients (inpatient and outpatient) and vice versa. These views are not consistent with the fundamental requirements of generalizability theory or the theoretical underpinnings of most statistical models.

Despite the fact that one should not expect nondepressed individuals to experience a decrease in depression following an exercise program, there have been studies published that indicate the converse. If an investigator does not control for expectancy effects, demand characteristics, pretest sensitization, the placebo effect, or response distortion, it is easy to understand why normals might become "more normal" following an exercise program. However, there is at least one additional possibility that was demonstrated dramatically in a report by Stern and Cleary (1981). Unlike the related study by Stern and Cleary (1982) indicating that 24 months of exercise does not lead to an antidepressant effect, their 1981 study reportedly showed that exercise produces a significant reduction in depression. This report has been cited uncritically as evidence for the antidepressant effect of exercise by a number of reviewers, but the effect was clearly influenced by the use of an inappropriate sample size. The mean score on the MMPI Depression scale fell from 22.1 to 21.3, and a reduction of 0.8 on this scale would be regarded as trivial by any standard. However, there were 784 participants in this study, and the "statistically significant" effect was simply due to the large and inappropriate sample size. The study was actually characterized by a number of additional methodological problems, which have been summarized elsewhere (Morgan, 1994b). Nevertheless, this study continues to be cited by reviewers as evidence for the antidepressant effect of exercise.

In addition to the problem of external validity resulting from the generalization of findings from nondepressed to depressed samples, and the trivial effects that are seen as significant because of excessive sample size, there is also the problem of regarding a clinically significant improvement as lacking statistical significance because of small sample size. Just how many subjects are needed in an experiment dealing with the psychological outcomes of physical activity? The answer to this question is dependent on a number of interrelated factors. A decision should first be made about the minimum number of participants needed in a study in order to demonstrate a psychological outcome effect that is significant from both a statistical and a practical or clinical standpoint.

Assume that an investigator is interested in evaluating the influence of aerobic exercise on mildly depressed outpatients who have a mean score of 50.0 ($SD = 10.0$) on a standardized self-report measure of depression. The investigator might elect to employ a conventional α level of .05 and a power (1-β) of .70. The investigator must decide a priori what sort of a decrease in depression would be regarded as significant from a clinical standpoint. Assume that a reduction of 10 units on this scale (i.e., 1 SD) is felt to represent a clinically significant antidepressant effect. In addition to exposing a group of patients to aerobic exercise, it would also be appropriate to employ a placebo group that receives an inert or passive treatment that will not produce improved levels of aerobic power, as well as a third group that serves as a strict control (possibly a wait-list control). The participants should be assigned randomly to the three groups, and a standard "before-after" design (Campbell & Stanley, 1963) might be employed as illustrated below. In the following designs R stands for randomization, O for observation, T for treatment, C for control, and P for placebo.

Before-After Design

$$R...O_1...T...O_2$$
$$R...O_1...C...O_2$$
$$R...O_1...P...O_2$$

The minimum sample size required for such an experiment is computed to be approximately 10 per group ($N = 30$) using procedures such as those described by Gordon, Primavera, and Allison (1995). In other words, for a given variance, α level, and power, the minimum sample size required to demonstrate a significant difference between treatments if, in fact, such a difference actually exists is calculated to be 28 in this case. However, if the desired level of power was increased to .80 or .90, the minimum sample sizes would increase to approximately 35 or 46, respectively. Furthermore, the minimum sample size required for this example would increase from 28 to 43 if the α level were changed to $p < .01$. It is also important to recognize that sample size should not be too large, and attention should also be paid to the matter of optimal sample size. Additional details concerning the estimation of sample size and statistical power can be found in the studies by Cohen (1988, 1992), and a statistical program has been developed by Gorman et al. (1995). This simple, interactive computer program enables one to compute effect sizes and power estimates, as well as estimates of sample sizes needed for various combinations of power, significance levels, and effect sizes.

The before-after design is probably the most frequently employed in the behavioral sciences where it is important to know from the outset whether or not the various groups differ on the dependent measure(s). This is especially true when it is not possible for some reason to assign participants randomly to conditions. However, if there is reason to believe that a pretest (i.e., O_1) might influence the posttest (O_2), it might be more appropriate to employ an "after-only" design (Campbell & Stanley, 1963). It is known, for example, that the before-after design can be problematic in the sense that pretest sensitization can lead to baseline suppression or amplification (i.e., distortion) on the part of participants.

After-Only Design

$$R...T...O_1$$
$$R...C...O_1$$
$$R...P...O_1$$

There is always a possibility that randomization does not result in the generation of three groups that are equivalent on the dependent measure at the outset, and this is particularly problematic when a small sample size is employed. An alternative to either of the above designs is the Solomon four-group design (Campbell & Stanley, 1963), which is actually the optimal approach when there are adequate resources and participants. This design is merely a combination of the before-after and after-only designs, and enables the investigator to assess the interactive effects of the pretest. However, this design requires doubling the total sample size, and an even greater increase is needed when the investigator elects to employ placebo groups.

Solomon Design

$$R...O_1...T...O_2$$
$$R...O_1...C...O_2$$
$$R..........T...O_1$$
$$R..........C...O_1$$

Another design that is often used in exercise science is the repeated-measures design in which the participant serves as his or her own control. This design has a number of obvious advantages such as the need for fewer individuals and reduced variability. The inherent danger in employing such a design, however, is that participants often become cognizant of the hypothesis being tested, and they might attempt to respond in such a way as to comply with the demand characteristics operating in the experimental milieu (Orne, 1962). One way of quantifying the extent to which such an effect occurs in a repeated-measures design is to employ a counterbalanced or random order of testing. The order of treatment (i.e., ABC, BCA, CAB, BCA, BAC, and so on) should be assigned randomly to test participants, and *post hoc* assessments should quantify the extent to which order effects did or did not take place. Regardless of the experimental design employed, it is important that minimal or optimal sample size be calculated from the outset. Actually, in some respects, the design one elects to employ might be governed in part by the number of individuals estimated to be needed for each group.

Summary   It is clear that some investigators have failed to observe significant psychological outcomes in exercise studies for a number of reasons. One obvious problem has been that samples have often scored in the normal range on various affective measures, and it has been unreasonable to expect these samples to change following exercise interventions. It is also apparent that some exercise studies have been associated with statistically significant changes merely because large sample sizes have been employed, while other studies have failed to observe positive psychological outcomes because the sample size has been too small. It is imperative that investigators take the matter of optimal sample size into account during the design phase of studies, and it is equally important that individuals involved in the review of published research consider the interrelated factors of sample size, statistical power, and trivial versus meaningful differences in concert with the tradeoff between committing Type 1 and Type 2 errors. Finally, the extent to which sensitization effects due to testing per se are known or suspected to influence behavior is an important consideration in adopting the most appropriate experimental design.

META-ANALYSIS

A great deal has been written in recent years about the advantages and limitations of meta-analysis. It seems reasonably clear that meta-analysis can be a powerful and effective methodology when used appropriately. One of the best examples of how meta-analysis can be used in the study of psychological outcomes was illustrated by Greenberg et al. (1994) in a meta-analysis of all double-blind, placebo-controlled trials on the efficacy of the drug fluoxetine (Prozac). While this drug had been accorded "wonder drug" status by the media, the meta-analysis revealed that effect sizes were not greater than those observed for other commonly employed tricyclic antidepressants. This finding alone can be viewed as a significant observation, but Greenberg et al. (1994) also considered the possibility that outcome ratings may have been influenced by systematic bias. Earlier research had suggested that a greater frequency of side effects can "unblind" study participants, and these investigators decided to study the relationship between effect sizes and reports of side effects. It was found that both patient and clinician ratings of outcome were significantly correlated with the report of side effects. This meta-analysis clearly raises questions about the influence of side effects on psychological outcomes in drug research.

The results of the meta-analysis by Greenberg et al. (1994) are significant for a number of reasons. First, these investigators demonstrate in a rather compelling manner that meta-analysis per se can be misleading unless relevant methodological issues are taken into consideration. Second, the efficacy of meta-analysis in attempting to understand the complex nature of antidepressant medication is quite apparent. Third, the importance of blinding investigators and study participants in drug research is reinforced.

Some authors who have written reviews dealing with the mental health benefits of physical activity have pointed out that methodological factors can create problems in outcome research, but these same individuals have made the implicit assumption that combining a large number of studies in a meta-analysis will serve to overcome methodological shortcomings. This is probably true in the case of *random error*, but it is probably not true in the case of *systematic error* of the type associated with numerous behavioral artifacts discussed throughout this chapter. Consider, for example, the obvious problem associated with the use of "transparent" self-report questionnaires designed to measure constructs such as anxiety, depression, or self-esteem. It is quite easy for study participants to "fake good" or "fake bad" on such variables in an intervention study designed to quantify the efficacy of any intervention (e.g., physical activity). It is also possible that demand characteristics (Orne, 1962) operating in a given experiment might produce both unintended and intended response distortion, and this possibility has been demonstrated effectively by Desharnais et al. (1993). While it is very clear that observed effects in many investigations may reflect the impact of demand characteristics, expectancy, and so on, the use of response distortion (i.e., lie scales) has been generally ignored in attempting to establish the psychological efficacy of physical activity. Meta-analysts in this area of inquiry have made the implicit assumption that study participants never lie, and as a consequence, the problem of response distortion has simply been ignored by investigators using this technique. However, as Dunn and Dishman (1991) have pointed out, "Contrary to the assumption of meta-analysis, the methodological problems of past research cannot be resolved by any type of review of the existing human literature on exercise and depression" (p. 48).

There are a number of pitfalls associated with the use of meta-analysis, as well as narrative reviews (Morgan, 1994b). It is obvious that the selective inclusion of studies in either case can be problematic, and it is apparent that meta-analysts have elected not to incorporate studies demonstrating that excessive exercise can lead to mood disturbance. This is somewhat surprising because there is now fairly extensive literature dealing with the impact of overtraining on affect (see chapter 9). This situation would be analogous to a drug researcher not including studies in a meta-analysis in which high doses of a drug resulted in undesired affective change. Part of the infatuation with meta-analysis stems from the mistaken belief that compiling a group of independent studies will lead to findings and insights that are not possible with a single study. However, the idea that a clear distinction can be made between the value of single-study statistical methods and meta-analysis is illusory according to Hoyle (1993), who argues for "the critical value of the primary research study and the traditional literature review in the enterprise of scientific psychology" (p. 1094).

There have been an increasing number of meta-analyses in the area of physical activity and mental health, but a number of these analyses have suffered from various methodological problems. An exception to this generalization is the monograph by McDonald and Hodgdon (1991). The limitations of meta-analysis in general have been articulated best by Eysenck (1994), and specific shortcomings in the area of exercise science have been addressed by Blumenthal (1989), Dunn and Dishman (1991), and Morgan (1994b).

It is not possible, of course, for any analysis of published research to deal adequately with the problem of data fabrication, or the more common problem known as "data torturing" (Mills, 1993). A distinction has been made between "opportunistic" and "procrustean" data torturing by Mills (1993). In the former case an investigator "can find significant results when none exist simply by making multiple comparisons" (p. 1197), while procrustean data torturing involves manipulation of the data in order to confirm the desired hypothesis by selective reporting of observations. While procrustean data torturing is more difficult to perform than opportunistic data torturing, its results are usually more believable and destructive (Mills, 1993). It is impossible for a meta-analysis, for example, to unearth effects due to the suppression of contradictory data. A book titled *How to Lie With Statistics* was published over four decades ago by Huff (1954), and meta-analysts, as well as those preparing narrative reviews, should become familiar with this book, as well as the more recent but equally instructive paper by Mills (1993).

Summary   There is good evidence that meta-analysis is a powerful and effective procedure when used appropriately, and the many pitfalls associated with this technique can be minimized or avoided by taking relevant methodological issues into consideration. However, there is an absence of compelling evidence at this point to suggest that meta-analysis has been more effective than traditional narrative reviews in attempting to improve our understanding of the relationship between physical activity and mental health. The important consideration in using both quantitative and qualitative review methods is to pay careful attention to relevant methodological issues, as well as including research data that refutes as well as supports the efficacy of physical activity in the development and maintenance of mental health.

OVERALL SUMMARY

It is noteworthy that a number of investigators have failed to observe significant psychological changes, as measured by standardized instruments that possess good reliability and validity (e.g., Profile of Mood States [POMS], Self-Rating Depression Scale [SDS], STAI) following exercise programs lasting 20 weeks or longer. This observation has been made consistently despite the fact that participants in these exercise programs report that they experience (a) an increased "sense of well-being" (e.g., Morgan, Roberts, Brand, & Feinerman, 1970; Morgan & Pollock, 1978), and (b) significant physiological improvements on various measures of physical fitness (e.g., Blumenthal et al., 1989).

The study by Blumenthal et al. (1989) is particularly instructive in a number of aspects, and it warrants closer examination. These investigators randomly assigned 101 men and women (mean age 67 years) to an aerobic exercise group ($n = 33$), a yoga and flexibility "control" group ($n = 34$), or a wait-list control group ($n = 34$). The randomization process resulted in the generation of three groups that were remarkably similar on a large battery of physiological and psychological measures, and this trial lasted for a 4-month period. The manipulation was effective from a physiological standpoint in that the exercise group experienced a 12% increase in aerobic power and a 13% increase in anaerobic threshold while the nonexercise groups did not change on either of these measures. One remarkable finding in this study was a reported adherence rate of 96% across the 4-month period. There were 48 men and 49 women at the close of the study. Of the 4 individuals who dropped out, 2 each were from the exercise and wait-list control groups. The issue of adherence is addressed by Dishman and Buckworth in chapter 4, and it is clear that an adherence rate of 96% is most unusual. Despite the physiological improvement, good adherence, and improved sense of well-being, there were no psychological changes noted by the objective measures of anxiety and overall mood employed in this study.

There are at least three possible explanations for the observation that individuals who improve physiologically following the adoption of an exercise program do not experience psychological changes as measured by standardized instruments. First, the participants in many of these studies fall within the normal range on selected measures of anxiety and depression, and this likely limits the possibility of anxiolytic or antidepressant effects. Second, it is possible that the enhanced sensation of well-being reported by these individuals reflects changes in psychological constructs other than those assessed in a given study (e.g., self-esteem). Third, it is possible that significant neurochemical and electrocortical changes occur in the brain, but existing psychometric tools are not sensitive to these alterations.

The possibility that changes in brain chemistry may lead to improved psychological function has been explored largely with animal models (Morgan, Olson, & Pedersen, 1982) up to this point, and this research is reviewed by Hoffmann in chapter 10 (e.g., endorphin hypothesis), by Chaouloff in chapter 11 (e.g., serotonin hypothesis), and by Dishman in chapter 12 (e.g., norepinephrine hypothesis). This research is very important because certain questions cannot be explored directly with humans. It is known that exercise can change the behavior of animals (Morgan et al., 1982), and animals differing in behavior patterns have been shown to differ in whole-brain levels of norepinephrine (Olson & Morgan, 1982). However, the question of whether changes in behavioral measures with exercise lead to alterations in regional or whole-brain levels of monoamines has not been addressed systematically.

It has been recognized for many years that muscle tension levels, as measured electromyographically, are associated with psychopathology (Morgan, 1968b). Furthermore, this neurophysiologic state was once thought to consist of "hyperactivity in neurons composing that portion of the nervous system which extends from the motor and premotor cortex to the peripheral musculature" (Whatmore & Ellis, 1959, p. 8). This condition has been labeled *hyperponesis*, and it has been reported that not only are depressed patients, for example, hyperponetic, but this patient group remains so following recovery. The more recent EEG work reported by Davidson (1994) and Davidson and Sutton (1995) indicates that individuals with extreme and stable left and right frontal activation differ on measures of depression (Beck Depression Inventory [BDI]), anxiety (STAI), and positive and negative affect as measured by the Positive and Negative Affect Scale (PANAS). The application of this work in research dealing with physical activity and mental health could prove fruitful. It would be interesting to see, for example, whether acute or chronic physical activity would have an influence on electrocortical and subcortical brain regions in depressed patients, as well as on peripheral measures performed on skeletal muscle. One intriguing observation made by Whatmore and Ellis (1959) is the report that neither electroconvulsive shock therapy (ECT) or tranquilizers produced any permanent changes in the hyperponetic states observed in depressed patients.

The idea that physical activity might result in reduced tension levels in skeletal muscle has been investigated by deVries (1987), deVries and Adams (1972), and deVries, Beckman, Huber, and Dieckmeir (1968). These investigations have shown that both acute and chronic physical activity leads to a reduction in the integrated EMG of the elbow flexor muscles. Furthermore, the tension reduction observed following acute exercise was found to be significantly greater than that observed following the administration of meprobamate, a commonly employed tranquilizer at the time the research was conducted (deVries & Adams, 1972). There is limited evidence that this effect may be mediated at a central level, but the mechanisms involved in the reduction of neuromuscular tension remain to be demonstrated.

There is also limited evidence that exercise deprivation can lead to EEG changes (Baekeland, 1970) and mood disturbance (Mondin, Morgan, Piering, Stegner, Stotesbery, Trine, & Wu, 1996), and this line of research could be fruitful. In other words, if physical activity actually causes physiological and psychological changes in habitual exercisers, these effects might be eliminated with exercise deprivation. However, it appears to be rather difficult to employ this type of protocol because habitual exercisers are reluctant to give up exercise even for short periods of time (Baekeland, 1970; Morgan, 1979a; Polivy, 1994).

There has been limited work carried out in an attempt to identify electrocortical correlates of improved mood following acute exercise (Petruzello & Landers, 1994). While this more recent work may eventually provide explanations about the mechanisms underlying the influence of exercise on affective states, it has been restricted to descriptive efforts up to this point. It is not clear whether physical activity reduces anxiety and the anxiolytic effect results in EEG changes, or if EEG changes cause the reduction in anxiety. It also remains to be demonstrated whether electrodermal measures obtained during and following exercise reflect changes in subcortical brain regions. Furthermore, there is an absence of research in this area dealing with concomitant measures of EEG and brain chemistry (e.g., monoamines, endorphins) during exercise. In other words, changes in the EEG may simply reflect alterations in brain chemistry, and there is a need for electrophysiological work during and following exercise in which attempts are made to manipulate outcomes experimentally rather than merely to describe observed changes.

Recent work by Davidson (1994) highlights the importance of individual differences in prefrontal electrophysiological asymmetries from the standpoint of both dispositional mood as well as reactivity to elicitors of emotion. This recent research also emphasizes the importance of cortical-subcortical interactions, and the efficacy of functional magnetic resonance imaging in place of older technologies is also noted (Davidson & Sutton, 1995). The use of functional magnetic resonance imaging should prove to be fruitful in future work dealing with the influence of physical activity on affect. While the existing EEG work has been limited to descriptive work, it has yielded some clues as to possible directions to be taken in future work dealing with the elucidation of electrophysiological mechanisms underlying affective change during and following physical activity.

Another line of research that warrants further attention is based on what has been termed the "distraction" or "time out" hypothesis (Morgan, 1981, 1982). It has been shown that simply resting in a quiet environment can lead to significant reductions in blood pressure (Raglin & Morgan, 1987), plasma levels of epinephrine and norepinephrine (Michaels, Hubert, & McCann, 1976), and state anxiety (Bahrke & Morgan, 1978; Stotesbery, Stegner, & Morgan, 1996; Wertz-Garvin, Trine, & Morgan, 1996). The reductions in these biochemical, cardiovascular, and psychometric measures of anxiety following quiet rest are comparable to those observed following vigorous exercise as well as meditation. The distraction hypothesis has been viewed as a psychological explanation because it argues that the anxiolytic effect observed following dissimilar activities such as exercise and meditation (cultic and noncultic) all have one feature in common—distraction from the cares and worries of the day. In other words, it is possible that individuals feel good after physical activity because they are distracted from various concerns while they are exercising. While this could prove to be a fruitful area of inquiry, this hypothesis suffers from the same problems described earlier for the EEG literature. It is descriptive in nature, and thus far investigators have not attempted to elucidate the mechanisms responsible for this effect.

The following chapters each deal with a specific topic judged to be of importance in the overall area of physical activity and mental health. While there is obvious overlap and interaction among various topics, each chapter addresses a unique part of the overall area. The methodological overview presented in this chapter is intended to provide a set of principles to be considered in evaluating the research and conclusions presented in each of the chapters that follow, and it is hoped that this summary will be of use to investigators in the design of future studies involving the influence of physical activity on mental health.

Chapter 2

Prevention of Sedentary Lifestyles: Rationale and Methods

Daniel S. Kirschenbaum

The prevention of a sedentary lifestyle is one of the goals of the helping professions. The importance of prevention is illustrated in the following scenario.

> Imagine that you are out for a picnic on a pleasant spring day with a group of friends. You have just set out a checkered tablecloth with all manner of your favorite foods. You have situated yourself by the bank of a river, and as you are about to bite into a sandwich a cry is heard from the river. "Help, help!" the screamer yells. Putting down your sandwich, you tear off your shoes and clothes and dive in to rescue a drowning victim, apply artificial respiration, and prepare to return to your picnic. Suddenly two people call out "help, help!" You dive in again and pull them out one on each arm. But as you return there are three or four others calling for help. Again you return, but this time, tired and overwhelmed by several people at once, you let a few slip away. Again, now in larger numbers, people call for help, but you cannot handle very many. You are only one person and you don't even swim very well yourself. Your friends don't swim at all, but as they watch you one has a bright idea. "Why not go upstream and find out who is pushing these people in?" (Recounted by Rappaport, 1977, p. 632, origin unknown)

The logic of prevention is well illustrated by this story of a somewhat strange spring picnic. Just what is the true benefit of the proverbial "ounce of prevention"? Can expenditures on before-the-fact preventive interventions be justified

This is a revised version of a chapter that originally appeared in Morgan, W.P., & Goldston, S.E. (Eds.) (1987). *Exercise and mental health.* Washington, DC: Hemisphere Publishing.

in this age of retrenchment in federal support? Even more to the point of this paper, can we justify expenditures to learn how to help people develop more active lifestyles—especially at a time when so many commercial enterprises (e.g., running shoe companies, athletic clothes manufacturers) seem to be doing just that and prospering?

The purpose of the first section of this chapter is to address the value of preventive efforts. Several examples from the medical arena are presented to document the remarkably potent effects of prevention. The second section considers the rationale for directing preventive interventions at *sedentarianism*—the sedentary lifestyle currently practiced by the majority of Americans. Having made what is hoped to be a convincing argument in support of *anti-sedentarianism* (the prevention of sedentary lifestyles), the next section presents concepts of prevention. In the final section, specific recommendations are reviewed that could facilitate the development of more effective research and intervention on anti-sedentarianism.

A RATIONALE FOR PREVENTION

Cleanliness Is Next to Healthiness

Many decades before medical authorities accepted the germ theory in the early 19th century, health officials took steps to eradicate miasmas, or noxious odors associated with sewage (Bloom, 1984). Even without the benefit of knowing that germs cause disease, the teachings of Hippocrates and others led to widespread acceptance of the belief that specific miasmas like the "bad air" (malaria) associated with swamps and sewage were responsible for most infectious diseases. These beliefs led to efforts to improve sanitation, which in turn greatly reduced the incidence of typhoid fever, yellow fever, tuberculosis, cholera, and infant and maternal mortality. For example, by 1800 maternal mortality had been lowered to one seventh of its 1750 level.

Of course, the improvements in sanitary conditions in the last 200 hundred years often occurred mainly in the living conditions of the wealthier classes. For example, consider the following graphic description of the unbelievable conditions in which many thousands of immigrants found themselves as they contributed to the industrial revolution in the middle and late 1800s in England:

> The infrequency of sewage and garbage removal . . . gave rise to the practice of using them as places of deposit for all the residents of a given court. As a result, there was scarcely a court that was not occupied by a communal cesspool or dunghill. . . . Instead of [bathrooms with toilets, most households used a] "necessary," a kind of tub that had to be emptied every morning. Even with this facility, the situation was grim. In one Manchester district the needs of some 7000 people were supplied by 33 "necessaries." (Rosen, 1958, pp. 205-206)

Vaccinations and Further Improvements in Sanitation in the 20th Century

In this century, many steps have been taken to improve sanitation across socioeconomic strata, to isolate disease carriers when treatments have been ineffective or long in duration, and to develop preventive medical vaccinations. Smallpox, diphtheria, diarrheal diseases of infancy, tuberculosis, influenza, measles, and poliomyelitis have been either completely eliminated or nearly so, or are much better controlled as a result of these efforts. For example, the *1979 Surgeon General's Report on Health Promotion and Disease Prevention* (Califano, 1979) clearly shows that the preventive medical efforts implemented during this century have paid off in the savings of literally millions of lives.

It is important to emphasize that these dramatic improvements resulted from improvements in hygiene, diet, and preventive medical care, rather than advances in biomedical knowledge regarding the treatment of infectious diseases (Leventhal, Zimmerman, & Gutmann, 1984; Thomas, 1977). Furthermore, we should certainly begin to recognize that the two major causes of death identified in the last year (and to date; cancer and heart disease) are unlikely to be "cured" by advances in biomedical research—at least in the foreseeable future. For people who develop most forms of cancer and heart disease, medical science can offer primarily technologies that decelerate disease progression (to minimal extents in many cases) or allow people to maintain a reasonable quality of life while moving inexorably toward an early death (Thomas, 1977). Paradoxically, the vast majority of dollars spent on health concerns goes to medical care for the sick.

Prevention by Legislation

Seven times as many people who are in motorcycle accidents get injured compared with injuries resulting from automobile accidents (Watson, Zador, & Wilks, 1980). There were more than 4,000 deaths and 350,000 injuries sustained in motorcycle accidents in 1977 alone (Bloom, 1984). In the mid-1970s virtually all states enacted laws requiring motorcycle riders to wear helmets. Approximately 30% fewer people died in motorcycle accidents in the year immediately after these laws were passed. However, lobbying by the American Motorcyclist Association and changes in federal mandates resulted in the repeal of these laws in 26 states between 1976 and 1978. The incidence of motorcycle fatalities and injuries rose by a substantial amount in 23 of the 26 states that had repealed the law. Watson, Zador, and Wilkes (1980) showed that there was a 38% increase in fatalities in those states that repealed the law compared with geographically and demographically similar states that retained the law. All of this makes a great deal of sense, given the evidence that mortality rates are twice as high in unhelmeted compared with helmeted accident victims. Many other examples also document the efficiency and effectiveness of a variety of preventive efforts (Bloom, 1984; Forgays, 1991).

Conclusions

It is very apparent that large-scale preventive interventions can be well worth the time and effort they require. What is needed to begin such efforts, in addition to an adequate level of funding and person-power, is a clear rationale for focusing preventive efforts on a particular behavior, problem, or aspect of living. The rationale must show a strong relationship between the proposed focal aspect of living and the health outcomes. Sanitary environmental conditions, vaccinations for various diseases, and the use of motorcycle helmets had all demonstrated their efficacy as preventive strategies before community- and society-wide preventive programs were launched. Let us now consider whether there is a similar empirical justification for advocating physical activity.

A RATIONALE FOR HABITUAL PHYSICAL ACTIVITY

> They are fatally mistaken who think that while they strive with their minds that they may suffer their bodies to stagnate in luxury and sloth. (Henry David Thoreau, 1840/1978, p. 42)

The wisdom of Thoreau is not an adequate reason to advocate the radical alteration of lifestyles as a means of preventing various health problems. Fortunately, data that provide more objective support for Thoreau's assertion have been accumulating rapidly .

Martin and Dubbert (1982a,1982b) summarized much of the available evidence on the effects on physical well-being of the practice of systematic, regular aerobic exercises (at least 15 min per session, 3 or more sessions per week, in which repetitive isorhythmic activities are focal). They reported that such exercise programs have improved cardiovascular efficiency and modified cardiovascular risk profiles in healthy people, as well as in individuals at high risk for cardiovascular disease and patients with CHD and borderline hypertension. Getting patients with heart disease to engage in regular and sustained exercise programs has also been linked with improvements in recovery, such as shorter hospitalization and decreased perceived exertion. All of these findings are extremely important in view of the increasing proportion of deaths in this country that are attributable to cardiovascular disease.

In 1988 an important international conference was held in Toronto, referred to in the scientific literature as the Toronto Conference on Exercise, Fitness, and Health (Bouchard, Shephard, Stephens, Sutton, & McPherson, 1990). A consensus panel was also convened in 1992 for the purpose of updating our knowledge regarding physical activity, fitness, and health (Bouchard, Shephard, & Stephens, 1994). These conferences were designed to establish a consensus about the current state of knowledge pertaining to the effects of physical activity. The participants in these panels consisted of international experts working on the cutting edge of exercise science, and they prepared written reviews of various aspects of the literature on physical activity. Their efforts represented the culmination of several years of preparation and the resulting books (Bouchard et al., 1990, 1994) include a very convincing analysis of the physiological and psychological benefits of regular physical activity. Very much in accord with Martin and Dubbert's (1982a, 1982b) analysis, the consensus statements clearly reinforce the importance of a physically active lifestyle.

It is clear that the consensus of scientific opinion very substantially favors the role of an active lifestyle in promoting physical and mental well-being. Additional evidence also supports even broader effects than those suggested by the consensus statements. For example, obesity has recently increased to an alarming degree in both children and adults (e.g., Kuczmarski, Flegal, Campbell, & Johnson, 1994). Specific evidence showing beneficial effects of exercise interventions for the treatment of obesity in both children and adults has been reported (e.g., Epstein, Wing, Koeske, Ossip, & Beck, 1983; Stalonas, Johnson, & Christ, 1978; Viegener et al., 1990).

Researchers have also begun to delineate the mechanisms for the beneficial effects of physical activity on treating obesity, using both animal and human research. For example, studies indicate that increasing physical activity in obese individuals can enhance metabolic rates (Donahoe, Lin, Kirschenbaum, & Kesey, 1984; Frey-Hewitt, Vranivan, Dreon, & Wood, 1990; Hill, Davis, & Tagliaferro, 1983; Mole, Stern, Schultz, Bernauer, & Holcomb, 1989; Van Dale, Saris, & Ten Hoor, 1990). Physical activity could also help facilitate fatty acid mobilization and produce other biochemical effects that should assist obese individuals in their attempts to lose weight (Bouchard et al., 1990, 1994).

In addition to establishing the real and probable benefits of physical activity, part of the rationale for the prevention of sedentarianism must include documentation of the pervasiveness of the problem. In other words, we must consider the extent to which people are currently sedentary. Martin (1981) appropriately characterized and summarized the current lifestyle practices in America:

> Studies have shown that virtually everyone believes that exercise, like democracy, is a good thing. Regrettably, the majority of individuals become merely approving spectators to each. . . . As poor as our voting participation is (65% of eligible Americans actually vote), our regular exercise participation in the U.S., (37%), is worse!" (p. 4)

More recent surveys continue to find sedentary lifestyles to be the dominant ones in the United States. Depending on the survey method and criteria, it appears that between 75% and 95% of the U.S. adult population does not engage in regular vigorous exercise (Armstrong, Sallis, Hovell, & Hofstetter, 1993). For example, telephone-interview data from over 17,000 respondents indicated that in the early 1980s only about 21% of the U.S. adult population engaged in 30 minutes of aerobic exercise at least twice per week (White, Powell, Hogelin, Gentry, & Forman, 1987).

Not only do most Americans fail to exercise regularly, a series of Harris polls (cited by Martin & Dubbert, 1982a, 1982b) indicate that 45% may not exercise at all. This percentage is particularly disconcerting when juxtaposed with the research showing the substantial benefits associated with even moderate levels of physical fitness (e.g., Blair, Kohl, Gordon, & Paffenbarger, 1992). Furthermore, approximately one half of the people who begin health-related exercise programs rejoin the ranks of their more sedentary peers within 6 months of beginning such efforts. The problem of exercise adherence is reviewed in detail by Dishman and Buckworth in chapter 4. This difficulty in "treating" sedentarianism suggests that preventive efforts may prove more cost-efficient than remedial efforts and that further developments in research and conceptualizations may be needed to advance both remedial and preventive approaches.

The final section of this chapter attempts to refine current views of the nature of the problem of sedentarianism, leading to practical suggestions for improving the efficacy of preventive programs targeted to anti-sedentarianism. Before providing those suggestions, however, it is necessary to review the options available for preventive interventions. For now, it seems safe to conclude that: (a) Prevention is a practical and very useful approach to reducing various health problems; and (b) sedentarianism is a health concern of sufficient impact to justify considering approaches to prevention that could reduce its prevalence in this country.

CONCEPTS AND APPROACHES IN PREVENTION

Three Types

There are many dozens of ways of operationalizing the basic concept of prevention. Gerald Caplan's book, *Principles of Preventive Psychiatry* (1964) brought the concept of preventive intervention into the modern mental health movement by defining the three major types of prevention.

He defined *tertiary prevention* as the reduction of problems in an entire community (i.e., large-scale amelioration) by intervening with people who have already developed serious problems in living. This idea is closest to traditional health care delivery or rehabilitation. However, one difference is that the term tertiary prevention directs attention to the impact on the community of such rehabilitative efforts. An approach to anti-sedentarianism that is an example of tertiary prevention is an exercise class provided for all patients with heart disease in a particular hospital who had practiced a sedentary lifestyle prior to their heart attacks. This large-scale rehabilitation effort might decrease the incidence of sedentarianism among the patients in the hospital and others in the community who observed the effects they achieved.

Secondary prevention refers to reducing the rate of problems in a community by intervening at the early stages of the development of problems in living. This could include, for example, providing young executives in a business with easy access to health club facilities, time off from work for exercise, and other encouragement for those at high risk for lifelong sedentarianism (e.g., young people who have already developed relatively sedentary lifestyles) to develop regular exercise habits.

Finally, *primary prevention* is the lowering of the rate of problems in a community "by counteracting harmful circumstances before they have a chance to produce illness" (Caplan, 1964, p. 26). Thus, the major difference between primary and secondary prevention is that the former acts before the fact (i.e., before the emergence of the problem), while the latter amounts to early intervention, usually with young people, after the problem has already emerged in an early stage. Primary prevention, therefore, can be (and often is) directed at high-risk groups.

Focus, Time Frame, and Target Population

The specific incarnation of a prevention program depends in large part on the central focus or goal of the intervention, the time frame used, and the dimension of the target population (Cowen, 1980; Jason & Glenwick, 1980). Table 1 presents a $4 \times 2 \times 5$ (Focus $\times$ Time frame $\times$ Dimension of target population) matrix of the variations in primary and secondary prevention programming that could be used in efforts to encourage anti-sedentarianism.

Focus   The focus dimension was distilled from a variety of papers on the extant practices and future possibilities for primary prevention (e.g., Cowen, 1980; Jason & Glenwick, 1980). Many programs have focused on methods of presenting information to individuals, groups, and larger segments of the population. These are sometimes referred to as educational programs or mass media campaigns. The users of this focus hope that the information will help people modify their behaviors or change their laws or environments to prevent specific problems from developing or worsening. Billboards and commercials warning us about the dangers of cigarette smoking, driving while drunk, and stress are common examples of this dimension of focus.

Prevention programs can also attempt to improve skills or competencies, such as social problem-solving skills or self-control skills. Programs have

Table 1   Key Dimensions in Primary and Secondary Prevention

	Focus							
	Provide information		**Improve competencies**		**Improve adjustment to stressors**		**Modify environment**	
Audience	**Acute**	**Chronic**	**Acute**	**Chronic**	**Acute**	**Chronic**	**Acute**	**Chronic**
Individual								
Group								
Organization								
Community								
Society								

attempted to train elementary school children in these skills, including several large-scale efforts directed at unselected groups of children and secondary prevention programs aimed at children with mild to moderate behavioral-emotional difficulties (Forgays, 1991; King & Kirschenbaum, 1992). In a related vein, programs have focused on helping people learn how to cope with impending or existing crises or stressors. These programs use known or specifically anticipated stressful events as the major impetus for the intervention. Thus, programs aimed at preparing children for hospitalization and surgery (e.g., Peterson & Shigetomi, 1981; Zastowny, Kirschenbaum, & Meng, 1986) and dental treatment (e.g., Kiorman et al., 1980) are not directed primarily at building general skills. Rather, they are aimed at reducing the potentially adverse impact of stressors.

Finally, preventive interventions can focus on modifying environments. Efforts could be directed toward changing the size of elementary school classrooms or using certain rules and organizational structures to reduce the frequency of classroom disruptions, enhance self-control, and improve affect (Humphrey, 1984). An example from a different domain of behavior concerns littering—a significant ecological problem. Geller, Mann, and Brasted (1977) rotated ordinary and artistically designed litter drums every 5 to 8 weeks for a year. The creative containers were shaped like birds, were brightly painted, and contained a litter-reduction message. These colorful containers attracted much more litter than the ordinary drums (15 vs. 9 lbs per week)—thereby effectively preventing a good deal of littering (approximately 312 lbs per year per container).

Time Frame   Preventive interventions can vary in duration as well as to focus. Bloom (1984) described the milestone approach to prevention as providing services to people "when they reach a particular, predefined point—or when they undergo some particular stressful life event" (p. 200). Examples of the milestone approach, which are always delivered in an acute, time-limited fashion, include preparatory programs for surgical and dental procedures (Kendall, 1979; Kiorman et al., 1980; Melamed & Siegel, 1975; Zastowny et al., 1986). These programs can focus on improving adjustment to stressors, but they can also focus on providing information, improving general competencies, and modifying environments. For example, most programs designed to prevent maladjustment among children undergoing hospitalization for surgery focus on providing information (Peterson & Ridley-Johnson, 1980).

Quite a few preventive interventions use a much more extended, or chronic, time frame. Many early secondary prevention programs for children, for example, attempt to build competencies and improve adjustment via therapy and consultation delivered over 1 year, and often several years (Forgays, 1991). Programs targeted to improve ecology and safety (e.g., litter reduction, recycling, seat belt usage) often include long-term interventions and evaluation (e.g., the attractive litter container mentioned earlier, Geller et al., 1977). The programs of longer duration often attempt to change more chronic or refractory conditions and tend to be more likely to evaluate such efforts for generalized effects (Geller, 1983).

Target Population Jason and Glenwick (1980) made it clear that prevention programs can be targeted to individuals, groups, organizations, communities, or societies. Many programs, especially competency building or adjustment programs, train individuals. However, a number of preventive efforts have targeted naturally interacting groups such as classrooms and families.

Organizations can also benefit from preventive interventions. Entire schools, companies, community mental health centers, residence halls, and hospitals have received interventions designed to improve attendance and job performance, and reduce the probability of a variety of disruptions (Jason & Glenwick, 1980). Many of these efforts focus on modifying environments. For example, Jason and Glenwick (1980) reviewed the results of two studies that modified nursing home environments. In efforts designed to prevent social isolation and concomitant mental or physical deterioration, or both, researchers placed puzzles, other equipment, and refreshments into lounge areas. These environmental changes effectively and sharply increased social interaction by the nursing home residents.

Even larger scale efforts have been aimed at entire communities or societies (Taylor & Stunkard, 1993). These efforts often involve mass media educational efforts designed to promote attitudinal or behavioral changes, such as decreasing smoking, decreasing littering, decreasing drunk driving, and increasing social support via volunteer work.

Guiding Strategy for Implementation

The foregoing analysis showed that some preventive programs can be described within a $4 \times 2 \times 5$ matrix (Focus $\times$ Time frame $\times$ Target population). Additional dimensions could be incorporated (Cowen, 1980), but the 40 types (cells) described in the present model provide a good sampling of the major options available to those interested in the primary and secondary prevention of sedentarianism.

Each preventive program, regardless of its specific focus, time frame, or target population, evolves within four stages of a general strategy (Bloom, 1984):

Stage 1. Identify a problem of sufficient importance to justify the development of a preventive intervention program.

Stage 2. Develop reliable methods for diagnosing the presence, absence, or degree of the problem so that target populations and the efficacy of interventions can be assessed accurately.

Stage 3. Using epidemiological, correlation, quasi-experimental, and experimental methodology, identify likely pathways of the origin and development of the problem.

Stage 4. Mount, evaluate, and then refine and further develop experimental preventive intervention programs based on the results of Stages 2 and 3.

Many efforts designed to prevent problems of all sorts have omitted one or more of these stages. Many expensive educational campaigns fill commercial television airways with ostensibly little regard for their actual effects on specific target populations. For example, some television commercial campaigns have

directed us to think of behavioral-emotional problems as diseases. This propaga-
tion of the medical model of psychological problems has persisted for two
decades, heedless of findings showing that such conceptualizations have adverse
effects (Farina, Fisher, Getter, & Fischer, 1978) and do not work (Morrison,
1980; Sarbin & Mancuso, 1970).

The next section of this chapter is devoted to an analysis of existing conceptualizations and interventions targeted at anti-sedentarianism. It is offered to help
avoid some of the mistakes made by campaigns for prevention launched in other
areas and possibly improve the efficacy of existing work on anti-sedentarianism.

TOWARD EFFECTIVE PROGRAMS
FOR ANTI-SEDENTARIANISM

It is important to consider the current status of anti-sedentarianism by using the
issues raised in Bloom's (1984) four-stage strategy for prevention. This analysis
will allow for consideration of which of the 40 cells of preventive programs are
being used currently and which could be developed or improved.

Stage 1: Is sedentarianism an important enough problem to justify the development of preventive intervention programs? Sedentary lifestyles are clearly
implicated in the development of cardiovascular problems, obesity, and perhaps
psychological difficulties (e.g., depression, anxiety, stress). Lifestyles that incorporate regular physical activity probably can help prevent these and other problems (e.g., behavioral-emotional troubles), while potentially promoting a higher
quality of life (Shephard, 1990). Certainly these are important goals. The first
section of this chapter further justifies work on anti-sedentarianism by demonstrating the cost-effectiveness of prevention programming.

Stage 2: Can we assess sedentarianism reliably and accurately? Articles by
Durnin (1990), Thompson and Martin (1984), and others (Skinner, Baldini, &
Gardner, 1990) document that a number of effective and efficient procedures,
several with existing norms, can be used to assess cardiovascular fitness. There
are also some questionnaires that have established track records for assessing rel-
evant cognitive aspects of sedentarianism, most notably the "Self-motivation
Questionnaire" developed by Dishman and colleagues (Dishman & Ickes, 1981;
Dishman, Ickes, & Morgan, 1980).

Stage 3: Do we know the likely pathways of the origins and development of
sedentarianism? We know surprisingly little about this crucial phase of prevention
applied to sedentary lifestyles. There have been some relevant, but largely correlational, studies that describe primarily who is likely to discontinue vigorous exercise programs, i.e., the development and maintenance of anti-sedentarianism
among high-risk adults. Because much of this work has been conducted by Dishman, and because this work is described in chapter 4, the summary presented here
is brief (see also Dishman, 1982, 1987, 1988a, 1990).

It seems that among the 50% of the population who are likely to quit their
exercise programs within the first 6 months, there is a disproportionate number of

people at high risk for significant cardiovascular problems (e.g., people who are overweight, who smoke, and who are less knowledgeable about health risks). Furthermore, various social-environmental and cognitive-behavioral factors contribute substantially to the likelihood of recidivism in such efforts (e.g., lack of social support; selecting unenjoyable, solitary, and inconvenient exercise programs; choosing only difficult and inflexible exercise goals and plans).

This work has led to a valuable realization that should be applied to conceptualizations of secondary prevention programs designed to change the physical activity habits of high-risk adults:

> Exercise can, perhaps, be likened in many respects to attempts at dieting, quitting smoking, reducing alcohol intake or other "New Year's Resolutions" by which people attempt to consciously change what has for them become a behavioral habit unconducive to their health or well-being! People start, but they don't finish up. (Dishman, 1984, pp. 2-3)

Stage 4: Do we know how to mount and evaluate experimental antisedentarianism programs based on extant knowledge of this problem? There are two answers to this bottom-line question. First, there are sufficient measures of physical fitness, as well as measures of related cognitive-behavioral variables (e.g., self-motivation, depression), to assess some key outcomes to which antisedentarianism programs are directed. However, the material regarding Stage 2 makes it clear that further work in this area is sorely needed. Second, regarding intervention, we know more about what not to do than about what to do at this juncture. The major realization derived from Stage 3 indicates that interventions that focus primarily on providing information should prove quite ineffectual in altering sedentarianism among high-risk adults. In fact,

> Previous research has indicated that well-conducted mass media campaigns directed at large, open populations can effectively transmit information, alter some attitudes, and produce small shifts in behavior, such as effecting choices among consumer products, but has failed to demonstrate that media alone can substantially influence more complex behavior. (Meyer, Nash, McAlister, Maccoby, & Farquhar, 1980, p. 130)

This conclusion does not mean that intensive public campaigns cannot produce benefits to some of the people some of the time. The evidence suggests that more intensive, group-targeted (rather than only community-targeted) health promotion campaigns can produce significant, usually small, improvements in various health risk factors (Meyer et al., 1980; Taylor & Stunkard, 1993). Perhaps people who are currently nonsedentary (e.g., children, nonobese casual exercisers) can be influenced to intensify their efforts via individual, group, or even community-society level campaigns. The question remains, nonetheless, how should secondary prevention programs for anti-sedentarianism be implemented? Further, what are some promising strategies for primary prevention?

RECOMMENDATIONS TOWARD
EFFECTIVE ANTI-SEDENTARIANISM

Primary Prevention

The very formidable costs and unproven effects of primary prevention for anti-sedentarianism justify secondary prevention efforts more easily. Likewise, risk profiles for cardiovascular disorders and depression help to establish more firmly that people who are currently rather sedentary and depressive (or anxious) are especially vulnerable to the very adverse effects associated with long-term sedentarianism. Thus, most attempts at anti-sedentarianism in the near future probably should focus on secondary prevention, using groups at high risk for sustained sedentarianism and likely to be affected adversely by the same.

This recommendation does not imply that primary prevention programming should cease entirely. It is very probable that some relatively inexpensive strategies could significantly deter at least some individuals from sedentarianism. Unfortunately, little extant empirical evidence is available to direct these efforts. It seems likely, for example, that certain media campaigns (i.e., those focusing on providing information) may prove effective for certain subpopulations, such as children or mildly to moderately active young adults. It would be very useful, therefore, to conduct analyses of the specific effects of various types of programs that provide information on sedentarianism to these subpopulations. This point advocates refined program-by-person analyses. It also calls for evaluations of preventive programming on those heretofore neglected subpopulations in addition to continuing studies in high-risk groups that are quite difficult to change (Meyer et al., 1980).

One focus for primary prevention programming has already demonstrated its promise as an efficient and surprisingly effective approach at least for inducing some changes in sedentarianism. Several clinical trials and at least one experiment have used environmental modifications targeted to communities (Brownell, Stunkard, & Albaum, 1980) and societies (Keir & Lauzon, 1980; see also Taylor & Stunkard, 1993). For example, Brownell et al. (1980) placed a large sign (3 × 3.5 feet) at several choice points at which pedestrians could take either stairs or escalators to reach their destinations. In their first of two studies, the sign more than doubled (i.e., significantly increased) the use of stairs by obese and nonobese white men and women both under and over 30 years of age. The use of stairs decreased to near-baseline levels when the sign was withdrawn, but stair usage significantly and immediately increased again on the first day the sign was returned. A replication again showed an immediate substantial impact of the sign that was largely maintained 1 month after withdrawal, but not at 3 months. Unfortunately, obese people did not respond differentially to the presence or absence of the sign in the replication study.

Perhaps such environmental changes could induce some people to lead more active lives. The previously noted findings on physical activity programs for high-risk adults (Dishman, 1984) make it unlikely that many high-risk people would change substantially as a function of such interventions (e.g., recall the nonsignificant effects for obese people in the Brownell et al. [1980] replication study). However, environmental modifications may be an inexpensive way to facilitate the effectiveness of more intensive individual- or group-targeted secondary prevention programs emphasizing "lifestyle exercising" (Epstein et al., 1983). These modifications could produce promising results even for high-risk groups. Furthermore, if communities embrace such concepts, a larger scale adoption of inexpensive but effective means to support anti-sedentarianism could be promoted. This could become operationalized in further environmental modifications. Thus, a more "anti-sedentary future" could include more attractive stairwells, perhaps with built-in sound systems, fewer escalators and elevators, tolls for using escalators and elevators, "park and walk" programs for commuters replacing extant "park and ride" campaigns, and so on.

Secondary Prevention

Most of what has been learned about sedentarianism can be used to develop potentially very effective secondary prevention interventions. The justification for such efforts has been established clearly with regard to physical health, and guidelines for target populations and focus on intervention are easily derived from a substantial empirical foundation.

Regarding the latter issues, the most appropriate dimensions for target populations are individual and group. The work of Dishman (1984, 1987) and others (Meyer et al., 1980) shows that promoting anti-sedentarianism to people at risk for early cardiovascular problems mandates new conceptualizations of the problem and the intervention. Instead of viewing anti-sedentarianism for this subpopulation as a problem that is modified readily via mass media campaigning, it should be viewed and treated as a highly refractory self-regulatory problem.

Viewing sedentary lifestyles as a self-regulatory problem means that we can apply the substantial literature accumulated on behavioral self-regulation to refine methods of improving and maintaining exercise habits. Exercising is a self-regulated problem because it involves regulating one's goal-directed behaviors without immediate external constraints (Kanfer & Karoly, 1972). Furthermore, for many individuals at high risk for coronary problems (e.g., obese, already somewhat sedentary, adults), improving physical activity habits presents a conflict between immediate short-term goals (e.g., staying relaxed and comfortable, time pressures, avoiding the stress of dieting) and long-term goals (e.g., sustained good health). This defines anti-sedentarianism as a special type of self-regulatory problem, the tolerance of noxious stimulation variant of self-control.

Self-control (and self-regulation, more generally) involves complex interactions between cognitions (e.g., goal-setting, planning, self-evaluation), affect (i.e., emotional states), physiology (e.g., strength), and environmental variables. Kirschenbaum (1984) described these complex relationships in five sequential phases: problem identification, commitment, execution, environmental management, and generalization. This analysis, based on work by Kanfer and Karoly (1972; Karoly, 1993) and others (Mahoney & Thoresen, 1974) can be applied directly to the problem of anti-sedentarianism. In so doing, it suggests appropriate foci, time frames, and target population dimensions for secondary prevention programming.

Problem Identification   It is probably necessary, but not sufficient, for individuals to realize the long-term impact of sedentarianism and, conversely, the many potential benefits of more active lifestyles, including effects on mood states. This information should be communicated clearly and dramatically, using statistics as well as personalized appeals (e.g., from patients with CHD who regret their histories of sedentarianism and individuals who have enjoyed several specific emotional as well as physical health benefits of active lifestyles).

Commitment   It is clear that the amount of expressed desire to improve physical fitness can predict perseverance in various physical activity programs and favorable beliefs about one's ability to do so (Armstrong et al., 1993). It may be helpful to incorporate "milestone" or acute time frames in preventive programs, in part because of these findings. People may be more likely to commit to a goal when they reach a certain milestone, like their 30th or 40th birthdays or a new, sedentary job.

Several persuasive tactics can also intensify that commitment. For example, Janis and Mann (1977) have had people complete "balance sheets" in which they identify many positive and negative outcomes that might result from achieving specific goals. This procedure seems to help people increase their commitment, thereby improving the likelihood of achieving desired anti-sedentarianism outcomes.

Execution   With a self-regulatory problem identified and a commitment developed to modify it, the active change process or execution phase begins. This process frequently is conceptualized in cybernetic terms (Carver, 1979; Kanfer & Karoly, 1972). Individuals are presumed, for example, to self-monitor (i.e., systematically attend to and record target behaviors), self-evaluate (i.e., compare performance to goals), self-consequate (i.e., self-reward if goals are achieved; self-punish if goals are not achieved), and, in so doing, continually strive to modify target behaviors.

Many studies have helped to refine these conceptualizations, thereby clarifying principles of self-regulation. For example, one important principle that has emerged is, "Differential expectancies and self-monitoring interact with task mastery to affect self-regulation" (Kirschenbaum, 1984). Studies have shown, for example, that self-monitoring successes, not failures, often improve performance of difficult tasks (Kirschenbaum & Karoly, 1977). This finding has been applied to sport contexts; the results indicate that when people are novices in sports like golf (Johnston-O'Connor & Kirschenbaum, 1986) and bowling (Kirschenbaum, Ordman, Tomarken, & Holtzbauer, 1982), they can maximize their performance if they keep records of successful execution of components of that performance. Related evidence from basic laboratory research also indicates that such positive self-monitoring of difficult tasks can sustain involvement or persistence in the task (Kirschenbaum & Tomarken, 1982). These results suggest that high-risk and sedentary adults may persist more effectively when they self-monitor positively as they begin their exercise and sport programs.

Environmental Management It is known that social-environmental factors can affect persistence in physical activity programs (see chapter 4). The degree and type of social support, whether the activity is social or solitary, and convenience factors all contribute to maintenance of physical activity programs. The self-regulatory perspective merely argues that the individual can learn to shape his or her environment in a proactive fashion to maximize the probability of goal attainment.

It is also noteworthy that the type of external feedback provided to exercise and sport participants is another important environmental contributor to fitness outcomes. Extremely negativistic coaches need to be avoided and replaced by coaches, playing partners, and team members who provide ample support and encouragement (Smith, 1993).

Generalization Anti-sedentarianism, by definition, encourages very long-term (chronic) lifestyle changes. Maintenance of change in refractory behaviors, like exercising, seems to require the development of an "obsessive-compulsive style of self-regulation" (Kirschenbaum & Tomarken, 1982). That is, the evidence suggests that a great many factors can deter sustained self-regulated behavior change. In order to avoid self-regulatory failure, it seems necessary to self-monitor target behaviors continually, without letting emotional stressors, depressive or negativistic thinking, physiological pressures, and other factors described elsewhere (Kirschenbaum, 1987) dismantle sustained and systematic attention to target behaviors. Research in sport psychology supports this conceptualization by showing that elite athletes often develop an obsessive-compulsive style of maintaining their efforts in their sports.

It is clear that relatively brief (acute) interventions and mass media campaigns should not be *expected* to produce substantial long-term change. Individual and small group interventions that are intensive, multicomponent in focus, involving, and long-lasting appear warranted (Kirschenbaum & Fitzgibbon, 1995; Meichenbaum & Turk, 1987). For example, the use of well-developed behavioral contracting could yield important, and as yet untapped, benefits (Kirschenbaum & Flanery, 1984). Contracting is a flexible, self-involving tool that people can implement largely on their own with brief consultation from others. Use of this procedure also helps to ensure that sustained self-monitoring will continue and provides a forum for explicit goal-setting, planning, and environmental management. In addition, relapse prevention training (Marlatt & Gordon, 1985) could be utilized effectively in conjunction with behavioral contracting when individuals and small groups are the targets for intervention.

SUMMARY

In sum, concepts and strategies of prevention appear useful when applied to the problem of sedentarianism. Issues pertaining to the focus, time frame, and target population must be considered when designing preventive interventions. Thus, certain programs that focus on environmental modification, as well as providing information, may produce some primary prevention benefits even when applied to organizations, communities, and societies. On the other hand, secondary prevention of sedentarianism with high-risk and already somewhat sedentary adults probably requires multifocused, intensive, and long-term interventions targeted to individuals or groups. The latter efforts also must conceptualize the target of intervention as a refractory self-control problem. Principles and procedures developed to ameliorate such problems seem highly relevant, and worthy of explicit application, to anti-sedentarianism.

Chapter 3

Exercise Prescription

Andrea L. Dunn and Steven N. Blair

Regular physical activity and exercise are linked to improved physical and psychological health through all human developmental stages in both normal and disordered populations. Experimental studies demonstrate that regular exercise improves risk factors for cardiovascular disease such as physical fitness, blood lipids, blood pressure, and body composition in children, adolescents, and middle-aged and older adults (Cauley et al., 1986; Jennings et al., 1986; Wood, Stefanick, Williams, & Haskell, 1991). Furthermore, exercise has an important role in the treatment of CHD, hypertension, non–insulin-dependent diabetes mellitus (NIDDM), depression, and anxiety. The preponderance of research has examined the relation between physical activity and cardiovascular disease and because of the strength of these studies, the American Heart Association issued a statement in 1992 recognizing physical inactivity as an independent risk factor for cardiovascular disease (Fletcher et al., 1992). Although not as extensive as the evidence for prevention of cardiovascular disease, regular physical activity is correlated with the prevention and treatment of other diseases including some cancers, obesity, osteoporosis, and depression (Bouchard, Shephard, & Stephens, 1994).

Less certain than the evidence linking physical activity to good health is what constitutes "appropriate activity." Since the publication of the ACSM position statement on "The Recommended Quantity and Quality of Exercise for Developing and Maintaining Fitness in Healthy Adults" in 1978, there have been important revisions and expansions of exercise prescription recommendations (ACSM,

We thank Melba Morrow, M.A., and H. W. Kohl, III, Ph.D., for editorial assistance. We also thank Jim Sallis, Ph.D., for his creative ideas about the integration of stages of change with exercise determinants. This work was supported in part by U.S. Public Health Service research grant AG06945 from the National Institute on Aging, and HL48597 from the National Heart, Lung, and Blood Institute, Bethesda, Maryland.

1978). For instance, in the 1990 ACSM position stand, proper exercise intensity guidelines were changed from 60% to 90% of maximum heart rate reserve to 60% to 90% of maximum heart rate (ACSM, 1990). Guidelines for exercise duration were changed from 15 to 60 min to 20 to 60 min per session. These 1990 recommendations further specified that the frequency, intensity, and duration of exercise needed for fitness were not equivalent to those needed for health. Recently, the CDC and ACSM issued a position statement aimed at expanding the traditional views of exercise prescription (CDC & ACSM, 1993). This statement encourages those who are physically inactive or inadequately active to accumulate 30 min of moderate-intensity activity on most, preferably all, days of the week. The major impetus for expansion of these guidelines is accumulating epidemiological and clinical data that indicate there may be no minimum threshold for obtaining some health benefit from regular exercise. Rather, most studies indicate a dose-response gradient and the greatest difference in risk of all-cause and cardiovascular disease mortality is between those who are least fit or least active and those who are moderately fit or moderately active (Blair, 1993).

Public health officials acknowledge that the prevalence of participation in regular physical activity has not increased since the mid-1980s. Current population surveys indicate that 24% of adult Americans are completely sedentary and 54%, while physically active, do not receive adequate amounts of physical activity (DHHS, 1990). Clearly, to reduce the public health burden of a sedentary lifestyle, we need a better understanding of how much exercise is needed for health. This chapter reviews representative research concerning the type and amount of physical activity needed for physical and psychological health. For more complete reviews on the effects of physical activity on physical health outcomes, the reader is referred to Blair et al., 1992; Bouchard et al., 1994; and Paffenbarger, Hyde, Wing, and Steinmetz, 1993. Specifically, we discuss the goals of public health policymakers and the epidemiological and clinical evidence that provides the foundation for these goals. We also address specific health outcomes and the evidence for the dose-response relation in terms of these outcomes. Finally, we discuss a new approach to increasing physical activity in sedentary adults that takes into account the flexibility of the expanded exercise prescription recommendations.

HOW MUCH EXERCISE IS NEEDED FOR HEALTH?

The majority of prospective studies examining the relation of physical activity or fitness to all-cause mortality or CHD demonstrate a strong inverse relation. An excellent review by Powell, Thompson, Caspersen, and Kendrick in 1987 analyzed 43 studies that were evaluated and classified as good, satisfactory, or unsatisfactory in terms of the physical activity assessment, CHD measure, and epidemiological methods. Physical activity was evaluated in terms of the clarity of the definition, whether reliability and validity data were available on the measure used, the dose of activity, and adherence to and standardization in data collection. Similar criteria were applied to CHD surveillance and epidemiological methods.

The relative risks were then tabulated for all studies and a total of 96 comparisons were made from these 43 reports. The criteria recommended for evaluating scientific literature for public policy decisions include consistency, strength of relation in terms of relative risk, whether the study is sequenced appropriately, whether there is a biological gradient, and whether results are plausible and coherent. The findings relative to these criteria are as follows: (a) Two thirds of the studies reported a statistically significant association demonstrating that inactivity is related to CHD; (b) The relative risks ranged from 1.5 to 2.4 (median 1.9); (c) Two thirds of the studies indicated that physical inactivity preceded the onset of CHD; (d) Increasing risk of CHD with decreasing activity was demonstrated in 68%; and (e) Plausible mechanisms included evidence that physical activity decreased blood pressure and plasma triglycerides. It should be noted that studies with good measures or methods had even higher percentages of agreement of increasing risk with decreasing activity (i.e., 73% to 88%). An evaluation of these criteria leads to the conclusion that sedentary habits are a cause of CHD.

Since Powell et al.'s review (1987), other prospective studies have consistently demonstrated the same strong inverse relationship. Selected studies are depicted in Figure 1 (Blair et al., 1989; Ekelund et al., 1988; Leon, Connett, Jacobs, & Rauramaa, 1987; Morris, Clayton, Everitt, Semmence, & Burgess, 1990; Paffenbarger et al., 1984). These studies have been reviewed elsewhere and the reader is referred to Blair (1994) and Haskell (1994a, 1994b) for further discussion.

What is striking about the relation depicted in Figure 3-1 is that the slope of most of the lines is greater on the left side of the figure than on the right. In other words, increasing from no (or very little) physical activity or fitness to light or moderate amounts is associated with lower mortality than the same difference between moderate to high activity levels or fitness.

These data are in agreement with clinical studies that demonstrate that moderate-intensity exercise can improve fitness, endurance, and related risk factors. This is surprising to many exercise scientists as well as to the general public who believe that exercising at a high intensity is required to improve fitness. This assumption is due in part to a misinterpretation of the ACSM recommendations (1990), which state that the intensity should be between 60% and 90%. Exercise scientists have focused on relatively high-intensity exercise, in part because of the now classic study by Karvonen, Kentala, and Mustala (1957), in which 3 male students who trained at 60% of VO_2max were compared with 4 male students who trained at 71% to 75% of their VO_2max. Both groups trained for 4 weeks for 30 min per day 4 or 5 days per week. Results showed that only one of the subjects who trained at the 60% intensity improved his submaximal running speed, while all four of those who trained at the higher intensity improved on this measure. Even though only 1 person from the lower-intensity group increased his running speed, 2 out of 3 increased VO_2max, and all 3 had lower resting heart rates and increased heart volume. These results indicate that important cardiovascular adaptations can occur at lower intensities even though the group who exercised at the higher intensity had a greater improvement.

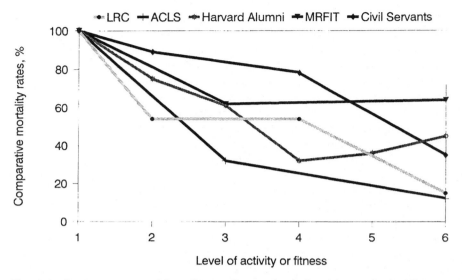

Figure 1 Data are presented from five studies on physical activity or physical fitness and coronary heart disease or cardiovascular disease: Lipid Research Clinics (LRC; Ekelund et al., 1988), Aerobics Center Longitudinal Study (ACLS; Blair et al., 1989), Harvard Alumni (Paffenbarger et al., 1984), Multiple Risk Factor Intervention Trial (MR-FIT; Leon et al., 1987), and Civil Servants (Morris et al., 1990). The vertical axis represents mortality rates, set at 100%, in the various physical activity and fitness categories as percentages for the least active and fit groups. The horizontal axis represents levels of physical activity or physical fitness. Credit for the concept for this figure is given to Dr. William L. Haskell of the Stanford University School of Medicine. It is modeled after a slide he presented at the R. Tait McKenzie Lecture at the American Academy of Physical Education. From *Physical Activity, Fitness, and Health: International Proceedings and Consensus Statement*, p. 583, by S.N. Blair, 1994, Champaign, IL: Human Kinetics Publishers. Reprinted with permission.

Exercise training studies in the 1960s and 1970s used similar protocols to the Karvonen study (e.g., subjects were male high school or college students, training programs lasted anywhere from 4 to 10 weeks, and exercise intensities ranged from 39% to 96%; Burke & Franks, 1975; Faria, 1970; Sharkey, 1970; Sharkey & Holleman, 1967; Shephard, 1968). In all of these studies, groups who trained at the lower intensities showed some improvement, although this was not always statistically significant for the lowest training intensity. However, considering the lack of statistical power due to small sample size, short-term training, and relatively high activity levels at baseline, a lack of statistical significance in some of the studies is not surprising. The major point is that evidence for a training effect from low- to moderate-intensity exercise has long been available, but has largely been ignored.

More recent training studies of sedentary and older men and women report significant improvements in VO_2max at training intensities as low as 40% (Gaesser & Rich, 1984; Gossard, Haskell, & Taylor, 1986). In a study conducted by Foster, Hume, Byrnes, Dickinson, and Chatfield (1989), 24 healthy older women (67 to 89 years of age) walked at least 3 days per week for 10 weeks after being assigned randomly to a group that trained at either 40% or 60% of their VO_2max. There was a significant increase in VO_2max in both groups after the 10 weeks of training; however, there was no between-group difference at the different training intensities.

Improvements in risk factors associated with regular physical activity also occur at moderate training intensities. Duncan, Gordon, and Scott (1991) assigned 102 sedentary premenopausal women to three different walking intensities of 8.0, 6.4, or 4.8 km/hr or a sedentary control condition. VO_2max increased in a dose-response manner, with higher intensities showing greater improvement; however, improvements in high-density lipoprotein (HDL) levels were the same for all three walking intensities.

In addition to these findings regarding the intensity of physical activity, other studies demonstrate that continuous exercise of 20 minutes or longer may not be necessary to achieve health benefits. For example, a number of epidemiological studies demonstrate that decreased risk of CHD is associated with the accumulation of moderate intensity activities performed on an intermittent basis. These include lifestyle activities such as walking, stair climbing, gardening, and housework in which the energy expenditure differences between sedentary and moderately active individuals range between 80 and 400 kcal/day (Paffenbarger, Hyde, Wing, & Hsieh, 1986; Rose, 1969).

Two other experimental studies demonstrate that intermittent activity can improve physical fitness and some of the risk factors associated with CHD. In 1990, DeBusk, Hakansson, Sheehan, and Haskell conducted an 8-week training study with 40 sedentary men (mean age 51 ± 6 years) comparing continuous versus intermittent exercise bouts on VO_2max. Continuous exercise consisted of a single 30-min bout of jogging at a training heart rate of 65% to 75% of the peak heart rate as determined by treadmill testing. Intermittent exercise was done at the same intensity, but consisted of three bouts of 10 min separated by at least 4 hours. Both groups experienced an increase in VO_2max (13.9% in the continuous group and 7.6% in the intermittent group). Other estimates of endurance fitness have demonstrated comparable improvements including reductions in heart rate at submaximal exercise intensities, increases in treadmill test duration, and similar amounts of weight loss. This study demonstrates that even short bouts of exercise improve fitness.

A second experimental study compared shorter bouts of exercise with longer bouts and examined changes in VO_2max and HDL cholesterol. Ebisu (1985) assigned 53 young male college students to one of four treatment conditions. One group served as a control and the other three experimental groups trained by running 3 miles 3 days per week. However, the first experimental group ran the 3-mile distance in one session, the second split the distance into two runs of 1.5 miles each, and the third split the distance into three daily 1-mile runs. After the program, which lasted for 10 weeks, all three experimental groups had increased their total mileage to 6 miles per day at the same running schedule. All experimental groups increased their maximal oxygen uptake by 8% relative to the control group, and there was no significant difference in maximal oxygen uptake between the three groups. HDL cholesterol also was measured, and only the group that ran three times per day showed a significant improvement.

The majority of epidemiological studies have shown an inverse gradient of risk of all-cause mortality and CHD for increasing levels of physical activity or fitness. Furthermore, the activity-related reduction in risk seems to be dependent on weekly habitual energy expenditure, and issues of frequency, intensity, and duration need to be examined further. Although the threshold dose cannot be specified, it is clear that some activity is better than none. This realization led the CDC and ACSM to issue their position statement encouraging accumulating 30 min of moderate-intensity activity on most, preferably all, days of the week. Considering that 20% to 30% of the population is inactive, these findings extend public health recommendations for increasing physical activity behavior in the population. Powell and Blair (1994) estimate that if half of those who do not participate in any leisure time physical activity would do *something* a few times per week, 20,000 fewer deaths per year would occur. The objectives of Healthy People 2000 are to decrease sedentary lifestyles to no more than 15% of the population and increase moderate daily physical activity to at least 30% of the population (DHHS, 1990). This would be a 38% decrease in the prevalence of sedentary lifestyle and a 36% increase in moderate activity levels for the U.S. population. These new guidelines provide greater flexibility in designing and implementing physical activity programs to reduce all-cause mortality and CHD. The dose-response relation to other specific physical and psychological health outcomes is less well known and are explored in the next section of this chapter.

PHYSICAL ACTIVITY NEEDED FOR SPECIFIC HEALTH OUTCOMES

Physical Health Outcomes

Physical activity has been studied in relation to the prevention and treatment of many specific health outcomes, including cancer, hypertension, stroke, NIDDM, osteoporosis, and weight control (Bouchard et al., 1994). Both acute and chronic physical activity may play a role in regulating the physiological mechanisms that play a role in these outcomes. In the case of diabetes, an acute bout of aerobic exercise has been found to enhance insulin sensitivity in skeletal muscle (Vranic & Wasserman, 1990). In patients with both insulin-dependent diabetes mellitus (IDDM) and NIDDM, blood glucose levels are lowered with a single bout of aerobic exercise and, with chronic training, glycemic control improves in patients with NIDDM. In the case of osteoporosis, physical activity with a sufficient mechanical loading on skeletal structure may reduce risk by boosting peak bone mass in young women and slowing the decrease in bone mass in middle-aged and older women, although findings are inconsistent (Snow-Harter & Marcus, 1991).

There is an inverse dose-response relation between physical activity and many chronic diseases and conditions. For example, evidence is accumulating that physical activity may provide some protection against colon cancer. Lee and Paffenbarger (1992b) show that men who expend 2,500 kcal/week have half the risk of developing colon cancer as men who expend less than 1,000 kcal/week. In the Aerobics Center Longitudinal Study, there was an inverse association between cancer mortality and maximal exercise tolerance on a treadmill test. In this study, 10,224 men and 3,120 women were followed up for 8 years (Blair et al., 1989), during which there were 64 cancer deaths among the men and 18 cancer deaths among the women. When age-adjusted analyses were performed to examine the relation between low, moderate, and high physical fitness and cancer, inverse trends were statistically significant across physical fitness categories. In the low, moderate, and high fitness categories, the age-adjusted cancer death rates per 10,000 person years were 20, 7, and 5 in men and 16, 10, and 1 in women, respectively. Although the numbers are small and must be interpreted cautiously, the trend suggests a dose-response relation.

Breast and prostate cancer also may be related to levels of activity. Frisch, Wyshak, Albright, Schiff, and Jones (1985) examined breast cancer prevalence in the perimenopausal years in former female collegiate athletes compared with nonathletes. Seventy-four percent of the athletes had maintained a regular exercise program compared with 57% of the nonathletes; and the risk for breast cancer was nearly twice as high in nonathletes. A more recent case-controlled study by Bernstein, Henderson, Hanisch, Sullivan-Halley, and Ross (1994) found that women who averaged at least 3.8 hours of physical activity per week were nearly 60% less likely to have breast cancer than their inactive peers. Studies by Lee and Paffenbarger (1992a) and Albanes, Blair, and Taylor (1989) suggest that higher levels of physical activity reduce prostate cancer risk. Findings for both of these types of cancer must be interpreted cautiously because of the small number of studies conducted, but it appears that higher levels of physical activity may lower the risk of these specific cancers.

Although these specific health outcomes indicate a dose-response relation, for other outcomes such as hypertension, not only is the amount of activity important, but the intensity may play a part as well (ACSM, 1993). In examining this relation across low to moderate to high intensities, moderate-intensity exercise was as effective, and perhaps more so, as higher-intensity exercise in the treatment of hypertension. The ACSM position statement (1993) on "Physical Activity, Physical Fitness, and Hypertension" reports that moderate-intensity exercise can reduce both systolic and diastolic blood pressure levels an average of 10 mm Hg in people with mild to moderate hypertension.

Psychological Health Outcomes

A number of reviews examining the relation of physical activity and mental health outcomes or psychopathology (i.e., general well-being or depression) indicate the need to better understand whether a dose-response relation exists for

Physical Activity and General Well-Being

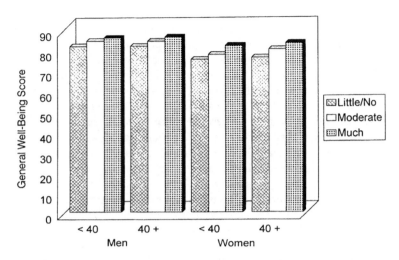

Figure 2 Data adapted from the work of Stephens (1988) indicates the relation between physical activity and general well-being in population survey data from the United States and Canada. The vertical axis represents the scores of general well-being, and the horizontal axis indicates gender and age categories. This figure indicates that general well-being increases with increases in physical activity. This is particularly true for women over 40 years of age.

these measures (Dunn & Dishman, 1991; Raglin, 1990). Few population-based studies that analyze the relation of physical activity and psychological outcomes are available. Stephens (1988) conducted several cross-sectional analyses examining the association among general well-being, levels of anxiety and depression, and positive mood by combining survey data from the United States and Canada. Increases in physical activity are associated with good mental health (defined as general well-being measures, an absence of symptoms of anxiety and depression, and positive mood). The data from this study indicate a dose-response relation for general well-being, particularly for women (Figure 2). However, the data for depression do not indicate the same graded response (Figure 3). Both figures indicate that benefits can occur with moderate levels of activity, particularly for women and older populations.

Three prospective studies examined the relation between physical activity and depression. Farmer et al. (1988) used data from the National Health and Nutrition Examination Survey (NHANES I) and found that low levels of recreational activity at baseline predicted depression 8 years later in white women who had not been depressed previously. Furthermore, this association was independent of age, chronic conditions, education, employment, and income. This relation was not found for previously nondepressed men who were depressed at

Physical Activity and Depression Scores

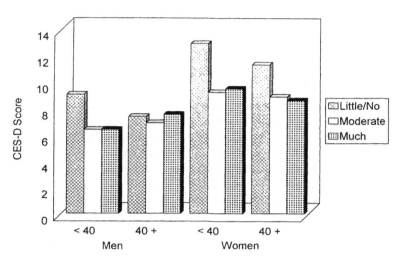

Figure 3 Data adapted from the work of Stephens (1988) from the same population as in Figure 2 shows the relation between physical activity and depression scores as measured by the Center for Epidemiological Studies-Depression Scale (CES-D). Scores on the CES-D are represented on the vertical axis, and gender and age categories are represented on the horizontal axis. This figure indicates that for women above and below 40 years of age and for men below the age of 40 moderate amounts of physical activity are associated with decreased symptoms of depression as measured by the CES-D scale.

follow-up; however, in men who were depressed at baseline, low levels of physical activity predicted their continued depression. Data from the Alameda County study also found evidence for an inverse relation between physical activity and depression (Camacho, Roberts, Lazarus, Kaplan, & Cohen, 1991). When the analysis was adjusted for sex, age, and health, the odds ratios for depression were 1.8 for men and 1.7 for women when inactive individuals were compared with their active peers. Although the increased risk for men is higher in this study (1.8) than in the NHANES study (1.3), it is not inconsistent with NHANES.

The most recent population-based study of Harvard alumni, conducted by Paffenbarger, Lee, and Leung (1994), indicates an inverse relation between physical activity and the risk of depression. These results showed that men who expended 1,000 to 2,499 kcal/wk in walking, stair climbing, and sportsplay had a 17% lower risk of developing clinical depression than their less active peers. Furthermore, the men who were most active, expending 2,500 kcal or more per week, were even less likely to develop clinical depression (28%).

Three meta-analyses also provide further evidence for a relation of physical activity to mental health outcomes. In one meta-analysis, depression scores decreased by about 0.5 SD in exercise groups compared with leisure activity, psychotherapy, and nonexercising control groups (North, McCullagh, & Vu Tran,

1990). A similar effect size was demonstrated for the impact of exercise on mediating mental stress (Crews & Landers, 1987) and a slightly smaller effect size was noted for anxiety (i.e., 0.25 to 0.33 SD) in normal populations (Petruzzello, Landers, Hatfield, Kubitz, & Salazar, 1991). Larger effect sizes for reductions in anxiety have been determined in populations who are highly anxious or who have low fitness levels. However, these meta-analyses have been characterized by a general failure to consider behavioral artifacts (see chapter 1), and therefore the results must be viewed with caution.

These studies indicate there may be an inverse relation between physical activity and some mental health outcomes such as general well-being and depression. Intensity of exercise has also been examined in relation to psychological outcomes, but studies of both acute and chronic exercise indicate that intensity may not be an important factor for psychological benefits. A short-term study conducted by Moses, Steptoe, Mathews, and Edwards (1989) compared moderate- to high-intensity training programs in sedentary adults and found that those who trained in the moderate-intensity program had greater psychological benefits than those who trained at the higher intensities. In a 1-year study, moderate-intensity exercise had effects similar to those of high-intensity exercise. Stewart, King, and Haskell (1993) found that the extent of participation in physical activity was related to better psychological outcomes, but the intensity or format of exercise was not. Furthermore, for individuals suffering from depression, exercise may not even need to produce a physiological training effect. Martinsen (1994) recently reviewed the effects of physical activity on depression and found that aerobic and anaerobic exercises are equally effective in the treatment of mild to moderate forms of unipolar depression. These clinical studies are reviewed more extensively in chapters 6 and 7 of this book.

NEW APPROACHES FOR INCREASING PHYSICAL ACTIVITY BEHAVIOR

Studies examining the relation between physical and psychological health outcomes with physical activity, when viewed collectively, suggest that sedentary individuals benefit from moderate-intensity activity. However, the numbers of people engaging in regular physical activity have not increased since the mid-1980s. These data suggest that new approaches are needed to increase physical activity in sedentary populations in order both to enhance psychological and physiological functioning and reduce mortality. New approaches to exercise prescription, which are based on methods we are currently using in the Lifestyle Exercise Trial (also known as Project Active), are discussed in this section. Project Active tests new approaches designed to encourage sedentary adults to adopt and maintain regular physical activity by incorporating the flexibility advocated in the new recommendations (CDC & ACSM, 1993). This approach differs from most traditional exercise programs in three important ways: by adopting a theoretical model to guide intervention; by teaching behavioral skills; and by encouraging lifestyle activity and its accumulation throughout the day. These three components expand the options for the individual and provide greater flexibility for sedentary people to increase their physical activity levels.

Historically, traditional exercise interventions were often atheoretical. The lifestyle approach in our study is based on the transtheoretical or stages of change model developed originally for smoking cessation programs (Prochaska & DiClemente, 1983). Using this as the foundation, individuals are classified according to their readiness to change the targeted health behavior, in this case physical activity (Marcus & Simkin, 1993; Prochaska, Velicer, DiClemente, & Fava, 1988). Readiness is conceptualized as a stage, and people are classified in one of the following five stages: precontemplation—not thinking about being physically active; contemplation—intending to be physically active but not doing physical activity; preparation—doing some physical activity but not on a regular basis; action— doing physical activity on a regular basis; and maintenance—maintaining regular physical activity. The strategies or processes employed to get them to adopt and maintain physical activity vary with whether they are trying to start or continue a physical activity program. In the stages of change model, these processes or behavioral and cognitive skills include consciousness-raising, dramatic relief, environmental reevaluation, self-reevaluation, social liberation, self-liberation, helping relationships, counterconditioning, contingency management, and stimulus control (Marcus, Rossi, Selby, Niaura, & Abrams, 1992; Prochaska et al., 1988).

In addition to these processes, other behavioral constructs such as decision making (Janis & Mann, 1977) and self-efficacy (Bandura, 1977) are incorporated into the stages of change model. Decisional balance helps to predict transitions across stages by examining the pros and cons of adopting the behavior (Marcus, Rakowski, & Rossi, 1992; Velicer, DiClemente, Prochaska, & Brandenburg, 1989). Self-efficacy, the cornerstone of social learning theory (Bandura, 1977), is the confidence individuals have that they can change their physical activity behavior and maintain it across a variety of difficult situations. Building self-efficacy is important through all the stage transitions.

These behavioral constructs and processes are utilized in different ways depending on the person's stage of change. For example, individuals in precontemplation often do not understand the benefits of being physically active. For these people, education or consciousness-raising about the benefits of physical activity and the risks of inactivity can help to move them from precontemplation to contemplation, i.e., a shift in the decisional balance to become physically active. Once individuals have moved into contemplation and have a better understanding of the benefits, they might again use processes such as consciousness-raising and self-reevaluation to examine their past attitudes and feelings about not being able to be physically active. They might also use environmental reevaluation to find opportunities in their environment to become physically active. As individuals find opportunities for doing some physical activity, they move into the next stage, preparation, in which positive feelings about one's ability to become more physically active increase self-efficacy. In addition, processes such as helping relationships and contingency management can be used to progress to the action stage by providing social support and rewards for regular physical activity. Self-efficacy is also important once individuals are in the maintenance stage because it enhances the person's confidence that they can be active in a variety of situations, thus reducing the potential for relapse.

The stages of change model has practical utility in getting sedentary individuals to change their physical activity behavior. Marcus and colleagues have developed measures to determine stages, processes, self-efficacy, and decision making for physical activity (Marcus & Owen, 1992; Marcus, Rakowski, & Rossi, 1992). They show that the behavioral and cognitive skills listed here are used in different ways depending on stage (Marcus, Eaton, Rossi, & Harlow, 1994). Self-efficacy and decisional balance also significantly differentiate stages in both cross-sectional and longitudinal studies (Marcus, Banspach, Lefebvre, Rossi, Carleton, & Abrams,1992; Marcus, Rossi, et al., 1992). Interventions based on the stages of change model increased the initiation, adoption, and maintenance of physical activity in a community intervention, a worksite intervention (Marcus, Banspach, et al., 1992; Marcus, Rossi, et al., 1992), and in Project PACE (Physician-based Assessment and Counseling for Exercise; Long et al., 1994). All showed increased physical activity in the targeted populations compared with standard control groups.

The stages of change model also complements what is known about determinants of exercise behavior. Exercise adherence research shows that multiple factors influence the adoption and maintenance of exercise behavior (Dishman & Sallis, 1994; King et al., 1992; Sallis & Hovell, 1993). Stages of change can be integrated with these determinants as shown in Table 1. For example, the exercise adherence literature demonstrates that confidence in one's ability to be physically active, health knowledge about physical activity, and perceived barriers and benefits of being physically active are important predictors of adoption of exercise. In the transtheoretical model, adoption corresponds to being in precontemplation, contemplation, or preparation. The behavioral change strategies that might be implemented for these stages might include (a) consciousness raising (i.e., increasing health knowledge); (b) self-reevaluation (i.e., understanding one's barriers to physical activity); and (c) increasing self-efficacy (i.e., experiencing success by incorporating multiple short bouts of physical activity into one's daily routine).

A similar scheme could be devised for maintenance of physical activity that parallels the action and maintenance stages in the transtheoretical model. The integration of the determinants of exercise adoption and maintenance as well as the processes of change are illustrated conceptually in Table 1. By integrating the stages of change with determinants, health professionals have greater flexibility in targeting the factors involved in adopting physical activity and greater ability to tailor the processes to meet the needs of the individuals. This is different from traditional exercise approaches in which the primary behavioral skills are learning how to monitor target heart rates and performing some aerobic activity for a certain period of time, and the intervention for each person is the same. While some traditional programs incorporate behavioral skills training such as goal-setting and self-monitoring, these are usually a secondary focus of the overall program.

Table 1 Integration of Stages of Change with Determinants of Exercise Behavior

Exercise stage	Stage of change	Determinants	Processes of change
Adoption	Precontemplation	Health knowledge	Consciousness-raising (e.g., learning about the benefits of physical activity)
	Contemplation	Perceived benefits and barriers	Feelings and attitudes toward physical activity (e.g., learning where activity fits into your day)
	Preparation	Self-efficacy	Contingency management (e.g., rewarding yourself)
Maintenance	Action	Social support	Helping relationships (e.g., eliciting support from family and friends)
		Behavioral skills	Stimulus control (e.g., having walking shoes handy)
	Maintenance	Access to facilities	Environmental reevaluation (e.g., learning about new physical activity opportunities in the community)
Resumption	Relapse	Injuries	Self-liberation (e.g., planning for relapse, transitions)

Note. This table depicts the theoretical integration of stages and processes of change with known determinants of exercise adherence. Credit for this concept is given to Dr. Jim Sallis of San Diego State University, Department of Psychology (personal communication).

In addition to the underlying theoretical approach and emphasis on behavioral skills training, the lifestyle approach also differs in the types and amounts of activity recommended. Lifestyle activity means that the individual looks for opportunities to expend energy, even in short bouts, with a goal of accumulating sufficient activity over the course of the day. Figure 4 depicts the lifestyle approach compared with sedentary activity and leisure-time (traditional) exercise. Because people have different work, family, and environmental situations, each person's lifestyle approach is unique. In our current study, several participants work for large corporations in tall buildings and sit at computers all day. They report they can take longer routes to the restrooms or coffee machines. They also have been able to incorporate some stair climbing and brief 10-min walks at lunch time. They found they could accumulate up to 40 min of physical activity over a workday. Others who have families with children find themselves incorporating more physical activity into the way they spend time with their children.

Theoretical Patterns of Physical Activity

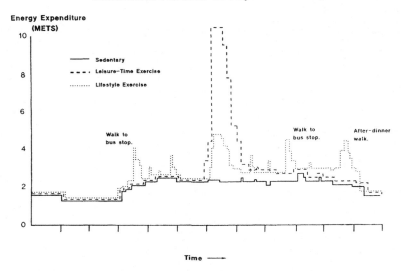

Figure 4 Three theoretical patterns of physical activity over the course of a day are depicted. Leisure time exercise is typical traditional exercise during leisure time, and lifestyle exercise includes accumulated short bouts of moderate-intensity activity that are integrated into daily life. Comparable health effects are expected for leisure time exercise and lifestyle exercise if the total daily energy expenditure is the same. From "Physical Activity and Health: A Lifestyle Approach," by S.N. Blair, H.W. Kohl, and N.F. Gordon, *Medicine, Exercise, Nutrition, and Health, 1,* p. 56. Reprinted with permission.

SUMMARY

The discussion of exercise prescription presented in this chapter intentionally differs from the typical approach to this topic. No mention was made of target heart rate, nor were specific recommendations presented for frequency, intensity, and duration of physical activity. Readers interested in these more traditional approaches to exercise prescription should consult the current edition of the ACSM book, "Guidelines for Exercise Testing and Prescription" (1995). We have attempted to describe alternate, and complementary, approaches to the prescription of physical activity, and we believe that technological advances in health change methods need to be applied to physical activity interventions. It is recommended that scientists and clinicians expand their definition of what exercise prescription means. Behavioral skill building and lifestyle approaches should be incorporated into more traditional exercise programs in order to encourage more individuals to become more physically active more of the time.

Chapter 4

Adherence to Physical Activity

Rod K. Dishman and Janet Buckworth

Only about 12% to 22% of adults in the United States engage in leisure time physical activity at recommended levels, and, depending on the strictness of the definition used, 24% to 60% are sedentary (Caspersen, Merritt, & Stephens, 1994). Furthermore, once sedentary individuals become active, the mean dropout rate from supervised exercise programs reported around the world has remained at roughly 50% over the past 20 years (Dishman, 1988a, 1994a; Morgan, 1977). In addition, the 1990 participation rate objectives set by the U.S. Public Health Service for vigorous and frequent leisure time physical activity (Powell, Spain, Christenson, & Mollenkamp, 1986) were not met (CDC, 1991). The midcourse review (DHHS, 1993) of the physical activity goals outlined in *Healthy People 2000*, the U.S. health promotion and disease prevention objectives for the year 2000 (DHHS, 1991), suggests that they too will not be met.

The failure of Americans to meet national physical activity goals is in part due to a lack of understanding with respect to the determinants of free-living physical activity and adherence to supervised exercise programs. Understanding the knowledge, attitudes, and behavioral and social skills associated with adopting and maintaining a regular exercise program is one research need identified in *Healthy People 2000*. No standardized protocol has been available for the assessment and counseling of physical activity habits. The influential Guidelines for Exercise Testing and Prescription (ACSM, 1991), and its resource manual, published by the ACSM, contain a practically oriented chapter on behavior change. However, there is no formal consensus by experts or a set of sanctioned and validated professional guidelines for interventions designed to increase and maintain exercise behavior.

This is an extensive revision and update of a chapter that originally appeared in Morgan, W.P., & Goldston, S.E. (eds.) (1987). *Exercise and Mental Health*. Washington, DC: Hemisphere Publishing.

One objective of this chapter is to summarize the determinants of adopting and adhering to leisure time physical activity in populations, communities, and supervised programs. We have borrowed from earlier, more detailed reviews (Dishman, 1994b,1994c; Dishman & Sallis, 1994) in order to provide a comprehensive synthesis. Determinants are categorized as characteristics of the individual, the environment, and physical activity. We also describe interventions for increasing physical activity and their effectiveness. Finally, we address some conceptual and measurement problems that have limited our understanding in these areas of research and application.

EXERCISE BEHAVIOR

Physical activity is a unique health behavior encompassing a wide range and complexity of dynamic behavioral demands. Planning for participation, initial adoption of physical activity, continued participation or maintenance, and overall periodicity of participation (e.g., relapse, resumption of activity, and seasonal variation) are characteristics of physical activity that can involve different determinants and warrant different interventions (Dishman, 1990). Physical activity is perceived as requiring more time and effort than other health behaviors (Turk, Rudy, & Salovey, 1984), and it is not correlated with most other health behaviors (Blair, Jacobs, & Powell, 1985; Norman, 1986). In a large population-based controlled trial in the United States, several health risk behaviors were influenced favorably by an educational media campaign, while self-reported physical activity remained unchanged (Meyer et al., 1980; Young, Haskell, Taylor, & Fortmann, 1996).

DETERMINANTS

The known determinants of physical activity can be categorized as past and present personal attributes, past and present environments, and aspects of physical activity itself (Dishman & Sallis, 1994). Few controlled studies have been conducted to manipulate experimentally variables presumed to operate as determinants, and no population trials have been completed. Therefore, we use the term "determinant" to denote a reproducible association or predictive relationship, rather than to imply cause and effect. In addition, it is believed that determinants may differ somewhat for supervised versus unsupervised settings and for adoption versus maintenance of a physical activity pattern (Dishman, 1982).

Table 1 presents a summary of studies of the physical activity determinants from 1988 to early 1991 compared with studies published before 1988 (Dishman & Sallis, 1994). Results from subjects in supervised versus unsupervised programs are reported separately. The small number of post-1987 studies with supervised samples reduces confidence in interpretations made from data.

Table 1 Summary of Physical Activity Determinants for Studies Conducted in Supervised and Unsupervised Settings

Determinant	Supervised: pre-1988 results	Supervised: 1988-1991 results	Unsupervised: pre-1988 results	Unsupervised: 1988-1991 results
Personal attributes Demographics				
Age	00	-	-	—
Blue-collar occupation	—	-	-	
Childless				+
Education	+		++	++
Gender (male)			++	++
High risk for heart disease	-	-	-	
Income/socioeconomic status			++	++
Injury history				+
Overweight/obesity	-	0	-	00
Race (nonwhite)			-	—
Cognitive variables				
Attitudes	0	+	0	
Barriers to exercise		-		—
Control over exercise				0
Enjoyment of exercise	+		+	0
Expect health and other benefits	0	+	+	+
Health locus of control	+	0		
Intention to exercise	0		+	++
Knowledge of health and exercise	0		0	0
Lack of time	—		-	-
Mood disturbance	-		-	—
Normative beliefs	0			0
Perceived health or fitness	++		-	++
Self-efficacy for exercise	+	+	+	++
Self-motivation	+	++	++	+
Self-schemata for activity			+	+
Stress				0
Susceptibility to illness				0
Value exercise outcomes	0		0	
Behaviors				
Alcohol				0
Contemporary program activity			0	
Diet	00		+	0
Past free-living activity during childhood			0	0

Table 1 (*continued*)

Determinant	Supervised: pre-1988 results	Supervised: 1988-1991 results	Unsupervised: pre-1988 results	Unsupervised: 1988-1991 results
Behaviors				
Past free-living activity during adulthood	+		+	++
Past program participation	++	+	+	
School sports	0		0	00
Smoking	—	-	0	0
Sports media use				0
Type A behavior pattern	-		+	
Environmental factors: Social environment				
Class size		+		
Exercise models				0
Group cohesion		+		
Physician influence			+	
Social isolation				-
Past family influences			+	0
Social support; friends/peers			+	++
Social support; spouse/family	++		+	++
Social support; staff/instructor	+	0		
Physical environment				
Climate/season	-		-	0
Cost	0		0	
Disruptions in routine	-			
Access to facilities: actual	+			+
Access to facilities: perceived	+		0	0
Home equipment				0
Physical activity characteristics				
Intensity	-		-	
Perceived effort	—		-	-

Note. + + = repeatedly documented positive association with physical activity; + = weak or mixed evidence of positive association with physical activity; 00 = repeatedly documented lack of association with physical activity; 0 = weak or mixed evidence of no association with physical activity; — = repeatedly documented negative association with physical activity; - = weak or mixed evidence of negative association with physical activity. Blank spaces indicate no data available. From *Physical Activity, Fitness, and Health*, pp. 223–224, by R.K. Dishman and J. Sallis, 1994, Champaign, IL: Human Kinetics Publishers. Reprinted with permission.

Moderate Versus Vigorous Physical Activity

Few studies have examined differences in patterns and determinants of moderate and vigorous physical activity. The marked decline in total physical activity with age is not seen with low- to moderate-intensity activities (Caspersen et al., 1994).

Studies reporting separate analyses for moderate-intensity activities have consistently noted increased levels with age (Hovell et al., 1989; McPhillips, Pellettera, Barrett-Connor, Wingard, & Criqui, 1989; Stephens & Craig, 1990). The most common and consistently reported form of moderate-intensity activity is walking (Stephens & Craig, 1990). While men have higher levels of total and vigorous activity, in at least two studies women reported more walking (Hovell et al., 1989; Stephens & Craig, 1990). Walking and other forms of moderate activity appear to have important health benefits (see chapter 3), and they may be more acceptable to older adults and to women.

Correlates of walking were examined in one sample that did not engage in vigorous exercise (Hovell et al., 1989). Psychological and social variables that were significant in relation to walking tended to have the same associations as with vigorous exercise (Sallis et al., 1989). However, the same determinants accounted for much less of the variance in walking. This may be due to error in measuring walking, or it could indicate that other variables not included in the study are important influences on walking.

Personal Attributes

Determinants that reside or originate in the individual can identify personal variables or population segments that may be targets for interventions to increase physical activity. Personal attributes include demographic variables, biomedical status, past and present behaviors, activity history, and psychological traits and states, such as knowledge, attitudes, and beliefs that are associated with physical activity.

Demographics   Demographic variables continue to have strong associations with physical activity. Education, income, male gender, and age are consistent and powerful correlates of physical activity habits. Because concomitant associations seen in the population for low activity with age, fewer years of education, and low income occur in cross-sectional comparisons, the degree to which they represent cause or a selection-bias effect remains unclear. Age is also unrelated to adherence to supervised exercise (Oldridge, 1982). Non-Hispanic whites appear to be more active than other ethnic groups, but in this case, it is difficult or impossible to disentangle the effects of ethnicity and socioeconomic status.

Smokers and blue-collar workers are likely dropouts from rehabilitative exercise programs following myocardial infarction (Oldridge, 1982), and are unlikely to use worksite exercise facilities. The robustness of these determinants for other supervised settings and the population is less clear, but blue-collar workers are less likely to be active when total leisure activity is considered.

Biomedical   Studies conducted prior to 1988 found that obese individuals were generally less active than those of normal weight and were less likely to adhere to supervised fitness programs (Dishman, 1981; Epstein, Koeske, & Wing, 1984). Overweight individuals were also less responsive to a public health intervention that included walking and climbing than were those of normal weight who were inactive. However, no association between obesity and physical activity has been a relatively consistent finding in more recent studies.

Cardiovascular disease and low metabolic tolerance for physical activity are not reliable predictors of adherence to clinical exercise programs (Oldridge, 1982), even though symptoms may prompt an individual to act on a physician's advice to begin an exercise program. Biomedical and demographic factors have low sensitivity for predicting behavior. In supervised settings, demographic and biomedical entry profiles can predict dropout for some groups, but not with the degree of accuracy required for diagnostic and screening purposes at an individual level (Dishman, 1981; Oldridge et al., 1983; Ward & Morgan, 1984). In addition, several factors that are useful for predicting dropout in some patient groups (such as smoking, blue-collar work status, obesity, and angina) are not prevalent in others, and therefore are not helpful for predicting dropout in those groups.

Activity History   If demographic or biomedical factors and other behaviors are found to represent selection biases rather than causes of physical activity, the importance of past activity history assumes great significance. Indeed, studies of social-cognitive correlates of physical activity indicate that habit is often as strong a predictor of physical activity as attitudes, self-efficacy about exercise, and intentions to exercise (Dishman, 1994b; Godin, 1994). In supervised programs in which activity can be observed directly, past participation in the program is the most reliable correlate of current participation. This prediction holds for adult men and women in supervised fitness programs, and is consistent with observations in treatment programs for obese patients and those with CHD.

There continues to be little evidence that activity patterns in childhood or early adulthood are predictive of later physical activity (Dennison, Straus, Mellits, & Charney, 1988; Dishman, 1988b). No prospective study has shown a relationship for adherence to cardiac rehabilitation exercise programs or for physical activity in the community at large with participation in interscholastic or intercollegiate athletics. This illustrates the need for cautious interpretation of the cross-sectional retrospective studies linking youth sport history with contemporary adult physical activity. However, a controlled prospective study of children from the Netherlands showed linear decreases in physical activity from ages 12 to 18 except in the most active 10% of the children, whose participation remained stable over time (Kemper, 1994).

Psychological Traits   Psychological constructs can account for variability in behavior within population segments that are demographically homogeneous and across settings that differ in place and time. While psychological traits are thought to be relatively stable, they can be changed under certain circumstances (see chapter 1). However, they are resistive to change over the narrow ranges of time, exposure, and settings characteristic of most medical and public health interventions.

A trait measure of self-motivation has been a relatively consistent correlate of physical activity (Knapp, 1988; Sonstroem, 1988). Evidence suggests that self-motivation may reflect self-regulatory skills such as effective goal setting, self-monitoring of progress, and self-reinforcement that are believed to be important for maintaining physical activity (Dishman, 1982). Successful endurance athletes consistently have scored high in self-motivation, and self-motivation has discriminated between adherents and dropouts across a wide variety of settings ranging from athletic conditioning, adult fitness, preventive medicine, cardiac rehabilitation, commercial spas, corporate fitness, and informal activity in college students (Dishman & Sallis, 1994; Knapp, 1988; Sonstroem, 1988; Steinhardt & Young, 1992).

Other studies have shown no differences between adherents and dropouts in self-motivation in adult fitness, dance exercise, and interscholastic sports (Garcia & King, 1991; Knapp, 1988; Sonstroem, 1988; Ward & Morgan, 1984). Psychological traits probably also interact with aspects of the physical activity setting to determine behavior. Strong social support or reinforcement in settings requiring low-frequency, low-intensity activity may negate differences in self-motivation (Wankel, Yardley, & Graham, 1985). The self-motivated individual might also leave a supervised program but continue a personal program of unsupervised activity.

Knowledge, Attitudes, and Beliefs   Knowledge, attitudes, values, and beliefs regarding physical activity have been modified in population-based educational campaigns and can influence the intention to be active. Intentions have accounted for about 50% of the variation in self-reported physical activity (Dishman, 1994b; Godin, 1994).

Those who perceive their health as poor are unlikely to enter or adhere to an exercise program, and those who do are likely to participate at low intensity and low frequency. There are mixed findings from both supervised and unsupervised settings about the roles of self-efficacy and outcome expectancies as determinants of physical activity. Specific efficacy beliefs about the ability to exercise have predicted compliance with an exercise prescription in patients with both heart (Ewart, Stewart, & Gillilan, 1986; Ewart, Taylor, Reese, & DeBusk, 1983) and lung (Kaplan, Atkins, & Reinsch, 1984) disease and unsupervised activity in a population-based study (Sallis et al., 1986). In young healthy adults, however, a belief in personal control over health outcomes predicts unsupervised (or informal) activity, but beliefs and values held specifically for exercise outcomes and personal ability to control them appear unrelated to both unsupervised and supervised physical activity. Self-schemata, expectation of benefits, and intention to exercise seem to be associated with physical activity in community samples. Perceived barriers to exercise, including lack of time, have been associated negatively in several recent community studies. Those with mood disturbances appear less likely to be active, but small numbers of studies preclude interpretations of other psychological variables. The lack of prospective studies that control for physical activity habits limits our confidence with regard to how much of the observed relationships of self-efficacy and intentions with physical activity is causal and how much reflects a selection effect. The reciprocal and causal nature of the relationships observed among contemporary physical activity, habit, and self-variables such as self-efficacy and outcome-expectancy values remains to be determined.

Environmental Factors

For the purpose of this discussion, environmental factors include variables such as access to facilities, time, and social support. Environments that promote increased activity, while offering easily accessible facilities and removing real and perceived barriers to an exercise routine, are likely prerequisites for successful maintenance of exercise behavior change.

Access To Facilities   Objectively measured, access to facilities is a reliable predictor of physical activity but the evidence on perceived access is mixed (Dishman, 1994b). In one population-based study of adults in southern California, a weak but significant association was found—after controlling for age, education, and income—between self-reported participation in three or more weekly exercise sessions and the density of commercial exercise facilities located within 1 km of the home addresses of participants (Sallis, Hovell, Hofstetter, Elder, Hackley, et al., 1990).

There is also some evidence that work environment may influence leisure physical activity. In one population-based study from the Swedish Central Bureau of Statistics Survey of Living Conditions (Johannson, Johnson, & Hall, 1991), monotonous job demands and lack of control over work processes were associated negatively with leisure activity for men and women workers 16 to 65 years of age after controlling for age and education level.

Time   A perceived lack of time is the principal and most prevalent reason given for dropping out of supervised clinical and community exercise programs (Dishman, 1982; Oldridge, 1982) and for inactive lifestyles. For many, however, this may reflect a lack of interest or commitment to physical activity. Population surveys indicate that regular exercisers are more likely than the sedentary to view time as an activity barrier. It is not yet clear whether time represents a true environmental determinant, a perceived determinant, poor behavioral skills (e.g., time management), or rationalization for the lack of motivation to be active.

Social Support   When social influences are studied, they are usually found to be associated with physical activity. Social support from family and friends is related consistently to physical activity in cross-sectional and prospective studies (Duncan & McAuley, 1993). Spousal influences on exercise appear to be reliable correlates of participation (Erling & Oldridge, 1985; Heinzelmann & Bagley, 1970). Group factors may be important in adherence to exercise programs as well. However, social influences on physical activity have received relatively little study. Influences by family and peers on social-cognitive mediators of physical activity are plausible but undemonstrated. Evidence in this area is sparse, and has been based largely on self-reports with few validation studies.

Physical Activity

Most studies of supervised exercise programs in adults do not show an association between dropout rates and exercise intensity or perceived exertion. However, intensity in these studies is usually relativized as a percent of maximum in an effort to minimize variation in physical strain and its role as a determinant. However, the goal may not be achieved for several reasons (see chapter 1). Unsupervised settings in which the energy cost of standard activities may require varying percentages of metabolic capacity, exertional perceptions and preferences (i.e., preferred exertion) may have an important influence on participation. In a study of California adults (Sallis et al., 1986), more men (11%) than women (5%) adopted vigorous exercise such as running during a year's time, but a comparatively higher proportion of women (33%) than men (26%) took up such moderate activities as routine walking, stair climbing, and gardening. Both sexes were more likely to adopt regular activities of a moderate intensity than high-intensity fitness activities. Adoption of moderate activities was associated with a dropout rate (25% to 35%) roughly one half of that seen for vigorous physical activity (50%; Sallis et al., 1986).

Injury There is a well-documented dose-response relationship between physical activity and orthopedic injuries (Macera, Jackson, et al., 1989). Injury rates may be as high as 50% per year in those who regularly engage in high-intensity physical activities such as running (Macera, Pate, et al., 1989; Pollock et al., 1991). Injuries from high-intensity running can lead directly to dropout, but it is likely that participants' subjective responses to injury can influence the probability of adopting or maintaining physical activity. Injury was the most common reason given for the most recent relapse from exercise in one investigation (Sallis, Hovell, Hofstetter, Elder, Faucher, et al., 1990). In another study, subjects who reported temporary injuries were less likely than healthy individuals to report vigorous exercise, but the injured reported significantly more walking for exercise (Hofstetter et al., 1991). This is consistent with previous findings that intensity of exercise is related to injury risk, and suggests that many injured people can still engage in regular walking. Injury appears to have a strong influence on maintenance or dropout from regular physical activity.

Summary

The research to date has demonstrated the multidimensional nature of physical activity determinants, and the need exists for comparisons of variables within and between categories at the various stages of exercise behavior. Progress has been made toward establishing that sport history (Dishman, 1988b) and age (Blair, Piserchia, Wilbur, & Crowder, 1986; Powell & Paffenbarger, 1985) largely represent selection biases, not true influences on contemporary physical activity. Family and peer influences, socioeconomic status, and education level may be selection bias effects but they have potential as true determinants. In addition, the construct validity of most of the social-cognitive variables studied as determinants of physical activity have not been established adequately in that these methods lack convergent and discriminant evidence (Messick, 1989).

Little or no progress has been made in understanding whether determinants and dispositions for physical activity differ or change at definable ages or lifespan stages. It now appears, however, that inactivity associated with age can be reversed in some groups. This priority has increased in importance due to increases in elderly populations as well as to the absence of demonstrated effectiveness of school-based curricula to increase children's leisure physical activity patterns outside of the school environment (Sallis, Simons-Morton, Stone, et al., 1992).

INTERVENTIONS

Because public health recommendations to exercise are not followed regularly by the majority of people, specific efforts to promote physical activity are needed. Numerous theories support different approaches to behavior change that can be applied to exercise behaviors. Reinforcement control and stimulus control strategies based on the traditions of behavior modification or cognitive-behavior modification have been implemented effectively with exercise. Other useful strategies include educational modeling approaches consistent with social-cognitive theory and health education techniques relying on health risk appraisals, fitness testing, and counseling (Parcel, Simons-Morton, O'Hara, Baranowski & Wilson, 1989).

Health Risk Appraisals and Fitness Tests

Early studies suggest that health risk appraisal and fitness testing might increase physical activity levels. These studies were uncontrolled, however, and the accuracy and validity of the self-reports of activity were not demonstrated (Dishman, 1991). Other investigators have examined the combined effects of health risk appraisal, fitness assessment, and educational interventions. There is generally some initial increase in physical activity, but little effect has been demonstrated after follow-up of 6 months or longer.

Because inconvenience and limited access to facilities have been cited repeatedly as reasons for dropping out of supervised cardiac rehabilitation exercise programs, several studies have used health-risk appraisal and health education strategies with home-based interventions. These studies have been limited by self-selected participants, lack of control groups, and unvalidated self-report of physical activity. Although some reports suggest that community and worksite (Blair et al., 1986) health promotions can increase physical activity, the collective evidence indicates only a small impact of health education promotions on the fitness or activity of adults.

Behavior Modification

Both reinforcement control and stimulus control strategies rooted in the traditions of behavior modification or cognitive-behavior modification have been implemented successfully with exercise (Knapp, 1988). Representative approaches such as written agreements, behavior contracts and lotteries, stimulus control, and contingencies have been used successfully in case and quasi-experimental studies (Dishman, 1991). Cognitive-behavioral approaches, including self-monitoring, sensory distraction, goal setting, feedback and decision making have appeared equally effective when used alone or when combined in intervention packages (Dishman, 1991).

A preliminary quantitative analysis of 20 studies of interventions to increase physical activity or exercise conducted from about 1988–1992 has been conducted (Dishman & Sallis, 1994). Results from the studies were transformed to a correlation coefficient (r) according to procedures outlined by Friedman (1968) and Rosenthal (1991). Population values approximating 0.10, 0.30, and 0.50 can be regarded as small, moderate, and large, respectively. The interventions typically were associated with effect sizes (unweighted for sample size) for frequency of physical activity that are small to moderate (i.e., rs approximately 0.15 to 0.20), with binomial effect sizes suggesting exercise programs that experience success rates (based on attendance) approximating 40% without a behavior change intervention might have increased success to about 60% with a behavior change intervention. A more recent quantitation synthesis of 127 studies found larger average effects ranging from 0.35 to 0.88 depending on whether sample size was considered (Dishman & Buckworth, 1996).

Some methodological limitations in these studies preclude a firm conclusion about the true size of the increase in physical activity due to interventions. In general, the size of effects is associated inversely with the scientific quality of the study. The effect size for uncontrolled studies is larger than of randomized or quasi-experimental studies. Most intervention studies in the past 5 years have used indirect measures of physical activity (e.g., self-report) or indirect estimates of physical fitness based on heart rate or treadmill time. The validity of these methods for measuring physical activity is not established (Ainsworth, Montoye, & Leon, 1994). Attempts to verify self-reports of activity with expected increases in fitness (e.g., VO_2max, weight loss, or decreased submaximal exercise heart rate) are few in number, and when this has been done the effects for self-reported physical activity were larger than effects for changes in VO_2max. The absolute levels of the increased activity in intervention studies often fall below the frequency, duration, and intensity required to increase physical fitness or to decrease markedly the risk for disease morbidity or all-cause mortality.

The majority of early research studies involving interventions designed to increase physical activity have relied on one-dimensional techniques and small numbers of highly selected subjects (Dishman, 1991). Because these studies relied on small, clinical, or otherwise homogeneous samples that were often in a restricted setting, the generalizability of the interventions to a community or a population was not possible. In a recent review of determinants (Dishman & Sallis, 1994), 24 of 33 studies published between 1988 and early 1992 used community or national samples, and both men and women were included in 26 of the studies. While a few studies included different racial and cultural groups, interventions typically have not included diverse samples. One strategy to intervention that potentially possesses more power involves the application of a community approach that spans multiple levels of analysis (e.g., personal, interpersonal, organizational/environmental, institutional/legislative) in concert with an aim to reach diverse segments of the population.

Relapse Prevention

Even among the habitually active, unexpected disruptions in activity routines or settings can interrupt or end a previously continuous exercise program (Sallis, Hovell, Hofstetter, Elder, Faucher, et al., 1990). Relocation, medical events, and travel can impede the continuity of activity reinforcement and create new activity barriers. It is believed, however, that interruptions and life events have less impact as the activity habit becomes more established (Dishman, 1982). Their impact may also be diminished if the individual anticipates and plans their occurrence, recognizes them as only temporary impediments, and develops self-regulatory skills for preventing relapses to inactivity (Belisle, Roskies, & Levesque, 1987; King & Frederiksen, 1984; Martin et al., 1984).

A popular example of self-regulation is relapse prevention, which was developed by Marlatt and Gordon (1985). The application of relapse prevention to exercise has been described thoroughly by Knapp (1988), who correctly noted that relapse prevention was designed for reducing high-frequency undesired addictive behaviors such as smoking and substance abuse, whereas exercise is a desired but low-frequency behavior for many. Thus the effectiveness of the relapse prevention model for increasing physical activity may require modification.

The relapse prevention model has received indirect support for guiding effective physical activity interventions (King, 1991). Successful interventions have incorporated parts of the model, particularly those dealing with planning strategies to avoid and overcome slips leading to relapse. However, the complete relapse prevention model has not been tested or validated for physical activity, in part because of a lack of validated measures of key components of the model, including lifestyle imbalances, dissonance, positive outcome expectancies for slips, high-risk situations for slips, and the abstinence violation effect. Thus, the prevalence and importance of these key components for physical activity cannot be determined.

Despite the intuitive appeal of relapse prevention for understanding adherence to physical activity, it is not known whether people naturally experience the cognitive processes outlined in the model when they attempt to change sedentary living. In addition, the absence of validated measures of the periodicity of exercise behavior itself has hindered compelling tests of the model in population-based studies.

Transtheoretical Model of Stages of Change

A number of early reviews of the exercise adherence literature have acknowledged the appearance of stages of exercise behavior (e.g., Dishman, 1982). It has become clearer during recent years that behavior change is dependent on the readiness of the individual for change to occur, and that exercise behavior involves different stages. A more articulate view of stages for behavioral changes can be found in extensions of the transtheoretical model (as discussed in chapter 3) for behavior change in smoking, weight control, and psychotherapy. The model proposes that when people try to change their behavior they move through stages of precontemplation, contemplation, preparation, action, and maintenance in a sequential manner. People often must make several attempts at behavior change, so the stages can be cyclical instead of always linear, and the processes of change presumably are unique to each stage.

A potential major contribution of the transtheoretical model for increasing and maintaining physical activity lies in its consideration of the readiness of individuals for change. Another is its capacity to bridge the use of behavior modification and cognitive-behavior modification traditions with population-based approaches to behavior change such as health promotion and education campaigns. Several of the processes of change proposed by the transtheoretical model require consideration of both cognitive (e.g., beliefs and values related to consciousness raising) and behavioral (e.g., stimulus control, reinforcement management, counterconditioning) variables. In addition, relapse cannot be understood or controlled without knowledge of the influence of past history on current physical activity patterns. Recent studies have extended the stage of change component of the transtheoretical model to exercise (Prochaska & Marcus, 1994; Sonstroem, 1988).

Integration of Adherence Interventions

Because exercise behavior involves different, and probably nonsequential, stages, determinants, and interventions should be considered in terms of stages. For example, decision-based theories and social marketing strategies appear helpful for increasing planning and adoption (Donovan & Owen, 1994). The goals of an intervention such as a media campaign will vary according to the individual's stage of readiness. The primary goal of a media campaign may be to capture the individual's attention and motivate him or her to contemplate the issue. For those who are already considering participation in an activity program, the desired outcome is to motivate them toward action by increasing the relevance of the behavior change or decreasing the barriers they perceive. For individuals in an action phase, the goal of the media campaign is diminished, but continued support and reinforcement should be provided to encourage continuation or maintenance of activity. Social support, self-motivation, self-regulatory skills, and interventions like relapse prevention seem necessary to maintain or resume a physical activity pattern.

It is becoming increasingly evident that one theory or type of intervention applied in general to all people will not solve the problem of sedentariness. For example, it is possible that some theories and technologies for increasing physical activity may be more or less effective depending on whether they are targeted to individuals with a lifetime history of inactivity, a history of sporadic activity, or a history of sustained activity with one or more periods of inactivity.

Until recently, most intervention studies have used single-dimensional approaches with small numbers of persons who were homogeneous in terms of gender, race, ethnicity, health status, and economic and educational status. Recently, community-based interventions have applied psychological and behavioral theories for behavior change. These approaches go beyond the traditional practice of individual counseling to include organizational (e.g., community recreation centers, churches, diffusion strategies through schools), environmental (e.g. facility planning), and social (e.g. family interventions) macro-changes; or they use cost-effective or pragmatically convenient avenues (e.g. mailings, telephone) to reach large numbers of individuals who might not be accessible or amenable to traditional clinically based interventions.

Project PACE is an example of an intervention that integrates other interventions, in light of the client's stage, by integrating stage theory and relapse prevention models. PACE employs a triage approach to assessment of activity history and readiness for physical activity and subsequent intervention (Pender, Sallis, Long, & Calfas, 1994). At entry, clients are given a screening questionnaire that focuses on the individual's current physical activity habits. The information obtained is used to classify the individual into one of three categories: inactive and not considering exercise; inactive and has considered exercise but has never exercised, or has exercised and ceased the activity; or presently active. The initial classification determines which of three counseling protocols should be utilized.

Project PACE is now being evaluated for effectiveness in the medical office, but it also offers a practical approach for face-to-face counseling by other health professionals such as physical activity consultants. Similar but unstandardized approaches have been effective in community-mediated approaches (Owen, Lee, Naccarrella, & Haag, 1987; King 1991).

MEASUREMENT ISSUES

Observations made by clinicians in practical settings can lead to functionally useful principles and interventions, but their validity and generalizability require empirical verification. Likewise, theoretical models may offer directions for successful programming decisions and interventions in practical settings, but such propositions require testing and confirmation. Natural science tradition based on quantitative assessment has been the approach taken by most investigators studying exercise adherence. The methods of qualitative assessment have been employed in only a few studies (Gauvin, 1989), and ethnographic approaches are more common in the social sciences (e.g., anthropology). However, the absence of uniform standards for defining and assessing physical activity, along with the determinants and the diversity of the variables, population segments, time periods, and settings sampled in published studies, make it difficult to interpret and compare results. Often only a few studies have been done in a particular area when this methodology has been employed. Most studies have used supervised settings, and relatively fewer population studies of determinants have been reported. Available population surveys have relied on the use of questionnaires with unknown reliability and validity, while generalizability to the population of the more controlled small sample results is also unknown in many instances.

Research on determinants as a whole is characterized by limitations of measurement methods (e.g., lack of standardized psychological variables), differences in sample characteristics, and the limited number of studies that have used the same variables, precluding the assignment of effect sizes to specific variables with confidence. The frequent use of self-reporting contributes to measurement problems in this area. For example, objective measures can provide different results from those obtained by self-reports to assess the same environmental variable (Sallis, Hovell, Hofstetter, Elder, Hackley, et al., 1990). When access to facilities has been measured by objective methods (e.g., distance), access typically has been related to both the adoption and maintenance of physical activity. When perceived access has been measured by self-report, it typically has not been related to the adoption and maintenance of physical activity. Studies attempting to assess and understand the effectiveness of community and population interventions are especially vulnerable to the measurement conundrum of using instruments designed for clinical purposes or validated for use with homogeneous samples of exercisers.

Physical Activity

The measures of fitness and physical activity used in past studies have usually relied on estimates rather than direct measures. Exercise programs and the methods used for assessing and defining exercise adherence, physical activity, and their correlates must be standardized if reproducible and generalizable results are to be obtained. Measures of physical activity have included job classification; retrospective self-reporting; daily self-recording; mechanical, electronic, and physiological surveillance; and observation. Although questionnaires validated against biological estimates of activity (e.g., metabolic tolerance) are useful in dichotomizing between highly active and sedentary individuals, they are less accurate in distinguishing between levels of activity intensity. Most studies of determinants have ignored the well-known problem of measuring physical activity in a population base (Ainsworth et al., 1994). The lack of uniform assessment methods for physical activity makes it difficult to evaluate whether determinants of physical activity truly differ across individuals, settings, and time. We do not know whether certain determinants, interventions, or theoretical models are associated with unique aspects of the physical activity, or if the various measures simply are each poor estimates of true physical activity. Therefore, both subjective and objective evidence of exercise behavior is necessary when direct observation is not feasible.

Problems in measurement of physical activity obviously affect theory and research in interventions. Nearly all of the available evidence supporting the validity of the theoretical models comes from self-reports of physical activity. Often the effect on fitness reported for behavioral interventions has not exceeded the measurement error of the fitness estimates employed. The exception is when attendance or another direct observation of behavior has been used. Concurrent validity for the various self-reports that have been used has not been established. It has also been reported that the relationship between social-cognitive variables and self-reported unsupervised physical activity does not generalize to physical activity estimated by a motion sensor (Dishman, Darracott, & Lambert, 1992).

Intensity of physical activity and perceived exertion during physical activity seem to be related negatively to participation, but there are not enough population-based studies on these topics to permit this conclusion. Assessing the intensity of physical activity is perhaps the most difficult, and as yet unresolved, of the many problems inherent with measuring physical activity in population samples (Ainsworth et al., 1994). Scales for perceived exertion have been validated as a surrogate of relative oxygen consumption for short-term, incremental exercise, but not as a measure of the absolute or relative metabolic intensity of exercise for use in population studies (Dishman, 1994b). Walking is a highly prevalent form of moderate intensity activity (Caspersen et al., 1994), but self-report measures of walking have not been validated for use in population-base studies.

Definition of Adherence

Widely varying definitions of exercise adherence have been used, making it difficult to compare studies. Some factors related to adherence early in a program are not related later on (Ward & Morgan, 1984), but unfortunately, attempts have been made to contrast studies in which the period of interest may range from less than 1 month to 36 months. Previous reviews (Dishman, 1990; Sallis & Hovell, 1990) have emphasized the need to distinguish adoption, maintenance, and resumption of physical activity, but virtually all studies have failed to discriminate between maintenance and adoption or the overall periodicity of activity patterns. Follow-up rates of physical activity after an intervention have been examined in some studies (Dishman, 1991; Dishman & Buckworth, 1996), but the natural history of physical activity has received very little attention (Kemper, 1994; Powell & Paffenbarger, 1985). There is at least one investigation that specifically assessed influences on resumption of exercise after dropout (Sallis, Hovell, Hofstetter, Elder, Faucher, et al., 1990). Adoption of vigorous exercise by a community sample of sedentary men during a 2-year period was predicted by self-efficacy, neighborhood environment, and age (negative), with younger men being more likely to adopt exercise. Adoption by women was predicted by education, self-efficacy, and friend and family support for exercise (Sallis, Hovell, & Hofstetter, 1992). In the same study, maintenance of vigorous exercise was predicted by some of the same variables. While some variables predicted both adoption and maintenance, it is interesting that the model was more successful in predicting adoption. An understanding of exercise adherence will depend on accurate measures of the resumption of activity following periods of inactivity or relapse. There is no measure of total activity history or periodicity that has been accepted by scientific consensus, and it is recognized that the validity of self-report methods of measuring physical activity are expected to be least accurate for persons who are active sporadically.

Defining adherence should take into consideration past exercise history, but no standardized and validated measure for assessing stage of exercise change has been reported. Furthermore, studies and applications of the transtheoretical model for exercise have used different measures to assess stage of change (Marcus, Bansphach, & Lefebvre, 1992; Marcus, Rakowski, & Rossi, 1992; Pender et al., 1994). Experimental studies have not validated the behavioral meaning of criterion groups formed from the various measures. Hence, it is not clear whether existing instruments for assessing stages of change measure distinct stages of exercise uniquely responsive to processes of change or to behavior change interventions, or are merely ordinal rankings of self-reported physical activity.

There is also a need to determine a reliable baseline expectancy for adherence to supervised exercise programs. Furthermore, uncontrollable factors such as injury can result in inactivity. Other developments such as conflicts in schedule or relocation can occur, and these events are often beyond the individual's control (Oldridge, 1982). However, these determinants of adherence are not explained adequately by most psychological theories.

SUMMARY AND CONCLUSIONS

Gains have been made during the past 15 years in understanding the determinants of physical activity, as well as appropriate interventions targeted to the initiation, maintenance, and resumption of physical activity. Determinants that reside or originate in the individual are important from a practical standpoint because they can identify population segments that may be responsive or resistive to physical activity interventions. Smoking, blue-collar occupation, ethnicity, low education and income levels, and obesity are examples of personal attributes that can present barriers to physical activity, and these factors can be viewed as sentinel markers of underlying habits or circumstances that reinforce sedentary living. There are not adequate numbers of studies available on children, the elderly, the physically challenged, or ethnic and minority groups, and few direct comparisons of men and women are available to permit conclusions about how determinants and successful interventions in these cases may differ from general observations. It is extremely important to identify unique circumstances and attributes that influence the adoption and maintenance of physical activity among population minorities that have different cultural values toward being active or special barriers to activity. Likewise, it is equally important to recognize that demographics such as gender, age, and race are not synonymous with ethnic or cultural values. Studies of the interaction of personal values with such demographics within the context of physical and social environment are critically needed.

Reconstructing past activity history is important for interpreting past and present determinants, designing and evaluating plausible interventions, and predicting future activity. However, there is currently no standardized method for assessing lifetime activity history or stage of behavior change. Attitudes, beliefs and expectancies, values, and intentions are amenable to change, but they do not predict behavior independently with sufficient accuracy for applied purposes.

Similarly, while traits such as self-motivation (Dishman et al., 1980) will not predict exercise behavior with sufficient accuracy for applied purposes, such measures may help explain why cognitive and attitudinal theories offer incomplete predictions of exercise. Furthermore, while constructs such as self-motivation are of limited value at a univariate level, traits of this nature have been shown to be effective when employed at a multivariate level (Dishman et al., 1980). Exercise programs with strong social support or reinforcement conducted in settings requiring low-frequency, low-intensity activity may offset differences in personality that might otherwise predispose a person to inactivity (Wankel et al., 1985). Logistical variables such as access to facilities and programs have not been widely studied, but these factors could potentially be just as important as altering knowledge and attitudes. They may also be moderator variables that are necessary for stimulating intentions into action.

Process-oriented interventions targeted to an individual's current stage of change have the potential to accelerate progress toward understanding and increasing the adoption and maintenance of physical activity. There has been no consensus with regard to which stages best explain sedentariness or habitual physical activity, nor is there much compelling evidence that validates the various stage models for explaining changes in exercise behavior. Advances in theory in this area cannot occur without standardized, validated measures for assessing stages.

It will continue to be important to identify psychological models that explain the various stages of participation in physical activity, and it is likely that different models may best explain different stages such as planning, adopting, and maintaining an activity pattern in supervised and unsupervised settings. Because of the substantial numbers of sedentary adults in the U.S. population and the assumption that multiple episodes of dropout and resumption are common, it is essential to study determinants in terms of adoption, maintenance, and resumption of physical activity.

The success of interventions probably depends on matching the appropriate attitudinal or behavioral approach to an individual according to his or her activity history and readiness for change. Modifying traditional exercise programming guidelines to deliver moderate-intensity activities, consisting of a broader variety of modes than traditionally employed, and tailored to individual or population-segmented preferences, based on formalized activity histories and goals assessments, represents a first step. This face-to-face approach can be implemented easily within the professional competencies of traditionally trained physical activity specialists with modest additional training (e.g., a course and practicum in exercise prescription). Population-based media campaigns in Australia and Canada as well as community-based clinical programs in the United States present good models for extending traditional fitness programming to a mediated counseling approach. Intervention strategies such as telephone prompts and mail-outs for education, monitoring, support, and problem-solving self-help kits appear to be just as effective as traditional full-fledged cognitive-behavior modification (Dishman, 1994b; Dishman & Buckworth, 1996) and are much more practical for fitness and health education personnel (King, 1991) to pursue and utilize.

Chapter 5

Drug Therapy
and Physical Activity

Egil W. Martinsen and Johan Kvalvik Stanghelle

Until the last two decades, most physicians have paid little attention to the lifestyles adopted by their patients. For many years, the most common advice to patients was to take it easy, and rest was considered the best way of preserving good health. Research has shown that there is an interaction between lifestyle and illness, and studies indicate that exercise can be an effective tool in the prevention and treatment of various diseases.

There was a pharmacological revolution in psychiatry during the 1950s with the introduction of phenothiazines in the treatment of psychoses and tricyclic antidepressants (TCAs) in the treatment of depressions, and a high percentage of psychiatric patients currently receive these and other psychotropic drugs. These two classes of drugs have a wide range of somatic side effects, the most important of which are their effects on the cardiovascular system. Like other health professionals, psychiatrists have paid little attention to their patients' passive, sedate lifestyles. In recent years, however, research has shown that psychiatric patients generally are in poor physical condition, and there is some evidence that regular exercise may lead to improved mental health (Morgan & Goldston, 1987).

Because many psychiatric patients are receiving psychotropic drugs, the following question arises: To what extent does the use of medication interact with the effects of exercise? Unlike the situation in cardiology and physical rehabilitation medicine, little interest has been paid to this issue by psychiatrists, and very little research exists on this topic. The importance and necessity of systematic

This is a revised version of a chapter that originally appeared in Morgan, W.P., & Goldston, S.E. (Eds.) (1987). *Exercise and Mental Health*. Washington, DC: Hemisphere Publishing.

research on this question becomes readily apparent when the increasing popularity of exercise therapy (Morgan & Goldston, 1987) is taken into consideration in concert with the widespread use of psychotropic drugs in the treatment of psychiatric patients.

This chapter focuses on selected problems in this area. The limited research involving the influence of exercise on patients receiving the most important groups of psychotropic drugs (i.e., major tranquilizers, TCAs, lithium, and minor tranquilizers), as well as the interaction between β-blocking agents and exercise are also discussed. β-blockers happen to be a very commonly used group of drugs: Many psychiatric patients receive these drugs for somatic disorders; and they seem to have effects on mental stress response as well (Jefferson, 1974). Finally, a review of case material involving the influence of exercise on patients receiving specific drug treatment at the time of exercise intervention is presented.

NEUROLEPTICS

Neuroleptics have a wide range of effects on the body, some of which interfere with the capacity and motivation to exercise. Drowsiness is a frequent complaint with high-dose phenothiazines. The effect is most pronounced initially, and will often be markedly reduced after the first 2 to 3 weeks of treatment. Parkinsonism, which reduces the capacity and ability for exercise, is another common side effect. Weight increase will, of course, reduce physical capacity, but exercise theoretically should be an effective way to deal with this side effect.

Neuroleptics, especially the high-dose compounds, have an adrenolytic and a less pronounced anticholinergic effect, which will affect the cardiovascular system and its response to exercise. Orthostatic hypotension is often seen initially in treatment with phenothiazines, and is particularly characteristic of treatment with the high-dose compounds. This effect often subsides or disappears after some time of treatment. Tachycardia often accompanies the hypotension, but may also appear as an isolated phenomenon. The phenothiazines have a quinidine-like effect on the ECG, but these changes rarely have clinical importance.

Long-term treatment with chlorpromazine results in a reduction of the mean arterial blood pressure in the upright position (Korol, Land, & Brown, 1965). Carlsson, Dencker, Grimby, and Heggendal (1968a) have performed several studies on the physiological effects of medication on patients receiving chlorpromazine (1.5 to 3.6 g/day). They found that large doses of chlorpromazine tend to reduce the stroke volume, leading to a reduction of cardiac output and arterial blood pressure during exercise. Carlsson, Dencker, Grimby, and Heggendal (1967) also reported that the concentration of noradrenaline in blood plasma and urine is increased with chlorpromazine treatment. This difference is present at rest, and is even more striking during exercise (Carlsson et al., 1967). The normal physiological response to regular exercise programs is altered by chlorpromazine use because the reductions of heart rate and blood lactate at a given work load are less consistent. After a period of systematic aerobic training, the high level of noradrenaline during exercise is reduced (Carlsson, Dencker, Grimby, and Heggendal, 1968b).

The small stroke volume and the fall in arterial blood pressure during exercise are factors that limit physical work performance. Some cases of sudden death among patients receiving phenothiazines may have been due partly to this maladaption of circulation. Another possible explanation may be the large increase in the blood level of noradrenaline during physical activity among physically inactive patients receiving phenothiazines.

It may be difficult for patients to exercise while receiving phenothiazines because of the side effects of drowsiness, orthostatic hypotension, and parkinsonism. Nevertheless, exercise is indicated for these patients, both to increase their physical work capacity and to reduce the level of noradrenaline in blood plasma.

At this time, it is not possible to draw any conclusions regarding the effect of fitness training on psychotic symptomatology (Folkins & Sime, 1981). However, these drugs are also used as tranquilizers for neurotic disturbances, and it is possible that regular exercise might have a tranquilizing effect comparable to that of these drugs. This hypothesis remains to be tested, and it is important to realize that studies addressing the effects of smaller doses of chlorpromazine and other neuroleptics on exercise performance do not exist at this time.

ANTIDEPRESSANTS

The structure of TCAs is similar to that of the phenothiazine group of the major tranquilizers (e.g., chlorpromazine), and their pharmacological actions are both anticholinergic and adrenolytic. These drugs have different adverse effects on the cardiovascular system. A common side effect of TCAs is increased heart rate, which is probably related to their anticholinergic effect on the vagus. Glassman and Bigger (1981) suggested that the only significant adverse cardiovascular effect of TCAs in healthy adults taking therapeutic doses is orthostatic hypotension. A decrease in blood pressure noted with TCAs is probably related to their noradrenergic blocking effect (Jefferson, 1975).

Veith, Raskin, and Caldwell (1982) found no change in left ventricular function in cardiac patients taking either doxepin or imipramine. There is little evidence indicating that TCAs in therapeutic doses reduce the mechanical function of the heart (Glassman & Bigger, 1981).

Some studies show that therapeutic doses of TCAs affect cardiac conduction, producing a significant prolongation of the QRS and PR intervals of the ECG (Vohra, Burrows, & Sloman, 1975). Veith, Raskin, and Caldwell, et al. (1982), however, did not observe such an effect. The TCAs are known to resemble quinidine with respect to their effect on cardiac rhythm (Glassman & Bigger, 1981). At therapeutic doses, both imipramine and doxepin have been reported to reverse some arrhythmias (Luchins, 1983).

Only a few studies of these drugs during exercise have been published. In a case-control study (Middleton, Maisley, and Mills, 1987), 7 female inpatients receiving various combinations of TCAs and tetracyclic antidepressants were compared with control subjects of identical sex and comparable age who were not on medication. All patients developed orthostatic hypotension, and there was a strong correlation between the dose of antidepressants and the severity of postural hypotension. Upon standing all subjects experienced an increase in heart rate with a subsequent slowing, but this increase was significantly larger among patients. During an isometric exercise test, the increase in heart rate was significantly larger among the controls than among the patients. Increases in systolic and diastolic blood pressure were significantly smaller among patients, and in some cases declines rather than increases were observed.

Gutrie, Grunhaus, and Danos (1991) followed the same line of research. They studied the effects of TCAs on heart rate and blood pressure following standing and a short walk in 21 depressed inpatients from 18 to 83 years of age. Patients were studied without medication and after having taken TCAs for 2 weeks. The use of TCAs caused an increase in supine heart rate, but did not affect the physiological increase in heart rate following standing up or walking. The physiological increase in diastolic blood pressure following standing or walking was either blunted or reversed.

Patients taking TCAs should be informed about the possibility of experiencing hypotension both when standing up and during exercise. These patients may have a higher risk of fainting or falling during exercise. Studies of the effect of these drugs during maximal exercise have not been performed (Powles, 1981).

As for the phenothiazines, drowsiness and fatigue are common complaints, especially at the start of the treatment, and this will reduce the motivation and ability for exercise. Another problem with these drugs is the associated increase in body weight.

Orthostatic hypotension is also a common side effect from the monoamine oxidase inhibitors, which is the other large group of antidepressants (Davidson, 1992). Over the past years selective, reversible monoamine oxidase inhibitors have been developed. These drugs generally have fewer adverse cardiovascular side effects, and should theoretically interfere less with exercise (Freeman, 1993). The influence of these drugs during exercise has not been studied in humans.

New classes of cyclic antidepressants have also been developed. The selective serotonin reuptake inhibitors in general have fewer adverse effects than the classical TCAs (Dechant & Clissold, 1991). In a placebo-controlled, double-blind study in 21 healthy volunteers, Juvent et al. (1990) studied the cardiovascular effects of therapeutic doses of tianeptine, one of these new drugs. Orthostatic hypotension, increased heart rate, or ECG changes were not observed, and cardiac output at rest and after bicycle exercise was not altered. This study indicates that these new classes of antidepressants will interfere less with exercise than did the older classes of drugs.

There have been attempts to explain the antidepressive effect of exercise on the basis of the mechanisms thought to operate with the TCAs, electroconvulsive therapy, and sleep deprivation. These explanations are usually based on the monoamine hypothesis (Morgan, 1985a) because exercise seems to have an antidepressive effect, and the effects of exercise on depression-related sleep disturbances resemble those of other methods for treating depression (Ransford, 1982). According to this view, one could speculate that exercise would potentiate the effects of TCAs and vice versa. On the other hand, TCAs seem to have the most potent effects on more severe depressions, whereas the antidepressive effect of exercise is best documented in patients suffering from moderate to mild depressions. Furthermore, patients with mild depression often do not respond well to antidepressant medication.

Studies comparing the antidepressive effect of exercise and TCAs on different types of depression have not been published. Two studies have addressed whether exercise and medication can potentiate each other. In the first study, Martinsen (1987a) found no synergistic effect of the combination of exercise and TCA, compared with exercise alone, in an exercise intervention study involving 43 inpatients with major depression as classified by the *Diagnostic and Statistical Manual of Mental Disorders* (3rd ed., 1980; *DSM-III*). In a second study involving 99 inpatients with *DSM-III-R* unipolar depressive disorders, there was a nonsignificant trend toward a larger reduction in depression scores in patients who received TCAs in addition to exercise, compared with those who only exercised (Martinsen, Hoffart, & Solberg, 1989a). These studies are reviewed in more detail in chapter 6. The studies have diverging results, and for the moment we do not know whether exercise may potentiate the effects of TCAs or vice versa.

LITHIUM

Lithium has well-documented effects in the prophylaxis of bipolar and unipolar depressive disorders and in the treatment of manic episodes. A common belief among clinicians has been that heavy sweating increases serum lithium levels due to sodium loss and hemoconcentration. There was some scientific evidence for this view from animal research; Smith (1973) found that renal lithium clearance was decreased in rats forced to exercise for 3 hr in a motor-driven activity wheel.

Recent empirical studies do not support this view. Jefferson et al. (1982) studied 4 healthy, well-trained athletes who were stabilized on lithium for 7 days and then ran a 20-km race under humid, hot conditions. The athletes became dehydrated, but their serum lithium levels still decreased. Their lithium concentrations in sweat were four times higher than in serum. Norman, Mathews, and Yohe (1987) studied an experienced male runner in his early twenties with bipolar disorder who completed a 5-mile (8 km) run. Before the run he had stable levels of serum lithium ranging from 0.9 to 1.0 mEq/l. After the run his serum lithium level dropped to 0.7 mEq/l, a value that remained stable the next day. Sweat lithium was 2.2 mEq/l, which is three times his serum lithium concentration. In other studies, human sweat obtained from pilocacpine stimulation

(Miller, Pain, & Skripal, 1978) and heat stimulation (Aref, El-Badramany, Hannora, et al., 1982) was analyzed, showing lithium concentrations two to four times higher than in serum.

During strenuous exercise with heavy sweating, serum levels of lithium will tend to decline rather than increase. The dosage may remain unchanged or may increase slightly, and careful monitoring of serum level is recommended (Jefferson, Greist, Ackerman, & Carroll, 1987).

Muscle weakness and fatigue are common side effects during lithium therapy. Tremor, dizziness, muscle twitching, and poor concentration may also be seen. Many patients gain weight (Gitlin, Cochran, & Jamison, 1989). These side effects may reduce the ability as well as the motivation for exercise, and are most problematic during the 1st year of treatment (Baandrup, Christensen, & Bagger, 1987). In patients without cardiovascular disease, therapeutic levels of lithium have only benign and reversible effects on the cardiovascular system (Baandrup et al., 1987). The physical work capacity does not seem to be attenuated during lithium therapy (Jefferson et al., 1987).

MINOR TRANQUILIZERS

Benzodiazepines may induce significant impairment in cognitive function, as well as various psychomotor skills such as reaction time and tracking test performance. It has been reported by Collomp et al. (1993) that administration of 1 mg of lorazepam 4 hr prior to completion of a Wingate test induced a significant decrease in postexercise levels of plasma epinephrine compared with placebo. Lorazepam administration was also associated with reduced end-exercise lactate and maximal blood lactate levels compared with the placebo trial. The acute administration of lorazepam did not influence the total work performed, but this drug did impair anaerobic peak power. Given the observation of reduced lactate and epinephrine, it would be interesting to know whether or not parallel shifts in perceived exertion took place. It would also be interesting to know whether or not this drug (and dose) has an influence on the anxiolytic effects known to accompany acute exercise. It should also be kept in mind that the test subjects consisted of healthy 27-year-olds, and the volunteers averaged 4 to 8 hr per week of physical activity. Hence, the results cannot be generalized beyond this population.

In a double-blind study of 5 nonanxious patients with chronic airflow obstruction who were 51 to 68 years of age, the administration of 7.5 mg clorazepate, a benzodiazepine, at bedtime for 2 weeks had no significant effect on exercise tolerance, arterial blood gases, pulmonary function tests, or self-rated breathlessness (Eimer, Cable, Gal, Rothenberger, & McCue, 1985). Eleven male patients 66 ± 4 years of age with chronic airflow obstruction and mild anxiety took part in a double-blind, placebo-controlled study of buspirone, a nonbenzodiazepine minor tranquilizer (Singh, Despars, Stansbury, Avalos, & Light, 1993). The authors concluded that the administration of 10 to 20 mg of buspirone three times a day had no significant effect on anxiety level or exercise tolerance. Whether these results may be generalized to patients with *DSM-IV* anxiety disorders remain to be studied.

Stratton and Halter (1985) studied 12 healthy male volunteers, 21 to 35 years of age, to determine whether alprazolam, a benzodiazepine, would inhibit sympathetic discharge during exercise stress. In the treatment group subjects had decreased catecholamine (epinephrine and norepinephrine) responses to exercise, but there was no significant change in exercise duration and only modest, probably clinically insignificant, decreases in heart rate and systolic blood pressure. Sympathetic outflow during stress is considered to be potentially harmful in patients with cardiovascular disease. Whether the same attenuation of sympathetic response to exercise has clinical benefits in patients with cardiovascular disease has not been studied.

Charles, Kirkham, Guyatt, and Parker (1987) studied psychomotor, pulmonary, and exercise responses to sleep medication. They compared two benzodiazepines (nitrazepam and temazepam) with placebo for 9 days in 27 physical education students 18 to 24 years of age. Psychomotor activity and pulmonary function were not affected by medication. Similar maximum exercise levels were obtained in all three conditions on Day 2, while those on nitrazepam reached significantly lower maximum exercise levels on Day 9, compared with placebo and temazepam. Thus, that the use of benzodiazepines may affect the performance of top athletes cannot be ruled out.

An important question is related to whether or not exercise can replace minor tranquilizers. DeVries and Adams (1972) compared the tranquilizing effect of single doses of exercise and meprobamate (400 mg) with respect to reduction of muscular action potential level and heart rate. These investigators reported that exercise had a significantly greater effect on the resting muscle action potential than did meprobamate. It has been shown in controlled studies that exercise is associated with reductions in anxiety levels (see chapter 7), but controlled exercise intervention studies in patients with *DSM* anxiety disorders have not been performed. It is therefore unknown whether exercise can replace drugs in the treatment of these disturbances. The widespread use of these drugs, and the risks of abuse, drug dependence, and other side effects certainly render this an important area for further studies.

β-ADRENERGIC BLOCKING AGENTS

The use of β-adrenergic blocking agents is now widely established in the management of a variety of conditions, such as angina pectoris, hypertension, obstructive cardiomyopathy, ventricular and supraventricular tachyarrythmias, and migraine. Long-term application of β blockers after myocardial infarction has been shown to reduce mortality and myocardial infarction rates, and these effects have further increased their use (Yusuf, Wittes, & Friedman, 1988; Kottke, 1992). Some authors report that β blockers are also effective in the treatment of emotional disturbances (Jefferson, 1974). However, mood disturbances such as depression, fatigue, and anxiety have been reported as side effects (Patten, 1990).

β-adrenergic blocking agents might, in theory, affect exercise capacity by several distinct mechanisms. First, they depress the total cardiac output by reducing the heart rate through antagonism of cardiac β_1 adrenoreceptors. Second, they impair the blood supply to the muscles by blocking the β_2 adrenoreceptors in the walls of the blood vessels. Third, they affect the metabolism of fatty acids and glucose, and they may have a direct effect on muscular contraction (Breckenridge, 1982).

The hemodynamic effects of β blockers have been studied extensively in normal subjects and in patients with heart disease. Propranolol is used frequently as a prototype agent. In normal subjects and in patients with CHD without heart failure, propranolol decreases heart rate moderately at rest (10% to 20%) and markedly during exercise. This heart rate reduction accounts for a great part of the observed decline in rest and exercise cardiac index, although left ventricular stroke volume also decreases (in up to 20%). In patients with CHD with depressed cardiac function (left ventricular ejection fraction 40%), the cardiac function will be depressed further after the administration of propranolol. Similar hemodynamic effects have been reported with other β blockers, although agents with sympathomimetic properties do not appear to be myocardial depressants. Sotalol also appears to have less of a myocardial depressant effect than conventional β blockers (Mahmarian, Verani, & Pratt, 1990).

Several studies have shown that β blockers improve exercise capacity in patients with chronic angina pectoris. Today, the combination of β blockers and calcium antagonists is often used in patients with angina pectoris. Amlodipine, a second-generation calcium antagonist, has been shown to have an additional effect on exercise capacity in patients with stable angina pectoris maintained on β blockers (DiBianco et al., 1992).

β-adrenergic blocking agents are also useful in controlling exercise ventricular rate in chronic atrial fibrillation, but often reduce exercise capacity when given alone or in combination with digoxin. Labetalol, a β blocker with α-blocking property, has been reported not to reduce exercise tolerance in these patients. Labetalol will also improve heart rate control in combination with digoxin, whereas digoxin alone is ineffective in controlling ventricular response during stress or vigorous exercise in patients with chronic atrial fibrillation (Wong, Lau, Leung, & Cheng, 1990).

Although different research reports provide somewhat conflicting results, it now seems generally accepted that β-adrenergic blocking agents impair exercise performance, and both endurance time and maximal oxygen uptake are reduced in patients taking these agents (Andersen et al., 1979). The size of the reduction varies from person to person and depends on the dosage of the drug given. A reduction in cardiac output of up to 22% has been reported in normal subjects at maximal work capacity (Epstein, Robinson, Kahler, & Braunwald, 1965).

Another important question is whether long-term β-adrenergic blockade affects the ability to obtain a cardiovascular training effect from an exercise conditioning program. The studies addressing this topic give conflicting results. One study has shown that aerobic exercise provided no increase in aerobic capacity in patients with coronary artery disease who were receiving β blockers (Malmborg, Isaccson, & Kallivroussis, 1974), while another showed that the use of β blockers markedly attenuated the cardiovascular conditioning effects of exercise in normal subjects, and the authors suggested that β-adrenergic stimulation is essential in exercise conditioning (Sable et al., 1982). There are at least four other studies of patients with CHD showing that substantial training effects can be achieved despite the use of therapeutic doses of β-blockers (Vanhees, Fagard, & Amery, 1982). This is important because the training heart rates are reduced consistently in patients receiving therapeutic doses of β-blocking agents. While there are diverging views, most experts today seem to think that training effects may be achieved while using β blockers.

A sensation of muscle fatigue while exercising is a common problem in patients taking β blockers, but the reason for this discomfort is not clear. One possibility is the decreased blood flow to the exercising muscles by blocking the β adrenoreceptors in the walls of the blood vessels. Metabolic changes with reduced substrate supply to the muscles is another. The blood levels of glucose and free fatty acids (FFAs) fall during exercise while using β blockers (Lundborg, Åstrøm et al., 1981). One study showed that β blockade influenced serum potassium levels during and after exercise (Carlsson, Fellenius, Lundborg, & Svensson, 1978), and there may be an effect directly on the muscles. Theoretically, β blockers may affect neuromuscular activity at the motor end place by virtue of their membrane-stabilizing action and this may contribute to muscle fatigue (Bowman, 1980). Hypoglycemia induced by exercise is another problem (Usitupa, Aro, & Pietkainen, 1980). The normal response of blood glucose to exercise as well as to hypoglycemia is reduced by β blockers, presumably by inhibition of the β_2 adrenoreceptor–mediated liver glycogenolysis (Bewsher, 1967). The reduction of warmth production by reduced lipolysis and reduced trembling may be of importance for maximal exercise, especially in cold climates (Aksnes, 1977).

An important applied question deals with the kinds of β blockers that are most comfortable for individuals performing various physical activities. Theoretically, selective β blockers might be expected to have an advantage, but this has been hard to prove in scientific research studies. An alternation in dose or a change of the particular agent may be beneficial in treating patients who report symptoms of undue fatigue and compromised exercise performance. At this time β blockers will have to be chosen on the basis of trial and error for patients receiving exercise prescriptions.

To conclude, the use of β blockers reduces the capacity to perform exercise in normal subjects, but improves exercise capacity in patients with chronic stable angina pectoris. The normal training effect does not seem to be attenuated by using these drugs. Common complaints are exercise-induced muscle fatigue and hypoglycemia, and patients performing endurance exercise while taking β blockers are advised to ingest suitable substrates for the muscles to prevent symptom-producing hypoglycemia.

CLINICAL EXPERIENCES WITH EXERCISE FOR PSYCHIATRIC PATIENTS RECEIVING PSYCHOPHARMACOLOGICAL TREATMENT

Martinsen has been engaged in the use of physical rehabilitation as a part of psychiatric treatment over the past 15 years in various psychiatric institutions. Approximately 300 patients have taken part in systematic clinical research studies, while a larger number have exercised as part of their therapy without taking part in scientific studies. The patients cover the whole range of psychiatric disorders, and patients have received the whole spectrum of psychotropic drugs, including major and minor tranquilizers, antidepressants, lithium, and anticonvulsants, in therapeutic doses.

Many patients are bothered by the side effects of medication, including orthostatism, tachycardia, dry mouth, drowsiness, and vertigo, but these side effects usually do not force them to reduce the intensity of exercise or to drop out of the exercise program.

Before patients are involved in systematic exercise, they should undergo careful medical screening. Patients with a history of cardiovascular disease, or those suspected of having cardiovascular disease, should not take part in exercise programs until they have been cleared for exercise by a cardiologist. Special care should be taken in exercising patients with CHD who are also receiving TCAs. Training intensity should be low while the doses of medication are increasing. Intensive exercise should only start when the patient has reached a steady-state level of medication and the circulation is reasonably well adapted to the medication.

SUMMARY

A critical review of the literature regarding the interaction between exercise and medication shows that our knowledge in this field is limited. The following conclusions seem justified at this point: (a) megadoses (1 to 3 g/day) of chlorpromazine tend to reduce cardiac output and attenuate the effect of training programs; (b) therapeutic doses of neuroleptics and TCAs often lead to a decrease in blood pressure; (c) the use of β blockers may lead to muscle fatigue and hypoglycemia during exercise and exercise performance is decreased, but normal training effects can be achieved while using them; (d) no serious complication to the combination of physical exercise and psychotropic medication has been published; and (e) physically healthy people who require psychotropic medication may exercise safely when exercise and medications are titrated under close medical supervision.

Part Two

Psychological Responses to Physical Activity

Chapter 6

Antidepressant Effects of Physical Activity

Egil W. Martinsen and William P. Morgan

Depression is a major health problem today, and the lifetime risk for having a major depressive disorder in the community has been estimated to vary from 10% to 25% for women and from 5% to 12% for men. In addition, the lifetime risk for dysthymic disorders is approximately 6% (APA, 1994). The standard forms of therapy are antidepressant medication or various forms of psychotherapy, or both, as well as ECT in severe cases. The costs for treating depression are escalating, and the health care system will never be able to meet the need for treatment presented by this large group of patients. Furthermore, many patients do not receive treatment. If a simple and inexpensive approach such as physical activity were shown to be effective in the treatment or prevention of depression, this could have a significant impact on public health.

Population studies have shown clear correlations between physical activity level and mental health at a given point in time (Stephens, 1988). Depressed patients are also characterized by reduced physical work capacity as compared with the general population (Morgan, 1969b, 1970b; Martinsen, Strand, Paulsson, & Kaggestad, 1989). This kind of correlational evidence, however, leaves open the question of causality. That is, are patients (a) depressed because they are unfit and inactive; (b) unfit because they are depressed; or (c) is there a third factor (e.g., genotype) that is connected to both reduced fitness and depression? The answer to these questions must await further intervention studies.

This chapter focuses on the antidepressant effects of physical activity, and its primary focus is the efficacy of this intervention in clinically depressed individuals. A secondary purpose is to consider the extent to which physical activity is effective in improving mood states of individuals who are either nondepressed or are experiencing mild depression. The first part of the chapter deals with research and applications involving clinical populations, and the second portion focuses on analogue research that has been carried out with individuals who have not been diagnosed as clinically depressed. While the use of such a dichotomy is somewhat arbitrary, it is clear that research and application with depressed and nondepressed populations has been characterized by different research methodologies (processes) as well as outcomes (products).

Assessment of Depression

Modern criteria-based diagnostic systems have greatly increased diagnostic reliability in psychiatry. Commonly used assessment procedures include the Research Diagnostic Criteria (RDC; Spitzer, Endicott, & Robins, 1978), *DSM-III* (APA, 1980), and *DSM-IV* (APA, 1994). These diagnostic systems make it easier to compare results across studies.

Several psychometric instruments have been developed to measure the level of depression, and the BDI (Beck, Ward, Mendelson, Mock, & Erbaugh, 1961) and SDS (Zung, 1965) are well validated self-report instruments. The Comprehensive Psychopathological Rating Scale (CPRS), depression subscale (Åsberg, Perris, Schalling, & Sedvall, 1978), and the Montgomery Åsberg Depression Rating Scale (MADRS; Montgomery & Åsberg, 1979) are frequently employed as well. Some of the scales (e.g., BDI and SDS) provide normal ranges for the item scores, and these instruments may be used to identify cases or patients. In many intervention studies involving the efficacy of physical activity, the scores on such scales serve as the only means of classification for a given patient, and formal diagnoses are not made. However, it is difficult to generalize the results of such investigations to other populations, and these studies have limited value.

CLINICAL STUDIES

Investigations dealing with the efficacy of physical activity that have begun to appear in recent years rely on the use of experimental and quasi-experimental designs, and these studies have been conducted with clinically depressed individuals. In some of these studies, there has been an effort to quantify the impact of various forms of physical activity (e.g., aerobic, resistive).

The first experimental study dealing with this topic was performed by Greist et al. (1979). Running therapy was compared with two forms of individual psychotherapy in 28 outpatients with RDC-classified minor depression. While significant reductions in depression scores were found in all groups, differences were not found in treatment outcomes for the various conditions after 12 weeks of intervention. In other words, the antidepressant effect of physical activity was comparable to changes noted for traditional psychotherapy.

Sime (1987) used a multiple baseline, single-case design in a study of 15 subjects with moderately elevated scores on the BDI. Depression scores were not changed significantly during a screening phase and a 2-week preexercise period, but scores dropped significantly during a 10-week exercise period. Doyne, Chambless, and Beutler (1983) used the same design in a study of 4 women with RDC-classified major depressive disorder. Significant reductions in depression scores were observed following 6 weeks of physical activity, and these reductions were significantly larger than changes noted in the preexercise screening phase.

Rueter, Mutrie, and Harris (1982) studied 18 subjects with elevated BDI scores who were assigned randomly to counseling alone or to supervised running in addition to counseling. The reductions in BDI scores were significantly larger in the combined running and counseling group than in the counseling alone group. However, because there was not a running group per se, it is difficult to ascertain the extent to which physical activity was responsible for the observed antidepressant effect.

In a study involving 74 patients diagnosed with major or minor depression (RDC), Klein, Greist, Gurman, Neimeyer, Lesser, Bushnell, and Smith (1985) randomly assigned participants to running, meditation and relaxation, or group psychotherapy. After 12 weeks, significant reductions in depression scores were observed in each treatment group, but there were no significant differences between the groups. However, the follow-up results indicated a better outcome for the exercise and meditation groups.

In a similar investigation, McCann and Holmes (1984) randomly assigned 41 women with elevated depression scores as measured by the BDI to either aerobic exercise, relaxation training, or a waiting list control condition. After 10 weeks there were significant reductions in depression scores in both treatment groups, but the reduction observed for the aerobic exercise group was significantly greater than that noted for either the relaxation or control groups.

Freemont and Craighead (1987) studied 49 individuals with elevated BDI scores who were assigned randomly to cognitive therapy, aerobic exercise, or a combination of cognitive therapy and aerobic exercise. Significant reductions in depression scores were obtained in all groups after 10 weeks, but there were no significant differences between the groups.

In a study of female and male inpatients diagnosed with major depression (*DSM-III* criteria), Martinsen, Medhus, and Sandvik (1985) randomly assigned patients to aerobic exercise and control groups. Patients in the physical activity group performed aerobic exercise (jogging and brisk walking) for 1 hour three times per week for 6 to 9 weeks, while those in the control group took part in occupational therapy that did not include vigorous physical activity. (The control group was actually a minimal treatment group from an exercise standpoint.) Both activities were performed in small groups under the supervision of professional instructors. Patients in both groups received individual and group psychotherapy, as well as milieu therapy. The group performing aerobic physical activity experienced a significantly greater increase in physical working capacity than did the controls Changes in depression were measured with the CPRS and BDI, and the exercise group experienced a significantly greater decrease in depression. In other words, the increase in physical fitness was associated with an antidepressant effect for the patients in the physical activity group. These results are summarized in Figure 1.

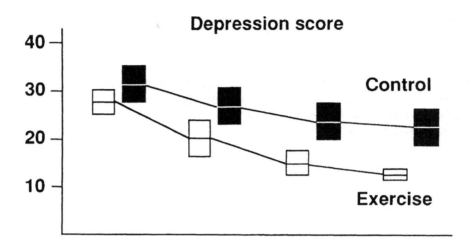

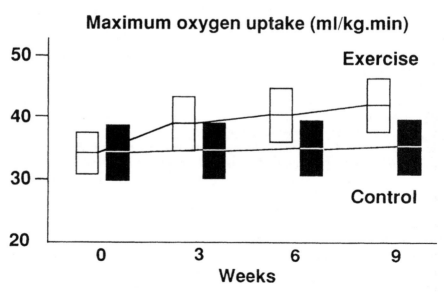

Figure 1   Mean depression score (Beck Depression Inventory) and physical work capacity, with 95% confidence intervals. From "Effects of aerobic exercise on depression: A controlled study," by E.W. Martinsen, A Medhus, and L. Sandvik, *British Medical Journal*, 1985, *291*: 109. Reproduced with permission.

Further analysis revealed that the antidepressive effect noted in this study seemed to be dependent on the degree of improvement in aerobic fitness. Patients in the physical activity group with gains in aerobic power of less than 15% had an antidepressive effect similar to that observed in the control group. Patients with moderate (15% to 30%) or large (>30%) increases in aerobic power had similar improvements in depression, and both of these subgroups had larger reductions in depression scores than those with small gains (<15%) in aerobic fitness as well as those in the control group. A correlational analysis using the Spearman ρ method revealed that gains in aerobic power and improvement in depression (BDI scores) were correlated at 0.40 ($p < .05$) in the male patients, but this relationship was not significant in the female patients.

In order to study these findings further, Martinsen, Hoffart, and Solberg (1989a) compared aerobic and resistive exercise in 99 inpatients with major depression (*DSM-III-R*), dysthymic disorder, or depressive disorder not otherwise specified. The patients were assigned randomly to either an aerobic exercise group, described earlier by Martinsen et al. (1985), or a resistive exercise group that included strength, endurance, and flexibility exercises. Patients in the aerobic group achieved a significant increase in aerobic power, while those in the resistance group did not. Both groups experienced significant reductions in depression as measured by the MADRS and BDI, but there was no difference between groups in the antidepressive effect. Unlike the earlier study by Martinsen and Sandvik (1985), patients in this study with substantial gains in aerobic power (>15%) had similar reductions in depression as those with little or no increase in aerobic power. Furthermore, the correlations between reduced depression (BDI scores) and improved aerobic power were 0.13 and 0.26 ($p > .05$) for the women and men, respectively. These results confirm the findings of the earlier study for female patients, but the previous report of a relationship between improved depression scores and aerobic power for male patients was not replicated. This issue warrants further attention because it is important to know whether a training threshold exists in order to ensure that an antidepressant effect will occur.

The research by Martinsen et al. (1989) represents one of the few studies in which investigators have attempted to compare different modes of physical activity. In a similar study, Doyne et al. (1987) randomly assigned 40 outpatients diagnosed with minor or major depression (RDC) to exercise groups involving aerobic (running) or resistance (weight lifting) training. Reductions in depression scores for both groups were larger than those observed in a waiting list control group. However, the improvement in depression for the two exercise groups did not differ significantly.

Most of the research in this area has involved supervised exercise programs, but it is often the case that exercise prescriptions are given to individuals who are expected to proceed on their own. Mutrie (1988) randomly assigned 24 individuals with elevated depression scores on the BDI to one of three groups. One group performed aerobic exercise, another engaged in a program that consisted of stretching and strengthening exercises, and a third group served as a waiting list control. The participants in the exercise groups trained on their own three times a week, and they met with a physical education specialist every 2 weeks for instructions and physical testing. Both exercise groups had larger reductions in BDI scores than the control group, but the only significant difference involved the comparison between the aerobic and control groups. These findings suggest that aerobic exercise is more effective in reducing depression than a program of stretching and strengthening when performed in a quasi-supervised manner. However, there are at least three problems with this investigation that limit interpretation or generalizability. First, the study suffers from the small sample size. Second, most investigations in this area have relied on training programs lasting from 6 to 20 weeks, and it is unlikely that meaningful effects can occur in a brief 12-session program carried out without supervision. Third, designs of this nature merely indicate that physical activity can be superior to nothing, i.e., an untreated control group. While it is sometimes difficult to create an adequate placebo group in such research, the problem of "any treatment versus no treatment" cannot be ignored. Alternatively, one can compare the psychological effects of physical activity with responses noted for minimal or traditional therapies (Greist et al., 1979; Klein et al., 1985).

Prevention

It appears that only two studies have addressed the question of whether physical activity can prevent the occurrence of depression in vulnerable individuals and prevent relapse for those who have recovered from a depressive episode. Gøtestam and Stiles (1990) studied Norwegian soldiers exposed to stressful life situations. Soldiers who engaged actively in sports were significantly less depressed 12 weeks after exposure to the stressful life situation compared with those classified as sedentary.

Martinsen, Sandvik, and Kolbjomsrūd (1989) found that previous adult experience with exercise and sports predicted less chance of relapse in nonpsychotic patients 1 year after discharge from the hospital, and further, that continuous exercise at follow-up was associated with lower symptom scores. Physical activity may have a prophylactic effect, but more evidence is needed before firm conclusions may be drawn.

Patient Perceptions

At 1 year follow-up Martinsen and Medhus (1989) asked patients to evaluate the usefulness of physical fitness training compared with other forms of therapy received during a hospital stay. Patients in the training group ranked physical fitness training as the therapeutic element that had helped them most, whereas those in the control group ranked psychotherapy as the most important. These results are summarized in Figure 2.

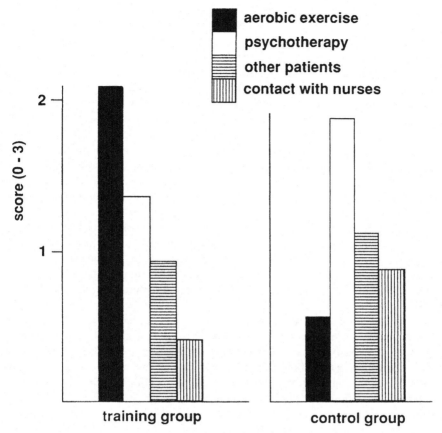

Figure 2. Patients' ranking of the most important therapeutic elements. From "Aerobic exercise in the treatment of nonpsychotic mental disorders," by E.W. Martinsen, L. Sandvik, and O.B. Kolbjomsrūd, *Nordic Journal of Psychiatry*, 1989, *43:* 411–415. Reproduced with permission.

The same trend was reported by Sexton, Mære, and Dahl (1989), who found many patients reporting that physical fitness training had helped them more than traditional forms of therapy, including psychotherapy and medication. While these studies give no proof for the efficacy of exercise treatment, the findings are of sufficient interest to warrant further research.

Summary

The results in these studies all point in the same direction. Aerobic exercise is more effective than no treatment, and it does not significantly differ from other forms of treatment, including various forms of psychotherapy. However, increases in aerobic fitness do not seem to be important because patients without physiological gains have similar psychological effects as those with improved fitness.

The studies reviewed here comprise outpatients and inpatients, men and women, and participants from 17 to 60 years of age. Exercise settings vary from home-based exercise performed alone to supervised exercise in outpatient and inpatient clinical settings. The same trends are seen across studies, indicating that the antidepressant effect associated with physical activity is general.

These results are limited to unipolar depressive disorders, without melancholic or psychotic features, that are commonly referred to as mild to moderate forms of depression. In the official American classification system, *DSM-IV*, this includes mild and moderate forms of major depression, dysthymic disorder, and depressive disorder not otherwise specified. Whether these results may be generalized to major depressive episodes in patients with bipolar disorder has not been studied systematically.

There are no well-controlled experimental studies addressing the value of physical activity in the treatment of severe forms of major depression. Clinical experience, however, indicates that exercise has limited value (Greist, 1987). Severe depression usually requires professional treatment, which may include medication, ECT, or psychotherapy, or some combination of the three, with exercise as an adjunct (Morgan & Goldston, 1987).

The question of exercise dose, or how much is needed in order to achieve an antidepressive effect, has not been addressed systematically. This issue has been pursued vigorously by exercise physiologists in recent years (see chapter 3), but the concern has been with health outcomes of a physical nature for the most part. One psychological study that dealt with this question in an indirect manner was reported by Sexton et al. (1989), who randomly assigned 25 inpatients diagnosed with unipolar depression (*DSM-III*) to physical activity groups involving walking or running. Both groups experienced significant reductions in depression scores, but there were no differences between the groups. This study would seem to suggest that walking is just as effective as running, but there is no evidence that either activity was responsible for the antidepressive effect reported. In other words, a group of untreated controls might have improved to the same degree, and it is also possible that the improvement was caused in part by other factors (e.g., drug therapy, psychotherapy).

There is also an absence of systematic research dealing with the value of physical activity in the prevention of relapse in bipolar disorder. Martinsen has personally followed 3 male patients with this disorder, all of whom were between 20 and 40 years of age and enthusiastic runners. All were lithium responders, but wanted to taper lithium and see whether daily running could replace it. Within 1 year all 3 patients had relapsed and had to resume lithium treatment. Physical activity may have various beneficial effects for patients with bipolar disorder, such as an improved sense of well-being and mastery, and improved self-esteem, but it is not likely to be effective in preventing manic or depressive episodes.

A few studies have compared physical activity with psychotherapy and counseling in the treatment of depression, finding them to be about equally effective (Freemont & Craighead, 1987; Greist et al., 1979; Klein et al., 1985). There have been many developments within the field of psychotherapy research in recent years, and many of the earlier exercise studies do not meet modern standards of psychotherapy research. Despite the methodological limitations of this research, the findings open up interesting perspectives, and these studies should be followed up with more rigorous investigations. Likewise, there have been no studies to date comparing the efficacy of physical activity and medication in the treatment of depression.

There has not been a great deal of research in this area, and many of the existing studies have methodological shortcomings. Some investigators have used single self-report measures of depression (e.g., BDI) for classification; while others have not described precisely the intensity, frequency, mode, and duration of exercise; and in some cases measures of fitness have not been employed. Hence, there is still a need for methodologically sound studies.

ANALOGUE RESEARCH

A great deal of the research involving the influence of physical activity on depression has not involved depressed individuals. Much of this research has dealt with nondepressed individuals, or samples of test subjects with mild or borderline levels of depression. This research has been summarized in a recent review by Morgan (1994b). In many respects this situation resembles the distinction that is often made between psychotherapy and analogue research. O'Leary and Borkovec (1978) have pointed out that "psychotherapy refers to psychological treatment of a clinical problem, that is, a problem that represents a real problem, in living for the client—for example, debilitating . . . depression" (p. 822). Analogue therapy, on the other hand, represents "psychological treatment of a problem that seldom or never causes concern to a client in his or her life and may or may not be relevant to a client's daily concerns, such as snake or rat phobias" (p. 822). However, O'Leary and Borkovec (1978) have also pointed out that psychotherapy and analogue therapy are not dichotomous; that is, clients often have problems that lie between these two extremes. At any rate, a substantial amount of the literature dealing with the influence of physical activity on depression has dealt with therapy and research, which falls under the *analogue* rubric. Examples of findings from this research literature are summarized in this section.

One of the first analogue studies dealing with the influence of physical activity on depression was reported by Morgan et al. (1970). In this study, 140 men ranging in age from 22 to 62 years (mean 39 years) served as volunteers. The subjects participated in one of eight exercise programs, and a sample of 16 individuals served as controls. The physical activities consisted of running, cycling, swimming, and circuit training. These activities were performed at approximately 85% of each subject's predicted maximal heart rate, and the frequency ranged from 2 to 3 days per week. Physical working capacity improved the most in the running groups, but each of the exercise groups had greater gains than the control group (Roberts & Morgan, 1971). The subjects in this study completed the SDS (Zung, 1965) before and after the 6-week intervention. None of the groups experienced a change in depression following the 6-week period, and none of the exercise groups improved more on the SDS than the control group. However, Zung (1965) has reported that individuals who score 53 or higher on the SDS possess depression of "clinical significance"; and 11 of the exercisers in the study by Morgan et al. (1970) scored above 53 at the outset. This subgroup experienced a significant decrease ($p < .05$) in depression. It was also reported that none of the nondepressed subjects became depressed, which argues against statistical regression as the reason for the antidepressant effect. A number of studies carried out over the subsequent two decades support the findings presented by Morgan et al. (1970). Research by Martinsen (1990), Morgan and Pollock (1978), and Stern and Cleary (1982) support the view that nondepressed subjects do not experience an antidepressant effect despite the observation that these individuals have gains in aerobic power with exercise training.

In a subsequent study, Morgan and Pollock (1978) randomly assigned 54 adult men either to aerobic exercise groups or to a control group. The subjects in the physical activity groups ran 3 days per week at an intensity of 85% to 90% of maximum heart rate for 20 weeks. The three exercise groups ran for 15, 30, or 45 minutes per session, and each subject completed a VO_2max test before and after the 20-week training program. The exercise groups improved in direct proportion to the training duration whereas the control group did not experience an improvement in aerobic power (Pollock, Gettman, Milesis, Bah, Durstine, & Johnson 1977). Depression was assessed before and after the 20-week training program with the POMS depression scale (McNair, Lorr, & Droppleman, 1992). None of the subjects in this investigation were depressed at the outset; none of the groups experienced a decrease in depression following 20 weeks of training; and the exercise and control conditions did not differ at any point. In other words, increased aerobic power following a 20-week running program was not associated with an antidepressant effect in these individuals who were not depressed at the outset of training.

The above findings were replicated and extended by Morgan and Pollock (1978) in a separate experiment involving an additional group of 54 nondepressed men. The duration of exercise was held constant at 30 minutes in this study, and the intensity ranged from 85% to 90% of maximum heart rate. The independent variable in this study was frequency, and subjects were randomly assigned to a placebo (minimal treatment) group or to groups that exercised 1, 3, or 5 days per week. Aerobic power increased in direct proportion to the frequency of exercise, and the placebo group did not change over the 20-week period (Pollock et al., 1977). The increased aerobic power was not associated with an antidepressant effect in these nondepressed subjects, which is in agreement with the observations made in the study by Morgan and Pollock (1978), in which duration of exercise served as the independent variable.

Reviewers such as Hughes (1984), Martinsen (1990, 1994), and Simons, McGowan, Epstein, Kupfer, & Robertson (1985) have pointed out that much of the research dealing with the antidepressant effect of exercise has relied on quasi-experimental designs as opposed to true experimental designs (Campbell & Stanley, 1966). However, in the experiments summarized earlier, Morgan and Pollock (1978) randomly assigned volunteers to the various exercise, control, and placebo groups. In other words, a true experimental design was employed, and despite the observation that a clear dose-response occurred in terms of training stimulus and gains in aerobic power, no antidepressant effect was observed regardless of exercise duration or frequency.

In many respects it is somewhat surprising that investigators would expect nondepressed individuals to experience an antidepressant effect following exercise, or any intervention for that matter. However, it has been reported widely in both the professional and lay literature that exercise reduces depression, and this view is seldom restricted to depressed individuals. Also, in reports in which meta-analysts have not controlled for various methodological issues such as demand characteristics, expectancy effects, response distortion, and so on, there has been a tendency to find that exercise leads to reduced depression in nondepressed individuals (North, McCullagh, & Tran, 1990). Other meta-analysts have arrived at a more conservative conclusion. McDonald and Hodgdon (1991), for example, have reported that the antidepressant effect of exercise was approximately 40% greater in depressed versus nondepressed groups. At any rate, unless meta-analysts and narrative reviewers alike control for the numerous behavioral artifacts known to influence outcome research, conclusions regarding the antidepressant effects of exercise must be viewed with caution. This matter is discussed at greater length in chapter 1.

Despite the fact that nondepressed individuals do not experience an antidepressant effect with exercise, these same individuals typically report that they "feel better" as a consequence of exercise (Martinsen, 1994; Morgan, 1994b). It is known that transient effects in anxiety occur following vigorous physical activity, and these anxiolytic effects persist for 1 to 2 hours (Raglin & Morgan, 1987). There is a possibility that transient effects in depression occur following acute physical activity. Morgan, Roberts, and Feinerman (1971), for example, randomly assigned 120 adult men to treadmill ($N = 60$) or bicycle ergometer ($N = 60$) exercise designed to evoke heart rates of 150, 160, 170, or 180 bpm. A posttest-only design (Campbell & Stanley, 1966) was employed in this study in order to control for pretest sensitization and expectancy effects (see chapter 1). Form A of the Depression Adjective Check List (DACL; Lubin, 1967) was administered to these subjects at approximately 5 min following the exercise. While the various exercise conditions did not differ significantly, all of the exercise groups had mean depression scores that fell below published norms.

In a more recent investigation Nelson and Morgan (1994) evaluated the influence of acute exercise on depression in depressed ($N = 6$) and nondepressed ($N = 6$) female college students. Depression was assessed with the POMS depression scale before, 0 to 5 minutes after, and 15 to 20 minutes after bicycle ergometer exercise performed at 40%, 60%, and 80% of estimated maximum heart rate on 3 separate days. The exercise intensity was counterbalanced and randomly assigned. Significant decreases in depression were observed following exercise at all intensities for the depressed subjects. This antidepressant effect was independent of exercise intensity, and was transitory. There were no changes in depression noted for the nondepressed group.

Summary

Analogue research dealing with the antidepressant effect of physical activity has not yielded a clear consensus, but it is possible to advance a tentative conclusion. It seems reasonable to conclude at this time that individuals with elevated scores on objective measures of depression (e.g., DACL, POMS, SDS) experience an antidepressant effect following acute and chronic physical activity of a vigorous nature. However, nondepressed individuals scoring in the normal range on these same measures of depression do not experience an antidepressant effect following exercise. It is also known that healthy, nondepressed individuals often experience elevations on standard measures of depression, and sometimes become clinically depressed when the volume of training becomes excessive. The psychological distress associated with overtraining can be viewed as a paradoxical effect, and this syndrome has been labeled as *staleness* in the sports medicine literature. In other words, it is not only the case that nondepressed individuals do not experience an antidepressant effect with exercise; it is possible for such individuals to actually become depressed when the training stimulus is excessive. This phenomenon is thoroughly discussed by O'Connor in chapter 9 of this book.

PRACTICAL MANAGEMENT

Several components in the depressive syndrome may make it difficult to exercise. Fatigue, lassitude, low self-esteem, and psychomotor retardation are common symptoms. Furthermore, for those individuals taking antidepressant medication, side effects such as dry mouth, drowsiness, and increased heart rate may cause additional problems. Because of these factors, many patients will need encouragement and support when starting to exercise.

The intensity of exercise should be no higher than patients can tolerate, and this is an important detail because most patients are unfit. During recent years

Martinsen has observed over 100 patients taking part in hospital exercise programs. This experience shows that it is possible to help a large proportion of depressed patients to initiate and maintain regular physical activity.

HYPOTHESIZED MECHANISMS

Physiological, biochemical, and psychological mechanisms have been suggested to explain how the psychological effects of exercise are mediated. The most compelling biological hypotheses at this time involve endorphin, norepinephrine, serotonin, and thermogenic mechanisms, which are discussed elsewhere in this book.

Several psychological hypotheses have been advanced as well. Bahrke and Morgan (1978), for example, have proposed that the psychological benefits associated with exercise may be due to mere distraction from the cares and worries of the day. Some have postulated that regular, monotonous exercise may be looked on as a kind of meditation or self-hypnosis, inducing an altered state of consciousness. Others claim that the important thing about exercise is the development of a positive addiction (Glasser, 1976). The concepts of competence and mastery (White, 1959) could easily explain the sensation of well-being that usually accompanies physical activity. Bandura (1977) has presented a self-efficacy theory, which specifies that a treatment will be effective if it restores a sense of self-efficacy by arranging self-mastery experiences, which could also explain the positive influence of exercise.

Different hypotheses are available, but the empirical evidence supporting them is limited. There is probably not only one mechanism mediating the psychological effects of exercise. Different mechanisms may work for different people, and biological, psychological, and social mechanisms may work in concert with one another in an interactive manner.

SUMMARY

In clinically depressed patients, aerobic exercise seems to be better than no treatment and not significantly different from other interventions, including various forms of psychotherapy. Aerobic and nonaerobic forms of exercise seem to be equally effective in treating depression. The results are restricted to mild to moderate forms of unipolar depression (*DSM-IV* mild to moderate forms of major depression, dysthymic disorder, and depressive disorder not otherwise specified). Patients appreciate exercise and find it to be a useful form of therapy. Physical exercise may be an alternative or adjunct to traditional forms of treatment in mild to moderate forms of unipolar depression.

There is less agreement regarding the influence of vigorous physical activity on depression in nonpatient groups. The results of this analogue research suggest that depression, as measured by standardized scales (e.g., BDI, SDS) is decreased in individuals with elevated depression scores, but antidepressive effects have not been noted consistently in groups scoring within the normal range on depression. In either case, definite effects of exercise are recognized and using this knowledge can help professionals modify the level of depression in clients and help them lead happier lives.

Chapter 7

Anxiolytic Effects
of Physical Activity

John S. Raglin

Mental illness is a major problem in modern society, and the various anxiety disorders represent the most prevalent forms of mental illness. In the United States it is estimated that approximately 7.3% of the adult population suffers from an anxiety disorder to a degree that warrants some form of treatment (Regier et al., 1988). Complaints related to the experience of stress-related emotions such as anxiety are even common among healthy individuals, and these problems often have consequences for physical health (Cohen, Tyrell, & Smith, 1991; Craufurd, Creed, & Jayson, 1990).

Physicians and mental health practitioners have a number of means to combat anxiety disorders, including various forms of psychological and psychiatric therapy and pharmacologic therapy. However, significant numbers of affected persons do not receive adequate treatment and up to 20% of those afflicted with mental health problems receive no treatment at all (Bloom, 1985). These figures clearly indicate that the scope of anxiety and other mental health problems is beyond the capacity of our current health care system. Furthermore, interventions such as psychotherapy can be expensive and time-consuming, and drug therapy is sometimes associated with after-effects and side effects as well as high costs. These problems are likely to be compounded by pressures for rationed care and other probable reforms, as well as increased calls for an emphasis on prevention.

Because of these issues there is interest in identifying and establishing alternative forms of preventing and treating anxiety disorders. Physical activity has been promoted as one means of enhancing and maintaining general emotional health (Hughes, 1984; Morgan & Goldston, 1987; Taylor et al., 1987). Unlike behavioral methods such as biofeedback, physical activity can be self-administered and can be a convenient, low-cost activity with minimal side effects. Regular participation in physical activity also results in various physical benefits such as enhanced physical capacity, altered body composition, and increased muscle tone, and these changes may impact on emotional health (Sonstroem & Morgan, 1989). Regular physical activity also results in reductions in risk factors for physical diseases such as coronary artery disease (Blair et al., 1989; Powell et al., 1987). Hence, habitual physical activity represents a behavior that has the potential to benefit both physical and psychological health.

Considerable research has been conducted on the psychological effects of physical activity (Hughes, 1984; Morgan & Goldston, 1987) and there is evidence supporting its benefit for various aspects of emotional well-being and psychological functioning (Morgan & O'Connor, 1988, 1989). However, basic issues such as causality remain unresolved, and some reviewers have questioned the validity of the published research because of various methodological problems characterizing this literature (Hughes, 1984; Folkins & Sime, 1981; Morgan, 1981; Morgan et al., 1990). The nature of these methodological problems is addressed in chapter 1. Moreover, a widely cited paper by Pitts and McClure (1967) emphasizes that vigorous physical activity can be a precipitating factor for panic attacks in anxiety neurotics as well as in some normal individuals. This report has undoubtedly impeded the study of exercise for persons with clinically diagnosed anxiety disorders, and this has resulted in a limitation of our understanding of both the potential benefits of physical activity for persons with clinical anxiety disorders as well as the actual risks of this intervention. Unfortunately, the paper by Pitts and McClure (1967) has serious methodological problems, and while these limitations have been pointed out by several investigators (Grosz & Farmer, 1969; Morgan, 1973c; Morgan, 1979b), the report continues to be cited as factual by authors in the fields of psychiatry and clinical psychology (Lader, 1985).

This chapter focuses on research evidence involving the anxiolytic effect of physical activity. Particular attention is paid to the effect of programmatic factors, and recent research involving the psychological effects of physical activity on persons with clinical anxiety disorders is examined. In addition, methodological problems that have hampered the growth of knowledge in this area of inquiry are addressed, and unresolved issues warranting future research are discussed.

DEFINING ANXIETY

Anxiety has been defined by Spielberger (1972) as an emotional response to stressors of either an objective or subjective nature that consists of combinations of feelings, cognitions, and physiological changes. Anxiety has also been conceptualized (Spielberger, 1972) as existing in state and trait forms. As discussed in chapter 1, state anxiety is a transient condition that may fluctuate rapidly within a span of time as short as a few minutes or even seconds, while the general tendency toward anxiety proneness is labeled trait anxiety. Trait anxiety indicates the general level of vulnerability to stress, and it is predicted that highly trait-anxious individuals will experience larger increases in state anxiety when exposed to a stressor than will those with low trait anxiety. The conceptualization of anxiety in this manner has been operationalized in the form of the STAI (Spielberger, 1983).

Most research involving physical activity has generally examined the concepts of state anxiety and trait anxiety separately. Changes in state anxiety have usually been studied in relation to either acute exercise or single sessions of physical activity. Acute physical activity has varied a great deal in the published literature, and ranges in duration from several minutes (Steptoe & Cox, 1988) to over 11 hours (Shimomitsu, 1993). Because trait anxiety usually does not change with transient stressors, its adaptations to regular participation in long-term or chronic physical activity programs has been of interest.

ASSESSMENT OF ANXIETY

Anxiety can be determined by a variety of methods including observational techniques, assessment of tonic levels or changes in physiological activity, or self-report. The use of observational methods is limited, particularly in research involving physical activity, because the behavior being observed must be interpreted according to its presumed relation to anxiety (Hackfort & Schwenkmezger, 1989). However, observational methods can be useful when applied to cases in which behavior is linked directly to anxiety, such as phobic behavior (Martinsen, Hoffart, & Solberg, 1989a). A more common means to assess anxiety involves the measurement of physiological variables such as heart rate, blood pressure, skin conductance or resistance, or hormonal (e.g., adrenaline, cortisol) responses implicated in the stress response. The use of physiological assessment has been promoted as being more accurate than self-report measures of anxiety (De Geus, Van Doornen, & Orlebeke, 1993; Hatfield & Landers, 1987) because these variables presumably provide greater objectivity, and in some cases continuous monitoring is possible. Unlike self-reports, physiological measures are not dependent on self-awareness or verbal ability, and presumably are not influenced by factors such as social desirability or demand characteristics, which are known to influence response distortion. Also, excessive physiological reactivity has been proposed to be an important causal factor in physical illnesses such as CHD (Matthews et al., 1986).

The underlying rationale for the use of this approach in measuring anxiety is based on the assumption that these physiological variables reflect the overall or global level of arousal, which itself is linked closely with anxiety (Duffy, 1962). Because global arousal is regarded as a nonspecific response, measures of physiological activity taken during arousal states should correlate closely. Under this assumption a single or limited number of measures of physiological activity could be used to determine changes in anxiety accurately. Yet evidence indicates that neither of these assumptions generally hold true. First, it has been found that the physiological response profiles for a given stressor may vary considerably among individuals, and physiological factors often display little covariance either at the interindividual or intraindividual levels (Lacey, 1967). Second, it is common for an individual to exhibit unique physiological response profiles to different stressors (Lacey, 1967). Moreover, there is only limited evidence that physiological responsivity is associated prospectively with increased risk of physical diseases (Manuck, Olsson, Hjemdahl, et al., 1992). Limitations could be circumvented if specific emotional states were identifiable by a characteristic set of physiological responses, but the reliability of such indicators is unclear (Stemmler, 1989). In addition, emotional profiles would likely be masked by the considerable physiological activity that occurs during the anticipatory period preceding the initiation of physical activity. These problematic phenomena have led Levitt (1980) to conclude that, "Physiological systems have not proven useful in the experimental measurement of anxiety" (p. 71).

The many problems associated with physiological measures of anxiety have resulted in the widespread use of self-report measures, and valid instruments such as the STAI usually present the most valid means of assessing anxiety in physical activity settings. Self-evaluation questionnaires have been developed for the purpose of measuring both labile aspects of anxiety (i.e., state anxiety) as well as the more stable form (e.g., trait anxiety). Several valid measures such as the STAI (Spielberger et al., 1983) and the tension/anxiety scale of the POMS (McNair et al., 1992) have been found to be particularly useful in physical activity settings (McDonald & Hodgdon, 1991; Morgan, 1994; Spielberger, 1989). In addition, research has found that postexercise decrements in self-reported anxiety correspond to reductions in stress-related physiological variables including blood pressure (Brown, Morgan, & Raglin, 1993; Raglin & Morgan, 1987; O'Connor & Davis, 1992) and central measures of activation such as the EEG (Petruzzello & Landers, 1994). Despite this evidence, it has been proposed that extant psychological measures can be misleading or even invalid when used to assess anxiety state during physical activity (Rejeski et al., 1991), and this contention has led to the development of alternative questionnaires.

It has been proposed by Rejeski et al. (1991) that the STAI should not be viewed as valid when used during physical activity because changes in anxiety are allegedly confounded with "psychological arousal" and, hence unduly influenced by physiological activity. It should be noted that this contention is not at odds with commonly accepted definitions of anxiety that include physiological activity as a contributing factor (Spielberger, 1972). Rejeski et al. (1991) assessed state anxiety in adult men before, during, and after 15 min of treadmill running at 75% of maximal heart rate reserve. Anxiety responses were contrasted with the Activation-Deactivation Adjective Checklist (Thayer, 1967), which was completed at the same time in order to contrast anxiety changes with perceived arousal. The results led the authors to conclude that "STAI data collected in conjunction with exercise is confounded by physiologic changes that occur during and possibly following exercise" (p. 70). However, anxiety responses were not contrasted with actual measures of physiological activity, but rather were limited to self-reports of perceived physiological activity. Moreover, the measurement of state anxiety during the exercise session used only 8 of the 20 STAI-Y1 items, and there was no indication that issues such as item content (i.e, anxiety absent or present) or item-intensity specificity were considered. State anxiety was measured following the 15 min exercise period during a 2-min active cool-down rather than during a more intensive phase of the exercise session. This research (Rejeski et al., 1991) is not compelling, and until a sound theoretical rationale and empirical evidence can be presented, it is proposed that anxiety continue to be measured during physical activity by means of existing measures such as the STAI (Spielberger et al., 1983) that are known to possess construct validity.

It should be recognized that self-reports are not without their limitations, and the validity and reliability of self-report measures can be limited by factors such as verbal ability and self-awareness. Various forms of response distortion can also influence outcomes in physical activity studies because of social desirability, expectancies, and demand characteristics. However, procedures such as the use of social desirability measures can be used to minimize or identify the occurrence of these problems (Levitt, 1980). In cases in which clinical samples are being studied, additional diagnostic criteria (e.g., *DSM-IV*) may be useful.

PREVIOUS REVIEWS

Numerous overviews of the literature dealing with physical activity and mental health have been published (Brown, 1992; Byrne & Byrne, 1993; Folkins & Sime, 1981; Hughes, 1984; Kerr & Vlaswinkel, 1990; Kugler, Seelbach, & Kruskemper, 1994; McDonald & Hodgdon, 1991; Morgan, 1979b, 1981; Morgan & Goldston, 1987; Morgan & O'Connor, 1988, 1989; Petruzzello et al., 1991; Plante & Rodin, 1990; Raglin, 1990; Schlicht, 1994). Although such a large number of reviews may imply that further examination of this literature is not needed, there are compelling reasons that support further review. It should be recognized that the field has developed and specialized to the extent to which there is a need for summaries on specific themes. Reviews of the literature on physical activity and mental health have spanned topics ranging from the influence of exercise on specific psychological variables such as anxiety (Kerr & Vlaswinkel, 1990; Morgan, 1979b; Schlicht, 1994) and depression (Dunn & Dishman, 1991), to overviews of specific populations (Brown, 1992), to the effects of particular forms of physical activity (Raglin, 1993). In addition, the literature on exercise and mental health does not come from a single discipline; research has been published in exercise science, sport psychology, general psychology, and medical journals. Hence, there is a need for summaries that effectively locate and consolidate these widely distributed findings.

Previous reviews of the physical activity and anxiety literature have generally indicated that both acute and chronic physical activity are associated with an array of psychological benefits, although excessive physical training (i.e., overtraining) has been associated consistently with undesirable psychological outcomes (see chapter 9). In the case of state anxiety, short bouts of vigorous aerobic exercise have been found to be associated with state anxiety decrements that may persist for up to several hours (Morgan, 1979b, 1981; Petruzzello et al., 1991). These reductions have been observed in persons with both normal and elevated anxiety levels (Morgan, 1973c), although specific information regarding the influence of particular types of physical activity or its efficacy for specific anxiety disorders has been lacking (Byrne & Byrne, 1993; Kerr & Vlaswinkel, 1990; Plante & Rodin, 1990).

Despite the finding that the majority of previous literature reviews indicate that chronic exercise is associated with improvements in trait anxiety (Kugler et al., 1994; McDonald & Hodgdon, 1991; Petruzzello et al., 1991), some reviewers have concluded that the psychological benefits are minimal or nonexistent for persons with normal to good mental health (Brown, 1992; Morgan, 1981; Raglin, 1990). Recent meta-analytic reviews are mixed on this point, and either support this contention (McDonald & Hodgdon, 1991) or indicate that psychologically normal persons also benefit (Petruzzello et al., 1991). However, another recent review contended that the anxiolytic effects may be limited only to middle-aged adults and are minimal at best (Schlicht, 1994). One of the explanations for the inconsistency in this area stems from the failure to consider the behavioral artifacts (e.g., expectancy effects, demand characteristics, response distortion).

In summary, a number of previous reviews of the exercise and anxiety literature indicate that acute and chronic physical activity significantly reduces anxiety. However, there is disagreement about who will or will not benefit psychologically from exercise, and some reviewers contend that previous findings supporting the palliative effects are unreliable. It is not immediately evident how these disparities can be rectified. Differences in the conclusions reached may be due in part to the choice of studies for review. In the case of meta-analytic reviews, it has been suggested that discrepancies in findings reflect the type of meta-analytic techniques used and differences in coding techniques (Schlicht, 1994). In addition, methodological issues not previously considered may be a significant factor in these inconsistencies.

Methodological Concerns

Both narrative and meta-analytic reviews have suffered from a number of methodological problems, and this has constrained our understanding of the psychological benefits of physical activity (Byrne & Byrne, 1993; Morgan, 1981; Morgan & O'Connor, 1989; Plante & Rodin, 1990). A variety of weaknesses noted in the earliest reviews (Folkins & Sime, 1981; Morgan, 1981) continue to be cited as concerns in reviews of more recent research (Byrne & Byrne, 1993; Plante & Rodin, 1990). Some of the most commonly cited problems include the lack of control or placebo comparisons, small sample size, nonrandom subject assignment, misuse of psychological inventories, or the use of dependent measures lacking construct validity. A common theme among these reviews is that methodological problems have handicapped our understanding of the psychological effects of physical activity.

In theory, weaknesses in flawed research should be surmountable by using meta-analytic techniques to review the literature (Glass, 1978). As discussed in chapter 1, it is not necessary in meta-analytic reviews to exclude studies because of problems such as inadequate sample size or poor design. In fact, methodological flaws can be coded and systematically analyzed to determine whether specific problems influence the psychological changes as measured by effect size or magnitude of difference equivalent to standard deviations units (Glass & Kliegl, 1983). Another advantage is that effect sizes can be averaged across published and unpublished studies to determine whether findings are influenced by publishing history. Hence, meta-analytic review techniques have the potential to surmount methodological inadequacies in the extant literature, and to resolve existing disagreements about the psychological benefits of physical activity. However, this is not the case when various behavioral artifacts lead to systematic error in a specific direction (e.g., reduced anxiety or depression) even though such a change does not actually occur.

In a comprehensive review of the anxiety literature, Petruzzello et al. (1991) found that physical activity resulted in significant reductions in state and trait anxiety as well as commonly assessed physiological correlates of anxiety such as blood pressure. Moderate effect sizes were observed for the influence of acute exercise on state anxiety (.24) and chronic programs on trait anxiety (.34). Additional analyses were conducted to examine the influence of factors including subject characteristics, programmatic factors, and health status. Although some significant differences were found for programmatic exercise factors, caution was given in interpreting these results in lieu of the small number of studies and potential confounds related to exercise variables or experimental design. Significant effect sizes were also found for the effects of physical activity on both state ($d = -.60$) and trait ($d = -.044$) anxiety in a meta-analysis performed by McDonald and Hodgdon (1991). However, in a more recent meta-analysis, Schlicht (1994) examined studies dealing with physical activity and anxiety published from 1980 to 1990. Nonsignificant ($p > .05$) effect sizes were found for acute and chronic exercise studies, indicating that physical activity was not associated reliably with significant reductions in either state or trait anxiety. A variety of potential moderator variables such as gender and exercise mode were examined in an effort to ascertain whether or not such variables had an impact on effect size, but none were statistically significant. These results stand in contrast to the meta-analysis conducted by Kugler et al., (1994), who found a significant effect size ($d = .31$; $p < .01$) for physical activity programs designed to reduce anxiety in samples of patients with CHD.

The lack of consistency of these reviews may be the result of a number of factors. Different meta-analytic techniques were used and the inclusion of studies for analysis was not consistent across reviews. Comparisons of various exercise types and regimens were limited. In terms of subject issues, contrasts with regard to the use or effectiveness of physical activity in persons with low, normal, or elevated anxiety were not made. Perhaps most important, there are methodological weaknesses related to the prescription of physical activity and fitness assessment that have garnered little concern in previous meta-analytic or narrative reviews. For example, in a recent narrative review of the exercise and mental health literature, Plante and Rodin (1990) excluded studies because of one or more basic experimental or methodological weaknesses such as the lack of control groups or use of random assignment in generating treatment and control groups. Despite this rigorous selection process, problems resulting from unreliable or inadequate measurements of physical fitness and control of the exercise stimulus were not considered. Studies that did not include the determination of fitness levels or the intensity of physical activity, or those in which these factors were calculated indirectly, were not excluded or analyzed separately. Among the four acute physical activity studies reviewed, three did not include the determination of fitness level or quantify the metabolic demand of the exercise intensity (Berger & Owen, 1983, 1988; Lichtman & Poser, 1983). In the remaining study (Steptoe & Cox, 1988), fitness levels were determined using an indirect method based on exercise heart rate, and it has been known for many years that heart rate before and during physical activity is influenced to a significant degree by psychological variables such as anxiety. Rather than regulating the intensity of physical activity on the basis of each subject's fitness level, absolute workloads were used in most of these studies.

The use of such indirect methods to determine exercise factors is widespread throughout the physical activity and mental health literature (McDonald & Hodgdon, 1991), yet such procedures routinely result in errors of estimation of as much as 20% when compared with accurate methods based on direct measurements (Åstrand & Saltin, 1961; Zwiren, Freedson, Ward, Wilke, & Rippe, 1991). This degree of error can result in inadequate control of the physical activity prescription. In practice, an intensity defined as moderate using these indirect methods can actually be low or high for some individuals. A high degree of accuracy is crucial in acute and chronic paradigms in which attempts are made to employ comparable intensity based on each individual's capacity (e.g., 60% of maximal aerobic capacity). Although reliable methods for determining fitness and controlling exercise intensity have been employed routinely for decades in exercise physiology research, their use in physical activity and mental health research has been far less common. Furthermore, while it is also recognized that perceived exertion can be an effective alternative to both direct and indirect assessments of maximal capacity, this heuristic methodology has seldom been employed in research dealing with the psychological effects of physical activity.

Accurate information concerning the relationship between programmatic factors such as the mode or intensity of physical activities and psychological outcome is crucial if this intervention is to be used effectively as a means of improving mental health. In enhancing and maintaining physical health and capacity, valid exercise prescriptions have been empirically established (ACSM, 1991). These guidelines have also been modified for exercise prescription for persons with various physical diseases, but prescriptions for psychological disorders do not exist. Moreover, there is emerging evidence that physical activities such as walking can result in reductions in disease risk factors (see chapter 3), but the impact of mild activity on anxiety or other psychological variables is uncertain.

In order to establish the psychological consequences of various forms of physical activity it is imperative that studies in this area employ accurate techniques to assess fitness and intensity of physical activity. Despite the recognized importance of these principles, there has been little attention paid to these issues in the published literature. Byrne and Byrne (1993) addressed the issue of properly quantifying fitness level in their review, but unfortunately they described outdated and inaccurate techniques for doing so. Of the recent meta-analyses only McDonald and Hodgdon (1991) contrasted studies that assessed fitness via tests of maximal aerobic power versus less accurate methods. However, their classification system did not differentiate between tests that measured oxygen consumption during maximal exercise protocols versus studies that used indirect and less accurate protocols. As a result of the widespread reliance on indirect estimates of important fitness variables many of the conclusions drawn concerning the influence of exercise intensity or particular forms of exercise must be regarded as tentative at best.

ACUTE PHYSICAL ACTIVITY

Aerobic Exercise

Most previous reviews dealing with acute physical activity indicate that vigorous bouts of aerobic exercise are associated with significant reductions in state anxiety (Kerr & Vlaswinkel, 1990; McDonald & Hodgdon, 1991; Morgan & O'Connor, 1988, 1989; Petruzzello et al., 1991; Raglin, 1990). Research has also shown that the psychological improvements associated with acute physical activity exceed decrements associated with control conditions (Crocker & Grozelle, 1991; Roth 1989) and compare favorably to quiet rest (Brown et al., 1993; Glazer & O'Connor, 1992; Raglin & Morgan, 1987) or meditation (Bahrke & Morgan, 1978; Crocker & Grozelle, 1991). Despite the consistency of the these findings the exercise intensity used across these investigations differed considerably, and the results may not be directly comparable. As a result, these findings do not indicate whether selected exercise dosages are more or less effective.

Initial research studies dealing with the influence of exercise intensity on anxiety indicated that low power outputs (i.e., below 60% of VO_2max) were not associated with reductions in state anxiety, whereas moderate or high power outputs did decrease anxiety (Morgan, Roberts, & Feinerman, 1971; Sime 1977). Moreover, the influence of physical activity on anxiety reduction was found to be independent of exercise mode in the sense that walking and running at the same power output had comparable effects (Morgan, Horstman, Cymerman, & Stokes, 1980). These findings suggest that physical activity should be of at least a moderate intensity to reduce state anxiety, but much of this early research did not employ direct methods to control exercise intensity. More recent work based on direct tests of VO_2max has been less clear about the effects of intensity. Farrell, Gustafson, Morgan, and Pert (1987) examined tension and anxiety reductions as measured by the POMS (McNair, Lorr, & Dropplemann, 1981) following acute bouts of treadmill running at intensities of 40%, 60%, or 80% of VO_2max. Significant reductions in tension and anxiety were noted following exercise at 60% and 80% of VO_2max, and the degree of improvement was equivalent between these intensities. However, exercise at 40% of VO_2max did not result in an anxiolytic effect. Although these results indicate that there may be a threshold effect that requires that physical activity be of at least a moderate intensity in order to provoke psychological benefits, the duration of the exercise sessions has differed across conditions in these studies. As a result it is unclear whether differences were due to intensity, duration, or a combination of both. In work in which duration and intensity were controlled, Raglin and Wilson (1996) observed similar reductions in state anxiety following 20-min bouts of stationary leg cycling at 40%, 60%, and 70% of VO_2max. State anxiety was reduced ($p < .05$) throughout a 2-hr assessment period following each condition, indicating that the degree of anxiety reduction was also independent of exercise intensity. The persistence of state anxiety was also independent of exercise intensity during the 2-hr postexercise period. Future research should include longer postexercise assessment periods in order to examine whether the mode, intensity, and duration of physical activity have differential effects on state anxiety.

Although previous findings indicate that vigorous aerobic physical activity is anxiolytic, some investigators have failed to find reductions following high-intensity exercise. Actually, several investigators have found that high-intensity physical activity is associated with significant elevations in state anxiety (Berger & Owen, 1992; Kerr & Svebak, 1994; Steptoe & Cox, 1988). Such findings have led Berger and Owen (1992) to propose, "it now seems that exercisers who wish psychological benefits should avoid exercising too intensely" (p. 81). The results of a study by Steptoe and Cox (1988) are in large part responsible for this viewpoint. These investigators tested 32 adult women before and after four 8-min bouts of stationary leg cycling performed at either a low or high intensity under music and no music conditions. All exercise was completed in a single session, and sufficient rest was provided between bouts to allow for recovery. The tension and anxiety levels were assessed before and after exercise using a modified version of the POMS. The results indicated that tension and anxiety decreased following the low-intensity session but increased following high-intensity cycling. These results were independent of the presence or absence of music. Unfortunately, absolute rather than relative workloads were employed, and differences in fitness levels were not controlled. An attempt was made to examine the influence of fitness, but aerobic capacity was predicted from submaximal exercise heart rate. As a consequence it is unclear whether the selected workloads were actually light or heavy for any given subject. In a follow-up study in which the exercise bouts were increased to 15 min, Steptoe and Bolton (1988) found that tension and anxiety were reduced significantly immediately following low-intensity stationary leg cycling, whereas these levels were elevated following high-intensity exercise. Tension and anxiety decreased over the ensuing 15 min following the high-intensity condition, suggesting that this effect was transitory. These results have been interpreted to indicate that high-intensity exercise does not benefit anxiety (Berger & Owen, 1992; Schlicht, 1994), but this interpretation is obviously not congruent with the reported findings.

Other studies have found an absence of anxiety reduction or other mood improvements following participation in active sporting events (Kerr & Svebak, 1994) or intense exercise (Berger & Owen, 1988, 1992). However, the fitness levels of the subjects and the exercise intensities, were either not determined (Kerr & Svebak, 1994) or were estimated using indirect methods (Berger & Owen, 1988, 1992). Some research has been conducted in which exercise intensity was determined or controlled using direct methodologies. High-intensity bouts of stationary leg cycling at 70% of VO_2peak (Raglin & Wilson, 1996), treadmill running at 80% of VO_2max (Farrell et al., 1987), road running at 84% of VO_2max (O'Connor, Carda, & Graf, 1991), and treadmill running to maximum (O'Connor, Petruzzello, Kubitz, & Robinson, 1995) have each been found to be associated with anxiety reductions similar in magnitude to moderate physical activity. These results are important because they indicate that high-intensity physical activity can reduce anxiety, as well as the fact that these intensities all fall above the anaerobic threshold for most individuals.

The discrepancy in the anxiety responses noted in the previous studies may be due to the timing of the postexercise anxiety assessments. During physical activity performed at 80% of VO_2max, state anxiety has been found to increase (Morgan et al., 1980). Accordingly, this increase may delay the reduction in anxiety commonly observed following less intense physical activity. Raglin and Wilson (1996) found that state anxiety increased ($p < .05$) immediately following 20 min of leg cycling performed at 70% of VO_2max, whereas reductions were observed immediately after exercise at 40% and 60% of VO_2max. However, the increase associated with the highest intensity was transitory, and at 60 min following exercise similar reductions in state anxiety were observed for all intensities. Similar delays in anxiety reduction with higher-intensity physical activity have been found in other studies (O'Connor et al., 1995; Steptoe & Bolton, 1988). Light to moderate exercise may not be sufficiently intense to evoke this response. Dishman, Farquhar, and Cureton (1994) found that state anxiety did not increase above baseline during 20 min of stationary leg cycling performed at 60% of VO_2max, and state anxiety decreased significantly immediately after exercise. These findings may be interpreted to indicate that sensations associated with exertion and postexercise fatigue following high-intensity activity delay, but do not eliminate, postexercise anxiety reductions. In the case of less-intense exercise, increases in anxiety may be modest or absent altogether during exercise, and thus postexercise anxiety reduction occurs more quickly.

Summary Acute bouts of aerobic physical activity are generally associated with reductions in state anxiety that may persist for up to several hours, although improvements may be delayed somewhat following higher-intensity exercise. While it has been proposed that exercise performed under competitive situations is not effective in reducing anxiety (Berger & Owen, 1988), there is research evidence indicating that exercise performed in competitive settings is associated with an anxiolytic effect (Morgan & Hammer, 1974; O'Connor, Carda, & Graf, 1991), which also appears to be independent of the time of day exercise takes place (O'Connor & Davis, 1992). Research is unclear at this point regarding whether or not exercise intensity consistently influences the degree to which anxiety is reduced following acute physical activity, and further study is needed using direct methods to control and measure exercise intensity. The majority of studies have examined the antianxiety effects of physical activity performed within the range of intensities (i.e, 50% to 80% of VO_2max) prescribed for improving cardiovascular fitness (ACSM, 1991). With the increased emphasis on "lifestyle" exercise prescriptions (see chapter 3), there is a need to determine the effects of walking and other forms of less vigorous physical activity on state anxiety.

It is also important to establish the time course of postexercise anxiety changes. Even if the degree of anxiety reduction is consistent across exercise intensities, it is possible that the duration of the reduction is dependent on intensity. There has only been limited research on this issue up to this point, and the stability of anxiety reduction also needs to be determined. Some research has examined the extent to which acute bouts of physical activity can depress physiological responses to standardized stressors after the cessation of exercise (Ebbesen, Prkachin, Mills, & Green, 1992), but little is known about the extent to which anxiety reductions remain in effect following such stressors. Even less research has been conducted to explore the influence of exercise duration on the persistence of postexercise anxiety reduction (Petruzzello et al., 1991). The potential influence of the individual's fitness level and exercise experience on anxiety change should be determined. There is some research indicating that both trained and untrained subjects experience similar psychological benefits following acute aerobic exercise (O'Connor et al., in press; Roth, 1989), whereas the results of other studies indicate that only experienced or trained exercisers show reductions in state anxiety following acute exercise (Boutcher & Landers, 1988; Dishman et al., 1994). The latter result has been presumed to be a consequence of the greater fitness levels in experienced exercisers, but the effect may simply reflect habituation or exposure. It has been shown by Brown et al. (1993), for example, that physically challenged adults with exercise experience but low fitness levels experience significant reductions in state anxiety following acute physical activity.

Resistance Exercise

The majority of exercise research on anxiety has focused on the influence of aerobic forms of activity (Petruzzello et al., 1991). This may be a consequence of the popularity of running at the time much of this research was conducted, as well as existing evidence demonstrating the physical health benefits of aerobic exercise. However, resistance exercise such as weight training has grown in popularity in recent years, and the physical health benefits of such forms of physical activity have also been documented (Dalsky et al., 1988). Resistance exercise differs from activities such as jogging in that it is intermittent rather than continuous, and often falls above the intensity or threshold for evoking "anaerobic" forms of metabolism. It should be noted that activities such as weight training may be performed at a low enough intensity to be primarily aerobic just as high-intensity interval running can be primarily anaerobic. Hence, exercise mode cannot be defined as aerobic or anaerobic simply on the basis of mode.

Some recent work has focused on the effects of acute sessions of weight training on state anxiety. Koltyn, Raglin, O'Connor, and Morgan (1995) examined the effects of acute weight training on state anxiety and blood pressure. College students enrolled in a beginning weight training class underwent a 50-min session of weight training performed at a self-selected intensity. The subjects were also allowed to choose their weight-lifting exercises. State anxiety and blood pressure were evaluated immediately before and after the exercise session. These variables were also assessed in control subjects who were seated during a 50-min lecture. It was found that state anxiety did not decrease following the weight training or control conditions. A significant trial by condition ($p < .05$) interaction effect was observed for systolic blood pressure, which increased following weight training and decreased following the control condition. Although the subjects had completed at least 8 weeks of training before participating in the study, it is possible that more experience is necessary before anxiolytic effects occur. Moreover, state anxiety was only assessed once following the resistance exercise, and it is possible that reductions in anxiety may be delayed just as investigators have noted for other exercise modes such as running, walking, and cycling.

Raglin, Turner, and Eksten (1993) examined the effects of bouts of cycling and resistance exercise in 26 trained college athletes, all of whom had several years of experience in such forms of training. Subjects underwent 30-min bouts of stationary leg cycling or weight training on separate days. The workload was controlled so that each activity was performed at an intensity between 70% and 80% of each individual's maximal capacity. State anxiety and blood pressure were assessed before exercising and during the 60 min following exercise. It was found that state anxiety and systolic blood pressure fell steadily following stationary cycling with reductions achieving significance ($p < .05$) by 60 min postexercise. In the case of weight training both state anxiety and systolic blood pressure were elevated significantly immediately following the end of the session, but these measures returned to baseline levels at 20 and 60 min postexercise.

The results of these studies indicate that acute weight training is not associated with reductions in state anxiety or related physiological markers of stress such as blood pressure. However, exercise intensity was not directly controlled in the Koltyn et al. (1995) investigation, whereas weight training was limited to high intensity by Raglin et al. (1993). It is possible that less strenuous weight-training bouts might have beneficial effects on anxiety. In an investigation that examined this issue, O'Connor, Bryant, Veltri, and Gebhardt (1993) evaluated 14 female college students before and after 30-min bouts of resistance exercise performed at intensities equal to

40%, 60%, or 80% of each subject's 10-repetition maximum for each exercise. State anxiety was assessed at baseline before exercise and periodically during the 120-min recovery period. Following exercise blood pressure was monitored continually via an ambulatory device. Significant state anxiety reductions were observed at 90 and 120 min following exercise performed at 60% of maximum, but there was no anxiolytic effect at any time for exercise performed at 40% or 80% of the 10-repetition maximum. Blood pressure reductions did not occur following any of the exercise conditions. The authors concluded that the reductions found following moderately intense weight training could not be attributed unequivocally to the exercise because the daily activities that took place during the postexercise assessments were not controlled. It should also be noted that the participants in this investigation had only minimal experience with weight training exercise.

Summary   In contrast to the extensive research literature indicating that state anxiety is reduced following vigorous aerobic exercise, this area of research indicates that reductions in state anxiety do not occur routinely following resistance exercise (e.g., weight training). It is not clear why this form of exercise fails to reduce state anxiety, but recent research (Wertz, Koltyn, & Morgan, 1992) indicates that postexercise lactate accumulation is not a contributing factor.

Different weight-training routines were used in each of these studies, and it is possible that the type of weight training could influence anxiety. Subjects were relatively inexperienced in two of the studies (Koltyn et al., 1995; O'Connor et al., 1993), whereas the results from Raglin et al. (1993) involved competitive athletes and may not be generalizable to populations of individuals who exercise for health or recreational purposes. Different methods were used to establish exercise intensity in these studies, and additional systematic research is needed in which these variables are controlled.

POPULATION ISSUES

Most of the existing anxiety research has focused on normal individuals with good mental health, and there is a relative paucity of data involving the psychological effects of exercise on persons with anxiety disorders (McDonald & Hodgdon, 1991). This is undoubtedly due in part to the results of earlier research conducted by Pitts and McClure (1967), who examined the effects of intravenous infusion of lactate, sodium DL-lactate with calcium, and a placebo (glucose) solution on anxiety in normals and anxiety neurotics under resting conditions. It was found that anxiety increased following the infusion of sodium DL-lactate in the anxiety neurotics, and anxiety attacks occurred in 93% of this group. Furthermore, symptoms persisted for 2 to 5 days in some of the cases. In addition, some of the normal subjects tested in this study also experienced anxiety following the infusions of sodium DL-lactate. On the basis of these findings it has been recommended that persons suffering from anxiety disorders should refrain from vigorous physical activity because this will lead to increases in blood lactate and consequently provoke a panic attack. Despite the influence this article has exerted on panic research, significant methodological problems were noted. Grosz and Farmer (1969) argued that the increase in blood lactate resulting from the infusion used by Pitts and McClure (1967) would be insufficient to raise blood lactate above preinfusion levels. The infusion would also result in plasma alkalosis, rather than the acidosis that occurs with vigorous exercise. Moreover, Pitts and McClure (1967) indicated that anxiety neurotics exhibit excessive lactate production during standardized exercise tests, but this has been shown to be a consequence of relatively poorer fitness levels in persons with anxiety disorder (Gaffney, Fenton, Lane, & Lake, 1988; Kellermann, Winter, & Kariv, 1969; Stein et al. 1992; Martinsen, Strand et al., 1989), rather than an excessive metabolic response to exercise itself. Most important, there is now compelling evidence that patients with clinically diagnosed anxiety can undergo submaximal or maximal exercise protocols with little or no risk of panic attacks.

In an investigation of panic during exercise and ambulatory settings, Taylor et al. (1987) compared treadmill exercise performance in 40 patients with panic disorder and 40 age-matched controls who were either physically active or inactive. Subjects underwent a symptom-limited maximal treadmill exercise test using a modified Balke protocol. The results of the exercise testing indicated that the patients with panic disorder had a significantly lower exercise capacity than the active controls but this did not differ from the inactive group. One of the patients experienced a panic attack during exercise, but continued exercising and reached a peak workload equal to that of the mean for the other patients and inactive control group (11 METs). Another patient experienced ischemia during exercise. The authors concluded that although there was evidence that patients with panic disorder were less fit than controls, there was no indication they were exercise intolerant. A trend for higher daily and sleeping heart rates was found in these patients, which the authors speculated was a consequence of fitness differences. In a related study, Gaffney et al. (1988) tested 10 patients with panic disorder and 10 healthy adults on a stationary leg cycling protocol designed to elicit a maximal effort. None of the patients experienced panic during the exercise testing, and cardiovascular and lactate responses to exercise were reported to be similar between patients and controls. The exercise test revealed that maximum oxygen consumption was significantly lower ($p < .05$) in the panic patients compared with controls (23.0 vs 31.7 ml/kg/min, respectively).

A comparison of 16 patients with panic disorder 15 healthy controls was carried out by Stein et al. (1992) who employed stationary leg cycling either to exhaustion or until a predetermined heart rate was reached. Venous blood was sampled before and twice after exercise in order to assess lactate accumulation. One of the 14 patients panicked during exercise, but lactate was not appreciably different in this individual compared with the remainder of the patients. However, there was a tendency for patients to terminate the exercise test sooner than controls, and this suggested that the panic group had a lower exercise capacity. The success of patients in tolerating the physical testing led Stein et al. (1992) to conclude that "moderate exercise is not contraindicated and should be encouraged in this patient population" (p. 287).

Summary   These results indicate that anxiety patients can undergo intensive physical activity without undue risk of panic. Their relatively lower performance appears to be due to a lack of physical conditioning rather than to exercise intolerance. However, some caution is needed in interpreting the fitness results based on leg cycling exercise (Gaffney et al., 1988; Stein et al. 1992). Leg cycling protocols may underestimate maximal fitness levels, especially in unfit subjects or in persons with little experience with vigorous exercise. The previous findings are promising, but the question remains whether patients with panic or other anxiety disorders experience reductions in state anxiety following physical exercise. Although this issue has not been examined there is some research indicating that clinical samples do benefit from aerobic exercise. Glazer and O'Connor (1992) found that a 20-min bout of walking at 70% of VO_2peak resulted in a significant reduction in state anxiety in bulimic women. The magnitude of this reduction was equivalent to that associated with 20 minutes of a passive resting condition.

CHRONIC EXERCISE

Previous narrative reviews of the exercise and anxiety literature suggest that participation in chronic exercise programs can benefit trait anxiety (Byrne & Byrne, 1993; Kerr & Vlaswinkel, 1990), whereas the findings of meta-analytic reviews have been less consistent. Three meta-analyses have led investigators to conclude that chronic physical activity is associated with significant improvements in anxiety for both normal populations (McDonald & Hodgdon, 1991; Petruzzello et al. 1991) as well as patients with CHD (Kugler et al., 1994). However, a reliable effect for physical activity was not observed in the most recent meta-analysis, and this led Schlicht (1994) to conclude that there was "only little support for the hypothesis that physical exercise reduces anxiety" (p. 285). One reason for this apparent disagreement could be the initial emotional health of the subjects studied. There is evidence indicating that significant benefits occur only in persons with some degree of disturbance (De Geus et al., 1993), and other research suggests that the degree of improvement is an inverse function of emotional health at the outset (Simons & Birkimer, 1988). Another factor may be the interaction between training intensity and initial exercise capacity. Some research indicates that improvements in anxiety occur following physical activity programs that involve light or moderate exercise but not high-intensity exercise. Moses et al. (1989) found that tension and anxiety were reduced significantly in sedentary adults following 10 weeks of a physical activity program involving moderate exercise performed for 30 to 40 min at 60% of maximal heart rate three times per week. No improvements were noted in a more intense exercise condition in which exercise was performed at 70% to 75% of maximal heart rate. However, in a study of adolescents randomly assigned to 10-week programs of flexibility training, at moderate or high-intensity levels, greater improvements in perceived stress were found for the high-intensity exercise condition (Norris, Carroll, & Cochrane, 1992). The authors noted that their high-intensity exercise program was similar to the one employed by Moses et al. (1989), and they hypothesized that because the subjects were younger, and presumably fitter than those studied by Moses et al., the high-intensity exercise was, in fact, moderate.

In cases in which participation in chronic physical activity programs results in significant anxiety reductions, the results have not generally supported the notion that the degree of psychological benefit is a function of improvements in fitness (De Geus et al., 1993; Kugler, Dimsdale, Hartley, & Sherwood, 1990; Martinsen et al., 1989a; Moses et al., 1989; Simons & Birkimer, 1988; Steptoe, Edwards, Moses, & Mathews, 1989) or initial fitness level (Kugler et al., 1990; Simons & Birkimer, 1988). In addition, the findings of one study indicate that tension and anxiety reductions are most pronounced for persons with both low fitness levels and elevated anxiety at the outset of the training program (Wilfley & Kunce, 1986).

Although the previous findings suggest that mechanisms other than those associated with fitness are responsible for the anxiolytic effects of exercise, it should be noted that much of the research that has examined the relationship between fitness changes and anxiety reduction has relied on indirect fitness estimates such as self-report of activity or submaximal exercise tests (e.g., Moses et al., 1989; Steptoe et al., 1989) rather than conventional methods of evaluating maximal capacity (e.g., VO_2max). Hence, the possibility that fitness changes contribute to psychological improvement cannot be completely ruled out. Subtle changes in physical capacity or other indicators of fitness and physical health may be associated with psychological improvement. For example, in a training study involving slightly obese women, Cramer, Nieman, and Lee (1991) observed a correlation ($r = .41, p < .01$) between improvements in general well-being and fitness, as determined by heart rate during submaximal exercise following 15 weeks of a moderate walking program. These changes occurred in the absence of improvement in maximal oxygen consumption. It has also been suggested that perceptions of changes in physical capacity or appearance, in the absence of physiological changes, contribute to psychological improvements (Sonstroem & Morgan, 1989), and there is some evidence to support this view (King, Taylor, Haskell, & DeBusk, 1989). Consequently, it is imperative that the most accurate and reliable protocols be employed when measuring fitness and regulating exercise intensity. Other health- and exercise-related variables (e.g., percent body fat, lean body mass) should also be assessed in order to quantify the impact of such changes on psychological improvement.

Summary   Research dealing with the chronic effects of physical activity on anxiety has shown that training programs can result in significant reductions in trait anxiety (Petruzzello et al., 1991), but benefits may be most pronounced for persons who have elevated anxiety levels at the outset. In studies in which improvements in anxiety have been observed, exercise programs have been found to be superior to placebo-control conditions (Moses et al., 1989; Steptoe et al., 1989) and comparable to other active treatments such as stress-inoculation training (Long, 1984). Moreover, benefits have been found to be independent of expectancy of psychological improvement (Long, 1984; Steptoe et al., 1989) or rated importance of exercise (Simons & Birkimer, 1988). Unlike the effects of acute physical activity on state anxiety, it appears that high-intensity aerobic exercise may be ineffective in reducing trait anxiety, at least in unfit or older subjects. Other research has shown that low-intensity training results in improved mood, whereas high-intensity training has worsened mood (Cockerill, Nevill, & Byrne, 1992). This finding is consistent with research involving endurance athletes that has found dose-response relationships between training load and mood disturbance (see chapter 9 and Raglin, 1993). It appears that if the intensity of training is too high, then improvements either do not occur (Steptoe et al., 1989) or detrimental changes result (see chapter 9 and Cockerill et al., 1992; Raglin, 1993), but a clear cutoff dosage threshold for beneficial and detrimental outcomes has not been established. It is likely that factors such as personality, psychological health, physical capacity, and degree of physical fitness may all play a role in the psychological response to high-intensity training. For most adults, mild to moderate aerobic exercise may be the most effective in reducing anxiety. Very light forms of exercise that primarily involve flexibility training appear to have less effect for healthy adults (Moses et al., 1989).

CLINICAL SAMPLES

Although research indicates that exercise may reduce anxiety in both normal individuals and those with elevated anxiety (Steptoe et al., 1989), studies using subjects with clinical anxiety disorders are notably absent in the literature (McDonald & Hodgdon, 1991). An important exception is the study by Martinsen et al. (1989b), who contrasted the psychological effects of aerobic and nonaerobic forms of physical activity in 79 patients hospitalized with anxiety disorders including panic and generalized anxiety. Aerobic capacity was determined prior to training using either submaximal or maximal exercise tests, and the patients were randomized to one of two exercise conditions. Exercise sessions were scheduled for 1-hr periods, with 30 min devoted to training. One group participated in sessions of walking or jogging for 30 min, and the intensity was approximately 70% of VO_2max. Patients in the nonaerobic group underwent low-intensity strength and flexibility exercises. Each condition lasted 8 weeks, and sessions were held three times per week. Anxiety was assessed with standardized clinical evaluations by clinicians who were blind to the exercise condition to which the subjects were assigned. The results indicated that the exercise conditions were associated with significant reductions in anxiety and phobic avoidance. No differences were found in the degree of psychological improvement between conditions, despite the fact that only the aerobic training group showed a significant increase in aerobic fitness. It is entirely possible, of course, that patients in the resistance training group had increases in muscular fitness (i.e., strength and flexibility). The dropout rate was low (11%), indicating that the exercise training was well tolerated by these subjects. It should be noted that the nonaerobic exercise used by Martinsen et al. (1989b) was not a form of anaerobic exercise but was more like the mild activity placebo-control condition employed by Moses et al. (1989). In other words, the observed improvements took place in the absence of high-intensity physical activity.

In another study involving clinical cases (Sexton et al., 1989), patients who were hospitalized for psychiatric disorders, including anxiety, underwent moderate- or low-intensity exercise training. Participants were assigned randomly to 8-week programs of either running or walking, and physical activity was performed three to four times per week for 30 min per session. The patients were instructed to run at a pace equal to 70% of predicted maximal heart rate, whereas those in the low-intensity group walked at a comfortable pace. The exercise was supervised while the patients were hospitalized, but some were discharged during the course of the study. These subjects continued to exercise without supervision at home for the remainder of the 8-week period. Significant reductions in trait anxiety (STAI) and general neurotic symptoms were observed in both groups, but the degree of improvement did not differ between conditions. The improvement in aerobic capacity was equal in the two conditions. Furthermore, analysis of a subsample of patients who exhibited the largest improvements in aerobic capacity ($>15\%$) revealed that psychological improvements were no greater in this subset. As in the case of Martinsen et al. (1989b) overall adherence was high (75%) and the dropout rate was significantly ($p < .001$) higher in the runners. Most of the runners discontinued exercise during the unsupervised exercise phase while at home, and the investigators hypothesized that the greater demands of running, coupled with a lack of supervision, were largely responsible for the elevated recidivism. At 6-month follow-up most subjects remained active, and the psychological and physical gains were maintained during this period. It was concluded that aerobic physical activity was an effective means of improving the psychological health of these patients. Because walking was found to be just as effective as more vigorous exercise, and because patients with the greatest gains in aerobic capacity exhibited no greater improvement, the authors concluded that exercise prescriptions based on lower intensities were preferable to more vigorous exercise.

Summary

The research reviewed in this section indicates that patients with anxiety disorders derive significant psychological benefits from physical activity. Moreover, it appears that exercise performed at low intensities is as effective as more vigorous forms of physical activity, and psychological benefits can occur in the absence of gains in aerobic power. However, even in the absence of increased aerobic power, improvements in other fitness factors (e.g., strength, flexibility) or perception of effort may well have occurred. These findings are important because there is evidence that mild forms of exercise result in fewer injuries and higher adherence rates (Pollock, 1988). However, additional research is needed to determine whether psychological improvements can be potentiated through the use of particular exercise modes and intensities. Although research on depression suggests that anaerobic and aerobic exercise each result in significant psychological improvement (Doyne et al., 1987), there is some evidence that aerobic exercise results in greater reductions in stress than anaerobic exercise (Norris et al., 1992) in healthy adults. On the other hand, Nelson and Morgan (1994) have recently reported that acute exercise performed at 40%, 60%, and 80% of maximum heart rate on a stationary bicycle ergometer led to comparable antidepressant effects in depressed college students. Similar comparisons should be made for clinically anxious groups.

OVERALL SUMMARY

Previous research has generally indicated that physical activity is associated with improvements in mental health, including reductions in both state and trait anxiety, but this statement must be tempered in light of the methodological limitations that have characterized much of this literature. In particular, the lack of quantification of fitness and exercise intensity, and the use of indirect estimates of these variables, have resulted in a lack of specific information with regard to the effects of exercise, and this in turn has contributed to inconsistencies in the conclusions drawn by various reviewers. Future research can minimize error by utilizing preferred methodologies for determining fitness and quantifying exercise intensity, as well as employing psychological measures that possess construct validity.

Although not entirely consistent, the extant evidence indicates that aerobic activity is associated with improvements in both state and trait anxiety. Acute benefits in state anxiety appear to be limited to aerobic forms of activity and have been observed following both light and heavy exercise. Persons with elevated anxiety have also been found to benefit, but there is a lack of systematic research with clinical samples. Available evidence indicates that acute bouts of resistance exercise such as weight training are not associated with reductions in state anxiety, but this finding may reflect the timing of postexercise assessments. Long-term physical activity programs appear to be associated with reductions in trait anxiety, although improvements appear to be most consistent in patients with elevated anxiety at the outset. The majority of evidence indicates that increased cardiovascular capacity is not necessary for reductions in trait anxiety, but these findings must be judged in light of the fact that most studies have used indirect methodologies to evaluate aerobic power. Unlike acute physical activity, in which benefits occur following high-intensity exercise, long-term programs that rely on high-intensity exercise prescriptions do not appear to be associated with improvements in trait anxiety. It is possible that age, initial fitness level, and exercise history may influence this relationship. Perhaps the most important finding to have emerged from the existing research concerns the effects of physical activity on patients with clinical anxiety disorders. Contrary to the traditional perspective that patients with anxiety disorders should not exercise vigorously for fear of experiencing panic attacks, recent evidence indicates that patients with anxiety disorders who are free of physical disorders (e.g., mitral valve prolapse) can perform vigorous or maximal exercise without undue risk of panic. Patients with clinically diagnosed anxiety experience substantial psychological benefits when exposed to mild exercise programs, and this type of exercise is well tolerated. There is good evidence that individuals regarded as clinically anxious, as well as those who fall within the normal range on standardized measures of anxiety (e.g., STAI), experience a reduction in anxiety following exercise.

Chapter 8

Physical Activity
and Self-Esteem

Robert J. Sonstroem

Reflecting about the self remains a familiar and favorite topic of many people. It is understandable, therefore, that the notion of a self-concept is grasped and appreciated so viscerally by the public. Additionally, the fact that clinical and research evidence has established self-esteem as the variable that is most indicative of life adjustment has not escaped attention. It follows that enhanced self-esteem is often operationalized in research to reflect the "feel good" phenomenon accompanying physical activity. Moreover, the symbiosis of physical activity and self-esteem has assumed reality in the minds of the public, the journalist, and the exercise leader.

The bulk of research in the area of physical activity and self-esteem has been singularly concerned with attempting to show that increases in self-esteem accompany physical training activities. It has not relied greatly on self-concept theory, and has often operationalized only a unidimensional global self-esteem. Therefore, research has been limited in terms of explaining why and how physical activity may influence self-esteem. Meanwhile, the general topic retains vital interest for members of the helping professions. A smaller segment of exercise psychology has been concerned with the development of newer models and measures designed to bring contemporary theory to the general area of exercise and self-esteem.

This chapter provides an updated review of our knowledge in this area by summarizing conclusions developed from both lines of research. Attention is focused on several questions endemic to the study of self-esteem, particularly as it relates to physical activity. Tentative conclusions, phrased as hypotheses, serve to summarize the chapter and bring newer theories and approaches to the study of self-esteem change through physical activity. It is hoped that this chapter will provide additional direction and hypotheses to a growing body of knowledge.

Life Adjustment Properties of Global Self-Esteem

There are major reasons why self-esteem is often identified as the most indicative variable of life adjustment. Low self-esteem repeatedly has been linked to psychopathology and to depression in Western societies (Wilson & Krane, 1980). Wylie (1979) observed that the large majority of psychotherapies set improvement of patient self-esteem as their number one priority. High self-esteem has been related to the possession of social skills and to the achievement of leadership status (Rosenberg, 1979). Hattie (1992) states that high self-esteem permits people to function better in society, provides them with greater adaptability and greater control over societal roles. Conversely, individuals with low self-esteem tend to adopt an external control orientation even to the extent of believing themselves to be at the mercy of social and environmental influences.

Multiple Self-Concepts

An emphasis on self-esteem components rather than on a single self-esteem represents current theory, which treats self-concept as a multidimensional construct (e.g., Harter, 1983; Marsh, 1990). People tend to think differently about their capabilities in different areas of life. By studying these more particular self-concepts, by noting the manner in which they covary, by systematizing their associations with global self-esteem and with the environment, we learn more about people and their perceptual self-systems than could be provided by a single univariate self-esteem. This is especially true with the utilization of a self component that is highly congruent with the behavioral focus of interest. Self concept is generally regarded as the collection of ideas one holds about the self or as the picture of oneself. Self-esteem is regarded as the evaluation one places on this picture and its various aspects. Because it becomes difficult to view the self without affect or evaluation, the two terms are often used interchangeably. A variety of physical self-concepts believed to be closely related to exercise and sport activities are discussed in this chapter. These physical self-concepts are regarded as components of global self-concept and are situated as mediators between the environment and global self-concept.

Interactions With The Environment

The interaction of self-esteem and the environment can be conceptualized as a two-way process. Successes and rewarding experiences in life tend to cause us to feel good about ourselves and to strengthen our feelings of competence. This is referred to as the *skill development hypothesis* of self-esteem (Marsh, 1990), and has been the focus of a majority of exercise and self-regard research. Alternatively, self-esteem is believed to be capable of influencing behavior in the environment. We tend to act as our conception of ourselves indicates, thus reinforcing the image. This is regarded as the *self-enhancement hypothesis* of self-esteem. Therefore, the relationship between self-esteem and the environment can be summarized under a bidirectional rubric. Experiences in the environment can impact self-esteem (skill development hypothesis) and self-esteem can in turn influence experiences in the environment (self-enhancement hypothesis).

THE EFFECT OF EXERCISE ON SELF-ESTEEM

An earlier review (Sonstroem, 1984) of 16 studies designed to test the hypothesis that participation in exercise programs improved self-esteem led to the conclusion that "Exercise *programs* are associated with significant increases in self-esteem *scores* of participants" (p. 138). This conclusion was based on a preponderance of positive results in the 16 studies, but it should be noted that the word "programs" is emphasized. It appeared that a majority of the investigators tacitly assumed that self-esteem change was caused by an agent of increased physical fitness. A study that directly tested this hypothesis failed to obtain support (Jasnoski, Holmes, Solomon, & Aguiar, 1981). The investigators concluded that self-esteem change scores were associated with feelings of social support emanating from group participation. These leaps of faith regarding the power of increased fitness were so pronounced that some of the studies did not even include tests of physical fitness. In actuality, many agents other than increased fitness appear capable of influencing genuine self-esteem change within physical activity programs. A nonexhaustive list of these program agents includes: (a) increased sense of competence, mastery, or control; (b) goal achievement; (c) feelings of somatic well-being; (d) social experiences; and (e) reinforcement by significant others. Additionally, there are nonprogram factors capable of biasing the scores obtained from self-esteem inventories, and that is why the conclusions presented in the earlier review (Sonstroem, 1984) emphasized the term "scores." These confounding factors include: (a) socially desirable responding; (b) perceived task demands; (c) expectancies (the placebo effect); (d) self-presentation strategies; and (e) perceived leader or group pressures. Marsh, Richards, and Barnes (1986a) speak of the postgroup euphoria felt by participants after intensive group experiences. These emotions probably contain certain of the biasing agents listed above and impair the assessment of genuine self-esteem change.

The considerations above would seem to imply that self-esteem is relatively easy to change. The facts present a distinctly different conclusion if one is ready to discount results when confounding nonprogram factors are not controlled for. Noted theorists have commented on the relative resistance of self-esteem scores to change (Wylie, 1979). The stability of self-esteem as well as proposed techniques for self-esteem enhancement with exercise programs has been described by Sonstroem (1995). The fact that response distortion factors have seldom been controlled in exercise studies leads to a consideration that reported self-esteem changes may be artifacts arising from faulty designs. Alternatively, research designs that operationalize the program agents discussed earlier could verify explanations of program effects capable of countering bias arguments.

A review of similar studies carried out since the earlier 1984 review was conducted by the author. The majority of these recent studies also report positive results. The purpose of the recent review was to identify newer information relating to four pervading questions involved in explaining how self-esteem changes. These questions were as follows.

1. *Are increases in self-esteem directly related to increases in physical fitness?* The earlier review (Sonstroem, 1984) led to the recommendation that statistically testing associations between self-esteem and fitness gains should be conducted as a method of examining causal relations. As indicated earlier, exercise science has supported the proposition that either directly or indirectly it is increased physical fitness that should produce enhanced self-esteem. Ossip-Klein et al. (1989) assigned depressed women to 8 weeks of either running or weight training. The exercise conditions were both associated with significant (and comparable) gains in self-esteem, and both exceeded controls. The authors concluded that similar mechanisms of psychological change were activated by weight training and running. However, subjects failed to display significant fitness improvements. Similar results have been reported by other investigators (Ben-Shlomo & Short, 1986; Hatfield, Vaccaro, & Benedict, 1985; Plummer & Koh, 1987). The first study attributed experimental effects to perceived task demands, whereas the second study invoked subject expectancies as the cause of self-esteem change.

Further evidence involving the causal effect of increased fitness on self-esteem is provided by a controlled study from King et al., (1989). Sixty male and 60 female employees of a large aircraft organization responded to company announcements regarding an exercise program. They completed 11 single-item self-perception scales, and were assigned randomly to training and control groups. Training consisted of 6 months of a home-based aerobics program. At the conclusion of this study the subjects in the exercise group, compared with controls, experienced improved ratings on 3 of the 11 scales. This included satisfaction with current physical shape and appearance, current physical fitness level, and current weight. These changes remained significant when controlled statistically for initial expectancies. The process of change was examined via biweekly assessment of subsamples. The exercise resulted in significant improvements in VO_2max of 15% in the men and 9% in the women. However, correlations between physiological and psychological changes were not significant. The investigators concluded that

> Our findings suggest that adoption of regular exercise in a healthy, initially sedentary population may influence largely those psychological variables associated with exercised-induced physical changes—that is, with changes in perceived fitness and satisfaction with physical shape and weight. The apparent rapidity of

these changes, as indicated by visual inspection of the graphs of the ratings suggests that factors (either psychological or biological) other than those stemming
from increased fitness are likely to be responsible. (King et al., p. 318)

While the author has long emphasized a reliance on physical self-perceptions (Sonstroem, 1978, 1984), it is the second part of the conclusion that is
stressed here. At this time it appears valid to conclude that higher levels of self-
regard following exercise intervention are based on perceptions of improvement
or other program or score factors rather than on fitness improvement itself.

2. *Are increases in self-esteem limited to those subjects with initially lower
self-esteem scores?* The recommendations presented by Sonstroem (1984)
included testing for subgroup changes. Past research has found that subjects with
lower self-esteem scores are those most likely to experience enhanced self-
esteem. More recently, Ossip-Klein et al. (1989) showed significant improvement
in self-esteem following exercise in 32 clinically depressed women. Because
depression is associated closely with low self-esteem, this sample may be
regarded as initially low in self-esteem. Other recent studies have supported a
conclusion that self-esteem gains through exercise are realized primarily by those
initially lower in self-esteem or its components (Ben-Shlomo & Short, 1986;
Rainey & Wigtil, 1985; Wilfley & Kunce, 1986).

It should be realized that significant improvements in self-esteem were also
obtained with "normal" samples of college students (Ford, Puckett, Blessing, &
Tucker, 1989; Plummer & Koh, 1987; Stein & Motta, 1992) and adult women
(Brown & Harrison, 1986). Therefore, it is incorrect to believe that enhancement
of self-esteem with exercise is limited to those with low self-esteem. At the same
time it would seem that those with "normal" self-esteem levels would find it
more difficult to increase self-esteem scores. Self-esteem norms generally produce a mean item endorsement value of approximately 80%, and across different
samples, item means of Harter's General Self-Worth Scale range from 3.18 to
3.40 on a scale of 4 (Messer & Harter, 1986). Attempts to increase normal self-
esteem scores must counter ceiling effects and perhaps the presence of statistical
regression. It would seem that theory as well as a preponderance of research indicate that probabilities of self-perception enhancement will be greatest in people
with initially lower self-perception values.

Many of the positive results in this area have occurred in volunteer groups
that were previously sedentary (Ben-Shlomo & Short, 1986; Brown & Harrison,
1986; King et al. 1989). Wilfley and Kunce (1986) found that increases in physical self-concept were significantly greater in normal adults with low fitness levels
compared with normal adults with high fitness levels after an 8-week individual-
ized exercise program. Based on this research and contemporary theory, the
author proposes an enlarged axiom to read: Probabilities for positive self-esteem
change are greatest in subjects initially lower in self-esteem and in subjects initially lower in fitness or ability who desire a change in some component(s) of fitness or ability which is important to them. The importance aspect is treated later.

3. *Are increases in self-esteem independent of confounding factors such as the placebo effect, response distortion, and social desirability?* Not all of the recommendations presented in the earlier review (Sonstroem, 1984) were utilized in more recent studies. Component importance ratings and response distortion scales were not employed. Nonuse of these scales is surprising because the often-used Tennessee Self-Concept Scale contains the self-criticism scale as a measure of defensiveness or conscious response distortion. However, several recent studies found that a variety of social desirability measures failed to extinguish relationships between physical self-components and performance (Sonstroem, Harlow, & Salisbury, 1993) or between physical self-components and measures of adjustment (Egleston & Sonstroem, 1993). King et al. (1989) formally assessed subject expectancies before program onset, then used these expectancies as covariates in analyzing perceptual change. As mentioned earlier, subjects improved in physical self-components even with expectancies statistically controlled. A recent study used an alternative procedure of establishing a distinct group in which expectancies for psychological improvement were induced by group orientation (Desharnais et al., 1993). Compared with a group ostensibly exercising for "physical benefit" alone, this "expectancy" group experienced significant improvement in self-esteem. Self-esteem also improved in the "physical benefit" group, but this gain was not significant. The use of component scales is seen as an additional method of partially discounting placebo effects. Marsh et al. (1986a) used the 13-scale Self-Description Questionnaire III (SDQIII) to separate experimental effects from postgroup euphoria at the conclusion of an Outward Bound program. They assumed that postgroup euphoria would affect all scales in an equal manner. They next hypothesized that scales more relevant to Outward Bound outcomes (e.g., self-concepts of physical abilities, honesty, problem solving) would show greater changes over time than less relevant scales (e.g., mathematics or academic self-concepts). While all 13 scales showed significant changes, changes were significantly greater in the relevant scales. The authors concluded that greater changes in these relevant scales provided evidence regarding genuine psychological benefits of Outward Bound.

4. *Are increases in self-esteem permanent or do they disappear after several months?* In the earlier review it was recommended that longer training periods with repeated assessment and follow-up testing be employed. Gains persisting over time and outside of the experimental setting provide evidence regarding the authenticity as well as the reliability of self-esteem gains. The entire field of self-concept and self-esteem research has devoted relatively little attention to this question. Ossip-Klein et al. (1989) used multiple measures across an 8-week program and found that improved self-concept persisted at 1, 7, and 12 months posttreatment. Twelve months after a 26-day Outward Bound course, self-concept scores of students remained significantly larger than their preprogram scores (Marsh, Richards, & Barnes, 1986b). A longer intervention period with repeated assessment tended to affirm the results of the King et al. (1989) study. None of the limited number of studies reviewed reported changes that failed to persist beyond the program. Additional research should provide us with knowledge of the manner in which self-esteem varies in people and over time.

RECENT MODELS AND MEASURES

Exercise and Self-esteem Model

A major recommendation of the earlier review (Sonstroem, 1984) cited the need for models to guide research in the area of self-esteem change via exercise. This need resulted in the development of the exercise and self-esteem model (Sonstroem & Morgan, 1989). Feelings of competence represent an integral part of self-esteem and are believed to form one of its two major dimensions (Harter, 1983; Wells & Marwell, 1976). Self-acceptance, or self-love, is regarded as another major dimension of self-esteem. It consists of the general regard people hold for themselves regardless of competence evaluations. A person may know that his or her motor skills are modest at best, yet still develops a personal fondness and regard for these skills. This model (Figure 1) posits that self-esteem change is caused by changes in perceptions of competence relating to the mastery of skills associated with the exercise or athletic situation. The most minute and specific self-perception level consists of *physical self-efficacies*, the expectations that, right now, one can perform particular skills or tasks within the training setting. The model calls for measurement of these skills (e.g., jogging distance, total

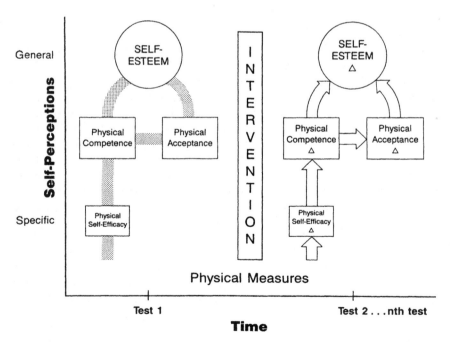

Figure 1 Exercise and self-esteem (SE) model. From "Exercise and Self-Esteem: Rationale and Model," by R. J. Sonstroem and W. P. Morgan, 1989, *Medicine and Science in Sports and Exercise, 21*, p. 333. Copyright 1989 by the American College of Sports Medicine. Reprinted by permission.

situps, batting average) as a means of studying the correspondence between physical and perceptual measures and their changes. The model proposes that changes in perceptions of specific competencies generalize to changes in broader self-constructs: first, *perceived physical competence* (PC), and, finally, *global self-esteem*. Perceived PC is defined as a general evaluation of one's overall physical abilities. It was measured in the initial validation study by combining seven items from the estimation scale of the Physical Estimation and Attraction Scales (Sonstroem, 1978) along with 10 new items assessing evaluations of stamina, strength, and physical condition. Items were selected based on relevance to the sample, which consisted of 145 adults in their middle and later years who were both physically active and sedentary. It should be mentioned that all empirical work to date has utilized only the competence dimension of the model.

The initial validation used confirmatory factor analysis and structural modeling to show that responses to seven scales were incorporated into three correlated but independent latent variables (self-efficacies, PC, and global self-esteem) as proposed by the model (Sonstroem, Harlow, Gemma, & Osborne, 1991). All model-fit statistics were excellent and included a root mean square residual of .04 and a Tucker-Lewis index of .94. Analyses supported proposed paths among latent variables. It was possible to obtain step test measures from 70 of the participants. These correlated significantly with the physical self-efficacies.

The longitudinal swim study, the second validation study (Sonstroem et al., 1993), utilized a longitudinal design (horizontal field of Figure 1). Male ($N = 93$) varsity swimmers from nine Rhode Island high schools completed inventories in November (preseason), January (midseason), and March (postseason). Within-time and across-time wave analyses employed structural modeling and a covariance matrix. Because of the exploratory nature of this study, both skill development and self-enhancement paths among variables were tested in the across-time wave analyses (e.g., from Time 1 to Time 2 or from Time 2 to Time 3 analyses). This swim study temporarily modified the exercise and self-esteem model in that self-evaluations of specific skills (e.g., start, arm stroke, turn) were substituted temporarily for self-efficacies and combined into a single measure labeled "SKILL." Performance was based on swim times combined across events and labeled "PERF" after standardizing to a mean of 0, and a standard deviation of 1 within swim events. PC was measured by a study-revised estimation scale, and self-esteem was assessed with the Rosenberg self-esteem scale. A path analysis across the three time waves documented the fact that data did not differ significantly from the model ($\chi^2 = 25.46, p >.15$, root mean square residual $= .04$, comparative fit index $= .99$). Subsequent addition of social desirability scores (Jackson, 1984) failed to greatly alter the data fit or variable associations. Social desirability is included in the path analysis of variables across the three time waves (see Figure 2).

While within-time wave synchronous associations and the very strong data fit provide excellent model support, Figure 2 indicates that only several across time associations between different variables were significant. (Note that only significant paths are drawn in Figure 2.) Most of these paths proved to be autoregressions (associations of the same variable across time), indicating the excellent

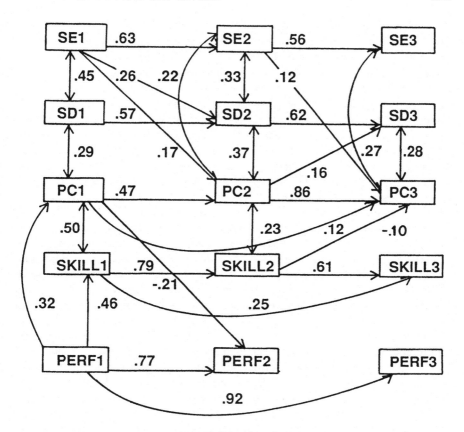

Figure 2 Path analysis of exercise and self-esteem model. (Values represent standardized coefficients). Self-esteem (SE), social desirability (SD), perceived physical competence (PC), perception of swim skills (SKILL), and swim performance (PERF) scores for November (Test 1), January 2 (Test 2), and March (Test 3). From "Path analysis of a self-esteem model across a competitive swim season," by R. J. Sonstroem, L. L. Harlow, and K. S. Salisbury, 1993, *Research Quarterly for Exercise and Sport, 64*, p. 350. Copyright 1993 by the American Alliance for Health, Physical Education, Recreation and Dance. Reprinted by permission.

reliability of measures. The model was developed initially to examine change mechanisms relative to the skill development hypothesis. Support for this hypothesis would specify significant associations between PERF1 and SKILL2 (PC2); between PERF2 and SKILL3 (PC3); between PC1 and SE2; and between PC2 and SE3. However, only several skill development (upward moving) paths are significant in Figure 2. This proved to be true even though both swimming performance and self-perception scores, including self-esteem, improved significantly over various testing intervals. After finding significant increases in performance and perceptual variables, studies have often concluded that the two increases are related (Sonstroem, 1984). This path analysis utilizing a model and repeated measures over time showed convincingly that such a conclusion was untenable.

Median PERF percent change across swim events over the two test intervals was 2.9%. It is possible that this value failed to achieve a threshold level necessary for perceptual change. Most of these young men had already been swimming competitively for 5 to 8 years. It is also possible that self-perceptions in the swimming area had stabilized or had become less sensitive to degree of performance change. Lacking additional information, it is inferred that a greater amount of swim improvement would have increased SKILL and PC scores, and eventually global self-esteem. Alternatively, it may have been that other program factors or extraprogram factors induced the perceptual change. This study can be considered meaningful for three reasons. First, the exercise and self-esteem model (slightly modified) was shown to fit the data extremely well over time and three consecutive testing sessions. Second, sport psychology has been criticized for its failure to study response biases (Morgan, 1978). Self-esteem research has also been doubted because of high associations between social desirability and self-esteem scores. In fact, Arlin (1976) found that early social desirability scores influenced later self-esteem scores, rather than vice versa. The addition of social desirability to the study analyses discussed here failed to alter associations among model variables. Additionally, social desirability failed to influence significantly any subsequent model measures. In across-time wave associations it was self-esteem and its component, PC, that significantly influenced later social desirability scores rather than vice versa (see Figure 2). Self-esteem scores obtained in November were correlated with social desirability scores measured in January and PC measured in January.

Finally, analyses were informative in identifying several significant self-enhancement paths. Self-esteem was associated ($p < .05$) with subsequent measures of perceived PC, and perceived PC scores obtained in November were associated ($p < .05$) with swim times measured in January. Furthermore, the relationship of the January PC scores and March PERF scores approached traditional significance levels ($p > .17$). These results are important in that they affirm the ability of a self-concept component to exercise the directive powers of global self-concept. Earlier research showed that estimation scores significantly predicted subsequent athletic participation (Sonstroem & Kampper, 1980). The study by Sonstroem et al. (1993) is more definitive, however, in that the statistical analysis controlled for the influence of associated variables such as global self-esteem and a form of social desirability on the physical concept's prediction of behavior.

Physical Self-Perception Profile

Recognizing that a multidimensional physical self-concept model possessed greater explanatory and discriminatory powers as compared with utilization of a single physical concept construct, Fox and Corbin (1989) developed the Physical Self-Perception Profile (PSPP). This model includes global self-esteem, along with two levels of physical self-perception based on scale specificity and generality. More specific subdomains include perceived sport competence (SPORT), physical condition (COND), attractive body (BODY), and strength (STREN).

The model defines physical self-worth as, "a superordinate representation of combined physical subdomain perceptions" (Fox & Corbin, 1989, p. 413). The net effect of the PSPP was to develop five "physical self-concepts." Preliminary validity for the model was provided by showing that correlations between physical self-worth and global self-esteem were greater than those between self-esteem and subdomains, which were smaller, also than the correlations between subdomains and physical self-worth. PSPP scales have displayed excellent reliability, and social desirability was unsuccessful at influencing their associations with other mental health variables (Egleston & Sonstroem, 1993). While the six-item scales were developed with college-age students, validity has been extended to adults in their middle and later years (Sonstroem, Harlow, & Josephs, 1994; Sonstroem, Speliotis, & Fava, 1992). The development and subsequent use of the PSPP has developed new knowledge and approaches to the study of physical activity and self-esteem, and these are reviewed in subsequent sections.

Physical Self-Description Questionnaire

A multidimensional Physical Self-Description Questionnaire (PSDQ) was recently developed by Marsh, Richards, Johnson, Roche, and Tremayne (1994). It contains a Self-Esteem scale, a General Physical Self-Concept scale, and nine subdomain scales: Strength, Body Fat, Activity, Endurance/Fitness, Sports Competence, Coordination, Health, Appearance, and Flexibility. Earlier, Marsh and Redmayne (1994) demonstrated convergent and discriminant validity for multiple physical self-concept scales by showing that they correlated most highly with physical tests of a similar nature.

Using confirmatory factor analysis, Marsh et al. (1994) showed factor stability for the PSDQ over two replications and across gender. A comparison of the PSDQ, the PSPP, and a Physical Self-Concept scale led to the conclusion that the PSDQ was the superior instrument in terms of breadth, reliability, and factor purity. However, it must be recognized that the PSPP was developed with US college students, whereas the Marsh et al. sample consisted of Australian high school students. Because PSPP reliability values (.77 to .79) are considerably lower in the Australian study as compared with five studies carried out in the United States, the possibility of both age and cultural differences must be entertained. The PSDQ offers outstanding opportunities for learning more about the perceptual world of active people.

Expansion of the Exercise and Self-Esteem Model

The development of the PSPP offered experimental opportunities in that it expanded the description of the physical self-concept and provided opportunities for testing convergent and discriminant validity. Sonstroem et al. (1994) tested an enlarged exercise and self-esteem model that replaced perceived physical competence with the two PSPP levels of physical self-worth (domain) and

SPORT, COND, BODY, STREN (subdomains). Figure 3 presents the hypothesized latent variables for the expansion of the competence dimension of the
"exercise and self-esteem model," labeled EXSEM. Self-esteem was assessed by
the six-item General Self-Worth scale (Messer & Harter, 1986). Self-efficacies
for aerobic dancing, jogging, and situps represented the three measures for the
latent variable, EFF. Subjects were 216 women involved in aerobic dance (mean

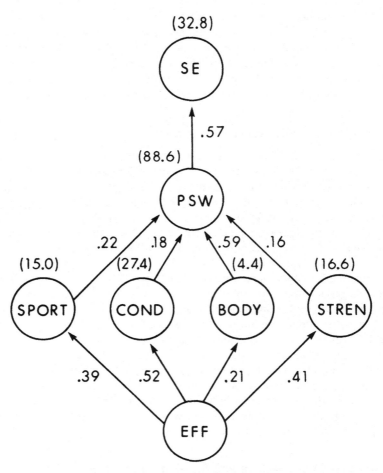

Figure 3 Standardized solution, test of expanded exercise and self-esteem model. Self-
esteem (SE), physical self-worth (PSW), sport competence (SPORT), physical condition
(COND), attractive body (BODY), strength (STREN), and physical self-efficacies (EFF)
were measured. Values beside paths represent standardized regression coefficients.
Values in parentheses represent variance percentages accounted for. From "Exercise and
Self-Esteem: Validity of Model Expansion and Exercise Associations," by R. J. Sonstroem, L. L. Harlow, and L. Josephs, 1994, *Journal of Sport and Exercise Psychology, 16,*
29–42. Copyright 1994 by Human Kinetics Publishers. Reprinted by permission.

age 38.4 years). Test of the measurement model indicated an adequate fit of data to the proposed model (root mean square residual = .05, comparative fit index = .91, parsimonious comparative fit index = .84). Structural modeling analyses testing paths among variables confirmed that the hypothesized paths of Figure 3 provided the best data fit. Additional analyses supported the necessity of including physical self-worth within the model as a mediator between subdomains and self-esteem.

Standardized solution statistics are presented in Figure 3. Values beside paths represent standardized regression coefficients and values in parentheses equal the amount of variance explained by EXSEM. Measures of self-efficacies are highly related to self-perception of physical condition by virtue of the coefficient of .52. Conversely, they are minimally (although significantly) associated with BODY (coefficient = .21), and they only explain 4.4% of BODY variance. It seems there are two forces operating in the model depicted in Figure 3. Self-efficacies are closely allied with exercise program activities, developing sizeable relationships with SPORT, COND, and STREN. While they fail to develop large associations with BODY, it is BODY that, of the four subdomains, develops the largest associations with physical self-worth and self-esteem. This latter observation replicates previous results in the literature (e.g., Harter, 1990). Physical attractiveness is the characteristic most closely related to favorable self-esteem in people across the life span, and this has major implications for the study of physical activity and self-esteem.

Directional Hypotheses for Exercise and Self-Esteem

After reviewing various aspects of the literature dealing with enhancement of self-esteem through physical activity and presenting newer theories and measures, certain conclusions can be advanced. Because of the scope and complexity of self-esteem and the lack of sufficient research, these conclusions are presented in the form of six hypotheses. Hopefully, they will challenge newer, more particular research, which will improve our understanding of the relationship between physical activity and self-esteem.

Hypothesis 1. Changes in self-esteem following physical activity interventions are not dependent on physical fitness increases. While minimal evidence for a linkage was found in the earlier review (Sonstroem, 1984), a significant association was not found in any of the five recent studies that directly tested this relationship. Additionally, both reviews revealed studies in which significant fitness improvements failed to result in significant self-esteem changes. Obviously, more research is needed in order to quantify which exercise program agents and nonprogram agents might influence self-esteem. From research and theory it seems quite possible that changes in higher-order self-esteem functioning must rely finally and more essentially on minute perceptual processes as opposed to relatively grosser and undefined increases in fitness. The exercise and self-esteem model is seen as providing preliminary structure for this line of research. Change in motor functioning (e.g., example, fitness) can be tested for its effect on physical self-concept with and without the presence of physical self-efficacies. Other program agents discussed earlier can be operationalized to examine their effect incorporated in the model.

Hypothesis 2. The use of relevant physical component scales will result in more meaningful results. This hypothesis follows a highly recommended tenet of contemporary self-esteem theory that discredits the use of a single global self-esteem as a means of studying self-regard relations. Sonstroem (1978) showed that it was estimation of one's physical abilities rather than global self-esteem that was related significantly to physical fitness. Marsh and Sonstroem (1995) found that the Condition scale of the PSPP was highly related to self-reports of degree of physical activity whereas global self-esteem was not. A comparatively large number of more recent studies testing the skill development hypothesis have used component scales. Unfortunately, the scale selected in 6 of the 10 studies was the Physical Self scale of the Tennessee Self-Concept Scale (Fitts, 1965). This underlines the importance of selecting a scale by the relevance of its items rather than by its title. A preponderance of Physical Self items refers to stimuli such as facial attractiveness, hair, eyes, teeth, and so on. More germane and recommended scales would refer to factors such as physical condition, strength, body fat, and health. Scales such as these develop tighter relationships and permit more meaningful inferences.

Other recent studies have tended to employ study-developed and even single-item scales, but these nonstandardized scales often lack reliability and fail to tap all aspects of a construct. These scales lack the nomological network and verified correlates that bring validated meaning to a construct. Use of the PSPP and PSDQ is highly recommended, because these scales represent developed instruments with a degree of past research. Continued use of these inventories will greatly increase our understanding of self-concept components as they relate to physical activity. At the same time, it is important to be aware of certain criticisms of the PSPP. Its scales are highly correlated, and subjects, particularly younger and older people, may have difficulty interpreting the forced choice response format (Marsh et al. 1994; Sonstroem et al., 1992, 1994).

Hypothesis 3. The physical self-concept and its components can predict exercise participation. This hypothesis is supported by the previously discussed swim study (Sonstroem et al., 1993) and by Sonstroem and Kampper (1980). In correlational research Fox and Corbin (1989) displayed PSPP discriminant validity in that only specific scales (e.g., SPORT and STREN) developed associations with self-reports of congruent activities (i.e., ball sports and calisthenics, respectively). Sonstroem et al. (1992) entered all 5 PSPP scales directly into a discriminant function analysis in predicting exercisers from nonexercisers. Prediction accuracy was 88.6% for women and 80.2% for men. While several scales were significant predictors in the two analyses, none approached the structural coefficient sizes of perceived physical condition (.97 and .88), which was hypothesized to be the leading correlate. When self-reports of activity were separated into quartiles, the PSPP was able to predict degree of activity significantly. The canonical *r*s were .73 for women and .64 for men. With a single exception the PSPP correctly classified subjects into the four categories above the base rate for each category and for each gender. Employing structural modeling, Sonstroem et al. (1994) found that the PSPP was able to predict 26.0% of the variance in aerobic dance attendance and 27.6% of the variance in exercise activities outside of class. Again, perceived physical condition was the best subdomain predictor of both activity variables with standardized regression coefficients of .69 and .51, respectively. Body was the only other subdomain to develop significant standardized regression coefficients with the two activity criteria ($-.29$ and $-.30$, respectively). These negative values indicate the presence of statistical suppression, and a substantive interpretation can be applied. Inspection of the data showed that many of the most active women in this sample had low ratings of their own body attractiveness and high ideal-body discrepancies. That is, on a 4-point category scale they rated the importance of body attractiveness as "4" (high) and evaluated their own bodies as "1" (low).

It appears that investigators have been concentrating on the skill development hypothesis of self-esteem at the expense of studying its self-enhancement hypothesis. Workers in the field of exercise adherence have been advocating a multidimensional approach for some time (see chapter 4). It is recommended that physical self components be utilized in future research in conjunction with barriers, self-efficacies, perceived benefits, and stages and processes of change.

Hypothesis 4. The use of component importance ratings will increase our understanding of the self in exercise. The contemporary emphasis on components of self-esteem rather than a unitary self-esteem has prioritized attempts to understand relations between the two. Theorists tend to agree that the contribution of any component to global self-esteem should be a function of the personal importance of that component to the individual. Methods of operationalizing this concept have included multiplying components by their assessed respective importances or by calculating discrepancies between importances and their respective components. Theoretically, the sum of components multiplied by their importance ratings should predict self-esteem better than the sum of components alone. This same approach to predicting physical self-worth by means of physical self-concept subdomains has been recommended by Fox (1990). The lack of success in better predicting self-esteem through component importances has been summarized by Marsh (1993). In addition, Marsh and Sonstroem (1995) were unsuccessful at increasing the prediction of physical self worth by means of weighting the importance of physical subdomains. This latter study, however, documented the fact that importance ratings were related to self-reports of physical activity and that the combination of importance ratings and their respective components made a small improvement over the use of components alone in predicting activity. It is possible that investigators have been pursuing the wrong dependent variable. An extension of the self-enhancement hypothesis would predict that people will engage in behavior that reinforces those self-concept components that are important to their identity. As indicated earlier, there is evidence that the discrepancy between the body's perceived importance and the ratings of one's own body was an important factor for women involved in aerobic dance. It should also be noted that the subdomains contained in the PSPP can be rated for importance by use of the Perceived Importance Profile (Fox, 1990).

Hypothesis 5. Physical self-concepts are associated significantly with favorable life adjustment. Physical self-concepts, considered as components of global self-esteem, experience a statistical association with self-esteem. It would seem, therefore, that they may possess some of the same life adjustment properties as self-esteem. An effort has been made to verify this hypothesis with 119 female and 126 male college students. Subjects completed the PSPP and four measures of life adjustment: positive affect, negative affect, depression, and health complaints (Egleston & Sonstroem, 1993). These students also completed two social desirability scales (Impression Management and Self-Deceptive Enhancement; Paulhus, 1991). Of the 20 correlation coefficients calculated between the five PSPP scales and the four measures of adjustment, 12 of 20 (range .24 to .51) were significant for the women and 16 of 20 (range .19 to .42) were significant for the men. Hierarchical multiple regression was employed to identify unique variance attributable to the association of adjustment scales PSPP variables. In hierarchical order, the two social desirability scales were entered first followed by self-esteem. The five PSPP scales were entered finally to determine whether they made a contribution to the prediction of adjustment beyond that provided by social desirability and self-esteem. The two social desirability scales were associated significantly with life adjustment variables in six of the eight cases for men and women, and all of the associations were significant except those with positive affect and depression for the women in this study. Self-esteem significantly improved this association with all four dependent variables across both samples. Above the contributions of social desirability and self-esteem, physical self-concepts significantly improved the associations in three of the eight cases. PSPP scales were able to increase variance accounted for by 16% in women with positive affect and by 8% in men with positive affect and the absence of health complaints. Three additional PSPP associations approached significance ($p > .13$). Size of subdomain standardized regression coefficients identified the perceived physical condition scale as the best predictor of life adjustment in women. Perceptions of sport competence performed a similar function for men.

It must be remembered that the total PSPP relationship with adjustment is increased further by indirect effects via the physical self-concept/self-esteem association. This conservative analysis indicates that physical self-concepts, devoid of social desirability and global self-esteem influences, are inherently associated with life adjustment variables, which supports earlier research by Sonstroem (1976). For skill development research it means that achieving increases in physical self-concepts by means of physical activity carries favorable life adjustment benefits, thus minimizing the necessity of including a measure of global self-esteem as the ultimate outcome variable.

SUMMARY

This chapter has focused on studies conducted since 1984 that tested the ability of physical activity to enhance self-esteem. While this summary agreed with the results of an earlier review (Sonstroem, 1984), efforts were made to identify principles and mechanisms of self-esteem change as developed both by this research and by contemporary theory and experimentation.

The research reviewed in this chapter leads to the conclusion that self-esteem change via physical activity does not rely on increases in physical fitness. A variety of possible change agents were identified. While the influence of social desirability on meaningful physical self-concept relationships tended to be discounted by limited research, its ubiquity is so great as to demand continued assessment and control in exercise and self-esteem research. This recommendation has added importance with regard to the study of expectancies and the placebo effect in research concerned with physical activity and self-esteem (Desharnais et al., 1993).

Newer models and scales emphasizing physical self-concepts were also reviewed in this chapter. Research has established that these constructs, considered to be self-esteem components, are more closely associated with exercise variables than is global self-esteem. Marsh and Sonstroem (1995) demonstrated that physical self-concepts, rather than self-esteem, were associated with physical activity involvement. Previously, Sonstroem (1978) demonstrated that physical fitness was related to physical self-concept rather than to global self-esteem. This chapter disclosed that perceived physical competence predicted subsequent swimming performance in varsity swimmers and that positive perceptions of physical condition and negative perceptions of possessing an attractive body (in certain women) were related to exercise participation in adult women. Additional reviewed studies documented the close correspondence between physical self-concepts and self-reports of physical activity in samples of varied ages. Research was presented that manifests a distinct association between physical self-concepts and contemporary indices of life adjustment in university students.

This chapter concludes that understanding of personal interaction with the physical activity environment can be greatly increased by employment of physical self-concept scales. It is hoped that this review and critique will open larger vistas to the investigator concerned with the skill development hypothesis. Perhaps it will be useful in promoting additional research in the exciting and promising area of the physical self-concept.

Chapter 9

Overtraining and Staleness

Patrick J. O'Connor

The dilemma of overtraining and staleness has been ignored frequently in discussions of physical activity and mental health (e.g., North et al., 1990; Seraganian, 1993). Not only are the detrimental psychological consequences of overtraining now well documented, but understanding this paradoxical phenomenon is important in efforts designed to explain the influence of physical activity on mental health.

The problem of overtraining and staleness has been addressed numerous times prior to the 1980s (Counsilman, 1955; Griffith, 1926; Karpovich, 1941; Kereszty, 1971; Mellerowicz & Barron, 1971; Michael, 1961; Parmenter, 1923; Westhall, 1863; Wolf, 1971); however, it has only been during the last 10 years that this topic has received significant scientific attention. A computerized (BIOSIS, Current Contents Plus, MEDLINE, & PSYCHINFO databases) reference list search of the published English language literature on the topic of overtraining and staleness from the years 1985 to 1994 revealed over 40 databased, peer-reviewed articles, approximately 75% of which were published in the 1990s. Reasons for the increased interest in overtraining and staleness are uncertain, but several papers published in the 1980s from groups in South Africa (Barron, Noakes, Levy, Smith, & Millar, 1985) and the United States (e.g., Dressendorfer & Wade, 1983; Dressendorfer, Wade, & Scaff, 1985; Guttman, Pollock, Foster, & Schmidt, 1984; Morgan, 1985c; Morgan et al., 1987; Ryan, 1983) helped to articulate the nature of the problem as well as hint at possible solutions. In addition, in the late 1980s and early 1990s the Sports Medicine Council of the United States Olympic Committee stimulated research by requesting and funding research proposals on the topic of overtraining and staleness.

This chapter has two foci. The first section introduces the concepts of overtraining and staleness, and the second summarizes research dealing with monitoring of mood state responses to overtraining as a way to prevent staleness. Readers interested in other aspects of overtraining and staleness are directed to the large number of prior reviews (e.g., Budgett, 1990, 1994; Dishman, 1992; Fry, Lawrence et al., 1993; Fry, Morton, & Keast, 1991, 1992; Hackney, Pearman, & Nowacki, 1990; Hendrickson & Verde, 1994; Kibler, Chandler, & Stracener, 1992; Kuipers & Keizer, 1988; Lehmann, Foster, & Keul, 1993; Levin, 1991; Newsholme, Blomstrand, McAndrew, & Parry-Billings, 1992; Raglin, 1993; Sharp & Koutedakis, 1992; Stachenfeld, Gleim, & Nicholas, 1992; Stone et al., 1991; Vailas, Morgan, & Vailas, 1990; Veale, 1991).

CONCEPTUALIZATION OF OVERTRAINING AND STALENESS

Overtraining

Overtraining is a type of physical training performed primarily by highly motivated athletes. The term "training" is a general one that refers to the completion of physical activity on a regular basis. For example, millions of people walk, jog, swim, or lift weights regularly (i.e., 3 to 7 days per week) to maintain or improve their health and physical fitness. Most of these individuals do not perform frequent (more than once per day), long-duration (more than 90 min per session), high-intensity physical activity on a daily basis. Some individuals, especially competitive athletes, engage in this type of physical training because of a belief that such training will maximize performance. In addition, a subset of noncompetitive athletes reportedly engage in physical activity in an obsessive-compulsive manner (Polivy, 1994).

Overtraining refers to a short cycle of training (lasting a few days to a few weeks) during which athletes expose themselves to increased training loads that are near or at maximal capacity. A training load that can be performed successfully for longer periods of time (e.g., approximately 1 month or more) is an insufficient exercise stimulus to be aptly termed overtraining. This definition of overtraining has three important features: (a) overtraining involves a series of acute exercise bouts; *it is a process*; (b) overtraining consists of *a significant increase in the training stimulus* compared with recent training history; and (c) overtraining involves exercise of a *high frequency* (often more than 1 session per day) with *an intensity-duration combination that is at or near maximal capacity*. It is important to recognize that exercise duration and intensity are inversely related; the lower the exercise intensity the longer the exercise can be sustained. In defining overtraining attention must also be paid to factors such as individual differences in performance capacity and exercise mode specificity. For instance, 10 days of swimming 10,000 m at 95% of VO_2max is not overtraining for the elite athlete who is accustomed to swimming 14,000 m per day at 95% of VO_2max. However, this would represent overtraining for a college swimmer accustomed to swimming 5,000 m per day at 95% of VO_2max. Consideration of exercise mode specificity requires an appreciation, for example, that 3 hours of running per day for 10 days at 70% of VO_2max is more likely to represent over-training than is 3 hours of daily swimming at 70% of VO_2max because long-duration exercise is tolerated better in non–weight-bearing activities such as cycling or swimming than in weight-bearing activities such as running.

It is widely believed that during each training season a period of overtraining is required if biological adaptations are to be maximized. Athletic performance improves because of complex biochemical, cardiovascular, neurological, and muscular adaptations, most of which are the direct result of increases in training load. For example, the increased aerobic capacity of muscle fibers is caused by an increase in both skeletal muscle mitochondrial content and the concentration of oxidative enzymes within the mitochondria, and these adaptations are criti-cally dependent on the total amount of muscle contractile activity (Holloszy & Coyle, 1984). Accordingly, it is axiomatic that progressive increases in training are required to produce biological adaptations that allow continued improvement in endurance performance. Competitive athletes are reluctant to restrain from progressively increasing their training because when the training load reaches a plateau, biological adaptations and performance also typically plateau. Equally unacceptable, however, is the situation in which progressive increases in training continue unabated and the training load reaches a point at which athletes become injured or stale. Thus, the scientific and artistic challenge for athletes and coaches is to titrate the training load so that optimal adaptations accrue and negative side effects such as injury and staleness are avoided. This notion dates from the earli-est of published references to the idea of overtraining. For instance, consider the writings of Charles Westhall (1863):

> . . . the man has had too much sweating and forced work, in consequence of which he is getting weak, and, in the professional term, "training off." This will easily be recognized by the muscles getting flaccid and sunken, with patches of red appearing in different portions of the body, and the man suffering from a continual and unquenchable thirst. These well-known symptoms tell the trainer that rest must be given to the pedestrian as well as a relaxation from the strict rule of diet. A couple days' release from hard work will in most cases prove suc-cessful in allaying the unwelcome symptoms, . . . (p. 35)

Westhall clearly recognized the usefulness of monitoring athletes in order to pre-vent the negative effects of excessive training. A primary focus of contemporary research has been to extend Westhall's idea by attempting to identify prodromal markers unique to staleness.

Staleness

The term staleness has been in use by sports medicine professionals in the United States for decades. In a discussion of chronic fatigue, Karpovich (1941) wrote, "Analysis of the situation discloses that in every case there was an outstanding factor of mental unrest. It was not the muscular work, but the mental anxiety, that brought about this condition, which is commonly referred to as staleness" (p. 418). Councilman (1955), an exercise physiologist who is also widely recognized as one of the world's foremost swimming coaches, defined staleness as:

> that condition under which the performance of the athlete is affected detrimentally for a more or less longer period of time. This decreased efficiency is believed to be due to overtraining or overwork. This decreased level of performance can be due to either physiological or psychological causes or to both. Perhaps the two types of staleness cannot be separated, for as one progresses so does the other. (p. 29)

The American Medical Association (1966), in its standard nomenclature of athletic injuries, included the term "stale" and defined it as "a psychological or physiological state of overtraining which manifests as deteriorated athletic readiness" (p. 126). Consistent with these early definitions, all of which incorporated mental health aspects of staleness, there continues to be a consensus that staleness is a psychobiological syndrome. However, the weight of the available evidence suggests that staleness presently is diagnosed most accurately from behavioral signs and psychological symptoms because physiological signs appear to be less sensitive and specific.

The principal behavioral sign of staleness is impaired athletic performance. The truly stale athlete has a significant reduction in performance (e.g., 5% or greater) for an extended period (e.g., 2 weeks or greater) that occurs during or following a period of overtraining and fails to improve in response to short-term reductions in training. When athletes compete infrequently, the impairment in performance often is first noticed during workouts. For example, a chronic (e.g., 1 or 2 weeks) inability to complete workouts that previously could be accomplished (i.e., in recent history) is a sign of staleness. Other behavioral signs such as insomnia are mentioned frequently as correlates of staleness but the presence of these signs is poorly documented. For instance, there is a complete absence of published data concerning the sleep characteristics of stale athletes using polysomnographic criteria (O'Connor & Youngstedt, 1995).

The principal psychological symptoms appear to be mood disturbances and increases in perceptual effort during exercise. Standard workouts are perceived as more effortful when athletes become stale, and workouts are completed only with extreme difficulty. Overall mood disturbances occur in association with staleness; however, depression appears to be the major mood malady. For example, it has been reported that approximately 80% of stale athletes are clinically depressed (Morgan et al., 1987).

Epidemiology   There has been no large-scale, systematic study of the epidemiology of staleness in athletes. Accordingly, it is not possible to make definitive estimates of its prevalence or incidence. Nevertheless, the available data suggest that the problem is not trivial. For example, 9 of 14 (64%) elite male distance runners reported experiencing staleness at some point during their careers (Morgan, O'Connor, Ellickson, & Bradley, 1988). Similarly, the lifetime prevalence of staleness was reported to be 60% in 15 elite female distance runners, a figure that was higher than the lifetime prevalence of 30% reported in a comparison group of highly trained distance runners who performed at a subelite level (Morgan, O'Connor, Sparling, & Pate, 1987). Given the likelihood that elite athletes endure cycles of overtraining that encroach on maximal limits, it is not surprising that they appear to be at increased risk for staleness.

The yearly incidence of staleness in athletes who overtrain while participating in endurance sports appears to range from 5% to 10% based on studies of approximately 400 college swimmers tested over a 10-year period (Morgan et al., 1987; Raglin & Morgan, 1994). Moreover, preliminary data suggest that one episode of the disorder is associated with an increased risk for a subsequent occurrence. Raglin (1993) has reported that 91% of college swimmers who developed staleness as first-year college students became stale again at some point during their sophomore, junior, or senior year. However, only 30% of those who did not become stale during their first year developed staleness during a subsequent college season. In addition, two of 14 (14%) elite male distance runners reported a regular yearly recurrence of staleness symptoms (Morgan et al., 1988). These studies suggest that certain athletes are particularly susceptible to developing staleness, and past episodes of staleness are accurate predictors for future development of staleness.

Semantic and Diagnostic Confusion   Perhaps the greatest barrier preventing greater progress in this area of research has been the confusion regarding terminology and the lack of a consensus about the diagnostic criteria for staleness. For example, some authors have incorrectly used the term "burnout" to refer to aspects of staleness (e.g., Rowland, 1986; Silva, 1990). However, as Raglin (1993) has made clear, burnout is a separate disorder that refers to the negative consequences of occupational stressors resulting in a lack of desire to continue in the occupation. In contrast to both burnout and chronic fatigue syndrome (Eichner, 1989), anecdotal and related empirical evidence suggests that motivation to train is maintained in stale athletes (Raglin, 1993). Further complicating matters, European authors have used terms such as "overtrained," "overtraining," "overstrain," "overload," "overreaching," and "overtraining syndrome" to indicate what North American researchers call staleness. Consider also the short-term condition of reduced performance that is less serious than staleness, which was labeled as "training off" by Westhall (1863). European authors currently tend to refer to this condition as "overreaching." Raglin and Morgan (1994) have termed it "training distress," and Hendrickson and Verde (1994) have labeled it "inadequate recovery syndrome." The need for unanimity about the language used to describe staleness (and its variants) is critically important. The current state of affairs is analogous to research and practice concerning mental disorders prior to the emergence of international and national agreements about diagnostic criteria (e.g., APA, 1994; Spitzer, Endicott, & Robins, 1978). Phenomenal progress in the understanding and treatment of mental disorders such as depression was made once researchers and clinicians agreed on what does (and does not) make up its formal diagnostic criteria. Because workers in the exercise and sport sciences have not yet taken this step, not only is it difficult to make meaningful comparisons between investigations, but the characteristics of stale athletes remain poorly described. For example, investigators have failed to report potentially important aspects of staleness such as the severity of the symptoms (e.g., magnitude of performance decrements), the mode of onset (e.g., fast vs. slow), the duration of the staleness bout, its progression, and whether it was a recurrent or a single episode. Moreover, inadequate attention has been paid to the possibility that another medical condition could have accounted for performance decrements in potentially stale athletes. Consider the case of a professional boxer who complained of chronic training-related fatigue. His trainers were concerned about his reduced performance and inability to complete workouts, and this boxer exhibited some of the classic symptoms of staleness. However, subsequent medical evidence led to a diagnosis of restrictive cardiomyopathy (White, 1994). This anecdote underscores the fact that athletes are not immune to serious medical problems. Similar cases occur regularly and include a documented myocardial infarction reported in association with overtraining in a college swimmer (Hanson, Vander Ark, Besozzi, & Rowe, 1982). Since chronic fatigue, depression, and reduced athletic performance can be caused by a variety of physical problems, it is especially important to rule out systematically medical conditions caused by cardiovascular, infectious, viral, sleep, immune, and endocrine disorders in order to make an accurate diagnosis of staleness.

Treatment   The generally recommended treatment for staleness is rest. Anecdotal reports indicate that a few weeks of reduced training or even complete rest is often inadequate for full recovery from staleness. Inadequate recovery has been reported after a rest period of 6 months (Barron et al., 1985).

Because many athletes who suffer from staleness are also diagnosed as depressed, it is possible that antidepressant medications might be effective in treating this syndrome. However, there have been no studies reporting the efficacy of antidepressant medications in the treatment of staleness. However, there is one anecdotal report involving a distance runner who achieved marked and rapid improvement in training and performance immediately following the use of fluoxetine (Burfoot, 1994). It has also been speculated that the cause of staleness involves dysregulation of the central nervous system (CNS) serotonin neurotransmitter system (Newsholme et al., 1992). This view underscores the conceptualization of staleness as an endogenous depression-like syndrome with biological underpinnings (Morgan et al., 1987), and there is a sound theoretical rationale for conducting experimental research dealing with the efficacy of anti-depressant medications in the treatment of staleness. In the meantime physicians and psychologists who treat individuals suffering from this malady should realize that staleness is a complex psychobiological syndrome for which there is no proven treatment other than rest. The solution to this problem is prevention, and professionals should counsel affected individuals about the importance of not training to the point where they become stale.

Etiology The causes of staleness are poorly understood because empirical evidence with stale athletes is sparse and inadequate. Barron et al., (1985) reported an impairment in hormonal responses to insulin-induced hypoglycemia in 4 stale athletes that abated following their recovery. The findings suggested that staleness is brought about by hypothalamic dysfunction; however, control subjects were not tested and the endocrine status of the athletes prior to their staleness was unknown. Future research aimed at understanding the causes of staleness is needed and should be guided by theoretical formulations concerning the etiology of staleness in order to generate and test plausible hypotheses (Dishman, 1992).

MOOD STATES AS MARKERS OF STALENESS

The dominant research paradigm used to identify early warning signs of staleness has been to measure a battery of putative markers in athletes prior to, during, and following a period of overtraining and then compare those athletes who develop performance difficulties with those who do not. Research of this type has been conducted with a range of performers including ballet dancers (Liederbach, Glein, & Nicholas, 1992), basketball players (Raglin, Eksten, & Garl, 1995), canoeists (Berglund & Säfström, 1994), judoists (Callister, Callister, Fleck, & Dudley, 1990; Murphy, Fleck, Dudley, & Callister, 1990), rowers (Cogan, Highlen, Petrie, Sherman, & Simonsen, 1991; Raglin, Morgan, & Luchsinger, 1990), speed skaters (Guttman, Pollock, Foster & Schmidt, 1984), swimmers (Morgan, 1991), and wrestlers (Morgan et al., 1987). However, the most conclusive research has employed physical activity modes such as running, swimming, or weight lifting, and these training modes have the advantage of permitting accurate and objective quantification of each individual's training regimen and performance level. In other words, research involving sports such as judo (Callister et al., 1990; Murphy et al., 1990) has focused on "overtraining," but there has been inadequate documentation of the training stimulus (e.g., metabolic expenditure) presented. Physical activities such as running and swimming, on the other hand, allow for the examination of dose-response relationships not possible in team sports or activities in which both training load and performance are judged in comparison to how well an opponent performs.

A plethora of variables have been employed as potential staleness markers, and these are summarized in Table 1. The complexity of this syndrome is best illustrated by the research findings involving endocrine responses. It has been reported that staleness is associated with elevated cortisol (O'Connor, Morgan, Raglin, Barksdale, & Kalin, 1989); reduced testosterone (Dressenforfer & Wade, 1991; Flynn et al., 1994; Griffith, Dressenforfer, Fullbright, & Wade, 1990; Roberts, McClure, Weiner, & Brooks, 1993); both elevated (Hooper, Traeger Mackinnon, Gordon, & Bachmann, 1993), and decreased (Lehmann, Schnee, Scheu, Stockhausen, & Bachl, 1992) norepinephrine; and both blunted (Barron et al., 1985) and augmented (Fry, Kraemer, Van Borselen, Lynch, Triplett, et al., 1994) hormonal responses to neuroendocrine challenges (e.g., insulin-induced hypoglycemia) and exercise.

Mood state responses to increases in training are effective in predicting the onset of staleness, and there is limited research indicating that monitoring of mood state can be an effective method of preventing staleness. Furthermore, mood states, unlike many physiological parameters (e.g., endocrine measures), are feasible in that they are relatively easy to obtain and noninvasive, with little associated cost. In addition, these measures can be obtained readily on a frequent basis, and this is important in any prevention effort. Finally, considerable research shows the following: (a) alteration in mood with increases and decreases in training are highly replicable; (b) some mood states are highly sensitive to

Table 1 Summary of Variables Employed as Potential Markers of Staleness

Measures	Investigators
Cardiovascular	Dressendorfer et al., 1985; Piepoli & Coats, 1994; Rusko, Härkönen M, & Parkarinen, 1994
Immune	Fitzgerald, 1991; Fry, Morton, Garcia-Webb, Crawford, & Keast, 1992; Peters & Bateman, 1983; Sharp & Koutedakis, 1992; Tharp & Barnes, 1990
Metabolic	Jeukendrup, Hessling, Snyder, Kuipers, & Keizer, 1992; Lehmann et al., 1991, Lehmann, Baumgartl, et al., 1992; Lehmann, Schnee, Scheu, Stockhausen, & Bachl, 1992; Snyder, Jeukendrup, Hesselink, Kuipers, & Foster, 1993
Dietary	Cogan et al., 1991; Fry et al., 1993; Morgan et al., 1988; Parry-Billings et al., 1992; Sherman & Maglischo, 1991
Neuromuscular	Costill, King, Thomas, & Hargreaves, 1985; Dressendorfer & Wade, 1983; Koutedakis, Frischkrecht, Budgett, Vrbova, & Sharp, 1993; Raglin et al., 1996
Endocrine	O'Connor et al., 1989; Hooper et al., 1993; Lehmann et al., 1992; Barron et al., 1985; Fry, Kraemer, Stone, et al., 1994; Fry, Kraemer, Van Borselen, et al., 1994; Dressendorfer & Wade, 1991; Flynn et al., 1994; Griffith et al., 1990; Roberts et al., 1993; Schnee, Schen, Stockhausen, & Bachl, 1992
Psychometric	Morgan, 1991; Morgan et al., 1987; Morgan et al., 1988

increases in training load (e.g., fatigue and vigor) while others (e.g., depression) seem to be more sensitive to the onset of staleness; (c) subjective measures of mood often covary with objective physiological markers of training distress, and (d) titration of training loads based on mood responses to overtraining appears to prevent staleness (Morgan, 1991).

Alterations in Mood With Overtraining

Cohen (1994) has reiterated the importance of findings that replicate in documenting meaningful progress in psychological science. The single most consistently replicated finding in the overtraining and staleness literature is that increases in training load are associated with shifts toward negative mood states while reductions in training load are associated with improvements in mood (Berglund & Säfström, 1994; Flynn et al., 1994; Goss, 1994; Gutman et al., 1984; Liederback, Glein, & Nicholas, 1992; Morgan et al., 1987; Morgan, Costill et al., 1988; Murphy et al., 1990; Newton, Hunter, Bammon, & Roney, 1993; O'Connor et al., 1989; O'Connor, Morgan, & Raglin, 1991; Raglin et al., 1995; Raglin & Morgan, 1994; Raglin et al., 1990; Raglin, Morgan, & O'Connor, 1991; Raglin, Stager, Koceja, & Harms, 1996; Verde, Thomas, & Shephard, 1992; Wittig, Houmard, & Costill, 1989). In the few cases in which small or nonsignificant effects of increased training on mood have been observed they appear to be explained easily by methodological concerns such as the imposition of trivial increases in training (e.g., Cogan et al., 1991) or the use of psychological measures that lack construct validity (e.g., Fry, Kraemer, Van Borselen, Lynch, Marsit et al., 1994).

Negative affect associated with overtraining is such a robust finding that it is observed even when investigators are not looking for it. Consider, for instance, a study that examined the influence of progressive increases in endurance running on racehorses (Bruin, Kuipers, Keizer, & Vander Vusse, 1994). Seven horses ran on a treadmill for 272 continuous days. Training alternated between low intensity endurance days (20 minutes of continuous running at a heart rate of 140 bpm) and high-intensity interval days (e.g., six 3-min runs at a heart rate of 200 bpm each followed by a 3-min rest interval running at a heart rate of 140 bpm). The interval training was made progressively more difficult, and every 2 weeks the horses completed graded maximal exercise tests to assess their running performance. Muscle biopsies allowed for an examination of muscle histology and biochemistry while intramuscular injections of ACTH were used to assess hypothalamic-pituitary-adrenal axis (HPA) alterations with overtraining. This investigation clearly showed that early warning signs of staleness can be produced in horses. For example, treadmill performance reached a plateau and the horses were unable to complete the prescribed training after the difficulty of the interval training and the relatively easy endurance days were both increased. Although mood measurements in the horses were not quantified, the authors concluded that, "The earliest sign of overtraining is the inability to complete the intensive training, with associated *increased irritability* and reluctance to exercise. The generally advocated blood chemical variables failed to demonstrate specific changes during overtraining in the horse" (pp. 1912–1913).

Research in human subjects frequently has quantified mood states using the 65-item POMS (McNair et al., 1971, 1981, 1992). The POMS yields scores for six individual mood states: tension, depression, anger, vigor, fatigue, and confusion. In addition, an overall mood measure can be computed by summing the five negative moods, subtracting the single positive mood (vigor), and adding 100 to avoid negative scores. High scores on the resulting overall mood measure indicate a global mood disturbance while low scores indicate a positive mood. There is a dose-response relationship between training volume and overall mood as depicted in Figure 1. That is, as the training volume increases progressive mood disturbances occur, and as the training volume is reduced overall mood improves.

Mood States Are Specific
To Overtraining And Staleness

Beyond the consistent association between training volume and overall mood, the analysis of individual mood states yields additional information that can be useful. As one might expect, the specific mood states that are most sensitive to increases in training (i.e., those that are first to be altered and show the largest change in magnitude) are fatigue and vigor (Morgan et al., 1987; Raglin et al., 1991). This concept is illustrated by a study in which 40 female and male college swimmers were assessed before and during a 3-day period in which their training volume was increased by 54% (from approximately 7,900 to 12,200 m/day). As shown in Figure 2, large increases in fatigue and large decreases in vigor were observed in association with the overtraining while little change in depression was exhibited.

When groups of athletes are studied, scores on anger, confusion, and depression show the smallest mean change in association with overtraining (Raglin et al., 1991). Nevertheless, increases in depression and anger scores appear to be one of the most effective markers of staleness. One piece of evidence in support of this idea is that stale athletes have scores on the POMS depression scale that are elevated when compared with those who have overtrained but are not stale. For example, Figure 3 presents POMS depression scores in female college swimmers who were classified as either stale ($n = 3$) or overtrained (i.e., completed the overtraining process without becoming stale, $n = 11$) during three phases of training: (a) at the start of the indoor training season when the training volume was approximately 2,000 yards/day; (b) at the end of a 3-week overtraining cycle during which the training volume was approximately 12,000 yards/day; and (c) following a 1-month period in which the training volume was progressively decreased to 4,500 yards/day. Not only were the POMS depression scores higher in the stale group immediately following the overtraining period but they remained so following the 4 weeks of reduced training. These data highlight the fact that once athletes

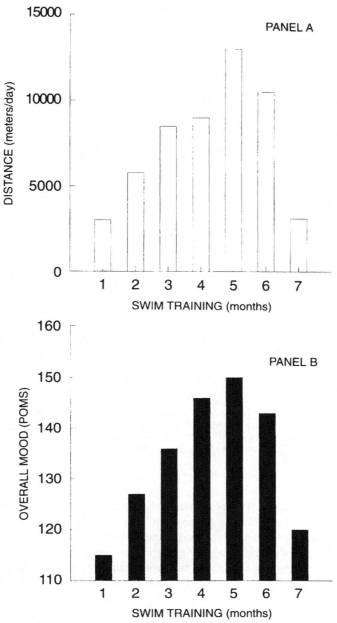

Figure 1 The change in training volume for 186 female and male college swimmers during swim training from September to March (top), and the associated change in overall mood as measured by the Profile of Mood States (bottom). Adapted from "Changes in Mood State During Training in Female and Male College Swimmers," by J. S. Raglin, W. P. Morgan, & P. J. O'Connor, 1991. *International Journal of Sports Medicine, 12*, p. 585. Reprinted with permission.

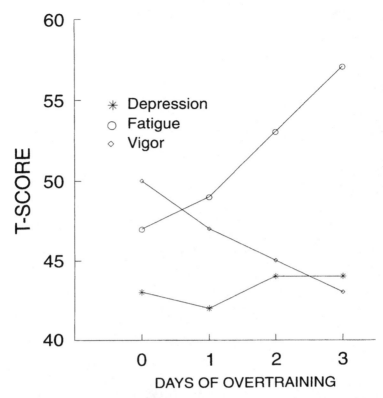

Figure 2 Change in Profile of Mood States depression, fatigue, and vigor T scores associated with 3 days of overtraining in 40 female and male college swimmers. Adapted from "Psychobiologic Effects of 3 Days of Increased Training in Female and Male College Swimmers, by P. J. O'Connor, W. P. Morgan, & J. S. Raglin 1991. *Medicine and Science in Sports and Exercise, 23*, p. 1058. Reprinted with permission.

becomes stale, they do not respond well to reductions in training. Additionally, resting saliva samples obtained at the same time as the POMS measurements showed that cortisol levels were elevated in the stale group compared with the control group following overtraining. Moreover, there was a significant correlation ($r = .50$) between resting salivary cortisol concentrations and POMS depression scores. Interestingly, these data imply a similarity between stale swimmers and depressed patients who also exhibit excessive activation of the HPA (Kalin & Dawson, 1986).

Additional evidence in support of the idea that increases in depression and anger scores are effective prodromal markers of staleness stems from the recently developed 7-item training-induced distress scale. Raglin and Morgan (1994) collected mood responses to overtraining in 70 female and 100 male college swim-

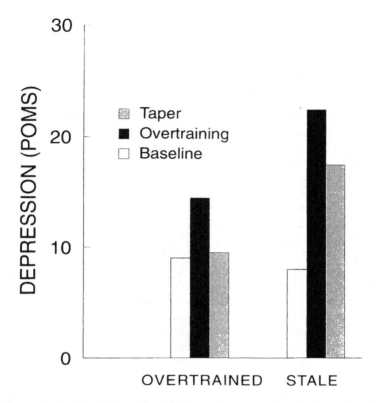

Figure 3 Profile of Mood States depression scores in stale (n = 3) and overtrained (n = 11) female swimmers during three phases of training (baseline, overtraining, and taper). Adapted from "Mood State and Salivary Cortisol Levels Following Overtraining in Female Swimmers," by P. J. O'Connor, W. P. Morgan, J. S. Raglin, C. M. Barksdale, and N. H. Kalin 1989, *Psychoneuroendocrinology, 14,* p. 303. Reprinted with permission.

mers over a 4-year period. Team coaches classified athletes as "distressed" if they exhibited overtraining associated performance decrements for several days or maintained performance only with increased difficulty. Athletes with extended and large (>5%) performance decrements were considered stale. Discriminant function analyses were conducted to learn which of the 6 POMS subscales and 65 individual POMS items best discriminated between healthy swimmers and those who were either distressed or stale. The resulting 7-item training-induced distress scale was found to be more effective in discriminating the healthy from the distressed or stale swimmers than either the 6 POMS subscale scores or the overall POMS mood measure. Five of the items that constituted the newly developed scale were from the POMS depression subscale and 2 were from the anger subscale. This psychometric scale development effort is a refreshing contrast to several crude instruments that have been employed ineffectively in overtraining studies (e.g., Fry, Kraemer, Van Borselen, Lynch, Marsit, et al., 1994; Lehmann et al., 1991).

Negative Mood and Measures Of Training Distress

Covariation between subjective mood states and objective physiological measures associated with athletic performance gives convergent evidence for the validity of mood as a marker of staleness. Collaborative research funded by the U.S. Olympic Committee provides a suitable illustration of this point (Costill et al., 1988; Morgan, Costill, et al., 1988). This study examined the influence of an abrupt increase in swim training (from 4,000 to 9,000 m/day at an intensity of 94% of VO_2max for 10 consecutive days) on putative physiological and psychological markers of staleness in 12 college swimmers. After several days, 3 of the swimmers were unable to tolerate the overtraining and were forced to swim at a slower pace. Deltoid biopsies revealed significantly reduced muscle glycogen levels in these swimmers. Without knowledge of the mood responses to overtraining, these swimmers were classified by the exercise physiologists on the research team as "responders" due to the adverse responses to training. Six other swimmers, classified as "nonresponders," were able to tolerate the increased training load and did not show reduced glycogen levels in their deltoid muscles. These classifications were compared with parallel classifications made by exercise psychologists who were blinded from the physiological and performance results. The classification of the swimmers as responders or nonresponders in this case was made on the basis of overall mood scores derived from the POMS. Four swimmers were identified as responders, and these athletes exhibited mean overall mood scores during overtraining that were elevated compared with the nonresponders (156 vs. 128, respectively). There was agreement in 8 of 9 cases (89%) between the physiological and the psychological classification schemes, and this percentage was significantly greater than chance agreement. These and related findings, such as the significant correlation during overtraining between POMS depression scores and resting cortisol (O'Connor et al., 1989) and between POMS overall mood scores and neuromuscular function (Raglin et al., 1996) lend support to the idea that mood states are related to physiological alterations that occur with overtraining.

Titrating Training Based On Mood Appears To Prevent Staleness

Two independent investigations using longitudinal paradigms have reported that the titration of training load based on mood responses to training was associated with a lack of athletic staleness. Berglund and Säfström (1994) administered the Swedish version of the POMS questionnaire to 14 elite canoeists on a weekly basis during 4 months of training preceding the Olympic Games. Weekly training was *reduced* for those athletes who showed both an overall POMS score that was elevated by more than 50% above their preseason baseline and a POMS fatigue score that was greater than the vigor score. These athletes were considered to be at risk for the development of staleness. Weekly training was *increased* for those athletes with overall POMS scores that were less than 10% above their own preseason overall POMS score. The authors reported that, "Titration of the training stimulus on the basis of POMS scores resulted in none of the canoeists developing signs of staleness in connection with the Olympics" (p. 1036).

Morgan, O'Connor, and Raglin (unpublished observations) provided mood state feedback to the coaches of 40 college swimmers (with the swimmers' consent) during a 17-day overtraining period in which the training volume was increased from 9,000 to approximately 14,000 yards/day. The training was *reduced* in those swimmers who developed overall mood disturbances that were 1.5 standard deviation units above the group average. In contrast, training was *increased* (to an even greater extent) in those swimmers who did not manifest any mood disturbance during overtraining. None of the 40 swimmers was judged to be stale at the time of the conference championships, but over the preceding decade, 12% ($SD = 3.0$) of athletes completing similar training in this same program had been judged as stale. These investigations (Berglund & Säfström, 1994; Morgan et al., unpublished observations) suggest that the titration of training load based on mood responses to training is an effective method of preventing staleness. While these exploratory investigations are promising, definitive conclusions await confirmation via randomized, controlled experimentation.

SUMMARY

There is now an extensive literature documenting that habitual physical activity is associated with positive mental health (Bouchard et al., 1994; Morgan & Goldston, 1987). There is also extensive support for this view throughout this book. Nevertheless, it is well documented that physical activity, when pursued at an excessive level (i.e., overtraining), can lead to mood disturbance. This paradoxical effect has been reviewed in this chapter, and a potential method of avoiding mood disturbances has been presented. Adverse consequences of overtraining such as injury and staleness are ongoing problems because athletes remain interested in achieving maximal performance. Scientific progress aimed at minimizing the problem of staleness will not be optimal until a consensus is reached as to its diagnostic criteria. An attempt has been made in this chapter to make the case that monitoring of mood state responses to training has great potential as a means of preventing staleness. There are several advantages to psychometric monitoring of overtraining. Unlike immune or hormonal assessments, the measurement of mood is relatively easy, inexpensive, and can be accomplished in a brief enough time to be useful to athletes and coaches. In addition, moods are sensitive to both increases and decreases in training volume, and mood responses to training are highly replicable. Limitations in the psychometric monitoring of mood states for the purpose of optimizing training and performance in athletes includes the possibility for response distortion and the lack of specificity. For example, it is possible for athletes to distort responses in order to avoid a rigorous workout if they know that test scores will be used to reduce training. However, the motivation for this is low when athletes recognize that accurate information may help them achieve their ultimate goals. With regard to specificity, depression and other adverse mood states can occur for various reasons, some of which are independent of athletic training. Accordingly, it is important for athletes to communicate with coaches or other professionals about salient life events that may influence their training and performance. Lastly, the arguments made here for the use of psychological monitoring to prevent staleness are not meant to call into question the potential efficacy of physiological markers. Psychobiological monitoring ultimately will provide the most accurate solution to the problem of staleness. Until more is known, however, psychological monitoring warrants attention as a means for the prevention of staleness.

Part Three
Hypothesized Mechanisms

Chapter 10

The Endorphin Hypothesis

Pavel Hoffmann

Aerobic physical activity can induce a sensation of well-being, as well as influence a variety of autonomic functions in the postexercise period. The discovery
of endogenous opioid peptide-containing neurons and opioid receptors in nuclei
of the CNS (where autonomic functions are modulated), as well as the elevation
of endogenous opioids in blood after exercise, has prompted research to elucidate
the role of opioids in behavioral regulation during and after exercise.

Habitual physical activity has been associated with increased physical, psychological, and mental health (Anthony, 1991; Bouchard et al.,1994; Stephens,
1988). Increased well-being, even euphoria, and decreased anxiety in the immediate postexercise period has also been reported (Farrell et al., 1987; Janal, Colt,
Clark, & Glusman, 1984; Raglin & Morgan, 1987). These postexercise effects
were found to be inhibited by naloxone (Janal et al., 1984) and further, the
increase in plasma β-endorphin levels during long distance running was correlated to the change in feeling of pleasantness after running (Wildmann, Krüger,
Schmole, Niemann & Matthaei, 1986). Thus, these effects have often been
referred to as "endorphin calm" or "joggers high." However, the positive mood
changes after exercise have not always been naloxone-reversible, and they have
often not been correlated to peripheral β-endorphin levels (Hatfield, Goldfarb,
Sforzo, & Flynn, 1987; Kraemer, Dzewaltowski, Blair, Rinehardt & Castracane,
1990; McGowan et al., 1993).

Animal studies have provided more direct evidence for activation of endogenous opioid systems by long-lasting exercise. Blake, Stein, and Vomachka (1984)
demonstrated an increased level of β-endorphin in specific brain regions, and an

This work was generously supported by Centrum för Idrottsforskning (CIF, no. 58/94) and by
the Swedish MRC (no. 4764 and 2855).

altered central opioid receptor occupancy after exercise in rats has been reported by several investigators (Christie & Chesher, 1983; Sforzo, Seeger, Pert, Pert, & Dotson, 1986). In recent studies from our laboratory an increased cerebrospinal fluid (CSF) β-endorphin concentration and an increased CSF dynorphin-converting enzyme activity has been shown after spontaneous running exercise in rats (Hoffmann, Terenius, & Thoren, 1990; Persson et al., 1993).

Yao, Andersson, and Thoren (1982a, 1982b) reported a poststimulatory analgesia and reduction in blood pressure in response to stimulation of the sciatic nerve in the spontaneously hypertensive rat (SHR). Interestingly, although it was not quantified, these investigators also described a behavioral calm after the sciatic nerve stimulation. These effects are similar to those seen after termination of exercise and thus suggest that the postexercise physiologic effects, including the "joggers high," may be elicited by afferent nerve signals from receptors in contracting skeletal muscles. Electrically induced, rhythmic contractions of skeletal muscles in rats also induce a poststimulatory reduction in spontaneous activity and calm, and these effects can be reversed by naloxone, thus suggesting an involvement of endogenous opioid systems (Hoffmann, Skarphedinsson, & Thoren, 1990).

The following key points are addressed in this chapter: (a) evidence suggesting the activation of circulating and CNS endogenous opioids by exercise; (b) involvement of endogenous opioid systems in exercise-elicited behavioral effects; (c) the fact that some opioid receptors are poorly antagonized by naloxone, which may explain why some investigators do not corroborate the involvement of endogenous opioids in exercise; (d) absence of support for the assumption that plasma opioid concentrations reflect changes in CNS opioid activity; and (e) evidence suggesting that prolonged rhythmic exercise can activate central opioid systems by triggering increased discharge from mechanosensitive afferent nerve fibers (Group III or A-delta) arising from contracting skeletal muscles.

ENDOGENOUS OPIOID SYSTEMS

Opiates have been used for thousands of years and their analgesic, euphoric, and addictive effects have been the subject of intense research throughout this century. Our understanding of the mechanism of action of opiates was greatly advanced by the discovery of the endogenous opioid receptors and peptides in the mid-1970s. Since then, research in this field has not only resulted in the identification of multiple peripheral and central endogenous opioid peptides and several opioid receptors, but also a wide range of biological functions has been suggested. Although they are in most situations "silent," unless challenged by a variety of stressors, the endogenous opioid peptides are considered to play an important role as neurotransmitters, neuromodulators, and hormones.

Being endogenous analogues of "opiates," the first (and most) studied role of endogenous opioid peptides was in analgesia and behavioral and affective disorders. Endogenous opioid systems also seem to be involved in addiction, cardiovascular regulation, respiration, appetite and thirst, gastrointestinal activity, renal function, temperature regulation, metabolism, hormonal secretion, reproduction, immunity, learning, and memory.

Endogenous Opioid Peptides

There are three major precursor molecules (or prohormones), stemming from separate genes, that give rise to three "families" of opioid peptides. An overview of each is presented in this section.

Pro-opiomelanocortin   When cleaved, pro-opiomelanocortin gives rise to several hormones with various functions. Thus, ACTH and three melanocyte-stimulating hormone (MSH)–like peptides possess nonopioid functions whereas β-endorphin has opioid activity (Akil et al., 1984). The location of β-endorphin–containing nerve cells within the CNS is distinct and limited to two major sites. The first is located in the arcuate nucleus in the hypothalamus and the second is found in the nucleus tractus solitarius in the brainstem. The β-endorphin–containing neurons in the arcuate nucleus have extensive projections throughout the brain, innervating many hypothalamic and limbic structures, periventricular thalamus, periaqueductal gray and the brainstem. From the nucleus tractus solitarius, the ventrolateral medulla is innervated (Khachaturian, Lewis, Schäfer, & Watson, 1985).

A second, independently regulated β-endorphin–containing system is found in the anterior and intermediate pituitary, where both β-endorphin, melanocyte-stimulating hormone, and ACTH are synthesized in corticotrophic cells and co-released into the systemic circulation. β-endorphin has also been found in peripheral tissues, mainly in the gastrointestinal tract (Hedner & Cassuto, 1987).

Proenkephalin   This precursor contains the sequence for seven opioid peptides with the enkephalin active core, four of which are met-enkephalin and one is leu-enkephalin. Proenkephalin-containing perikarya are distributed widely throughout the CNS and enkephalins are present at all levels of the neuraxis, from the cortex to the spinal cord (Akil et al., 1984). The enkephalinergic neurons mainly form short projections (Khachaturian et al., 1985), but their wide distribution gives the enkephalins the potential to influence a variety of CNS functions. Peripherally, enkephalins are present in several autonomic ganglia, such as the superior cervical, the mesenteric, and celiac ganglion. Enkephalins are also found in the adrenal medulla, where they are co-stored and released with the catecholamines in the gastrointestinal tract and in the heart and blood vessels (Hedner & Cassuto, 1987).

Prodynorphin   Prodynorphin yields several opioid peptides. Dynorphin is also widely distributed at largely all levels within the CNS. Thus, among other CNS nuclei, the striatum, amygdala, several hypothalamic nuclei, midbrain periaqueductal gray, brainstem nucleus tractus solitarius, and the spinal cord dorsal horn contain dynorphin perikarya (Khachaturian et al., 1985). Dynorphins are also present in the posterior lobe of the pituitary gland and in the gastrointestinal tract (Hedner & Cassuto, 1987).

In addition to the endogenous opioid peptides described, other peptides with less well-defined opioid activity are also derived from the three prohormones. Further, another group of opioid peptides is generated by hydrolysis of proteins derived from nonneuronal tissue. For instance, mitochondrial cytochrome gives rise to cytochrophins and hemoglobin to the hemorphins.

Opioid Receptors

The endogenous opioid peptides exert their function through stereospecific binding to membrane-bound receptors. As many as nine types of opioid receptors have been described but only three of these are widely accepted, the μ, δ, and κ receptors. Like the endogenous opioid peptides, the opioid receptors are distributed throughout the neuraxis, theoretically being able to influence several types of autonomic functions. Attempts have been made to correlate certain endogenous opioid peptides with a receptor, and it is considered that β-endorphin has high affinity to μ and δ receptors. The enkephalins preferentially bind to the δ receptor whereas dynorphin has highest affinity to the κ receptor. However, different peptides from the different precursor families can bind to μ, δ, or κ receptors (Mansour, Khachaturian, Lewis, Akil, & Watson, 1988).

μ **Receptor** The classical μ-receptor–mediated effects are analgesia, respiratory depression, bradycardia, miosis, hypothermia, and behavioral indifference and dependence; and the existence of multiple μ receptors has been suggested. The endogenous ligand with highest affinity to the μ receptor is β-endorphin, but met-enkephalin and some of its extended forms may also be agonists at this site. μ Receptors are present in several brain nuclei involved in pain perception, sensory integration, and autonomic nervous system control, including the neocortex, thalamus, hypothalamus, periaqueductal gray, locus coeruleus, raphe nuclei, and nucleus tractus solitarius, as well as in the dorsal horn of the spinal cord (Mansour et al., 1988). In the periphery, μ receptors are widely distributed, especially in the gastrointestinal tract (Hedner & Cassuto, 1987).

δ **Receptor** The endogenous opioid agonists for this receptor are leu- and met-enkephalin and β-endorphin. The δ receptor is thought to be involved in spinal analgesia and behavioral regulation (Jaffe & Martin, 1985). In the brain, δ receptors are found in the neocortex, nucleus caudatus, putamen, and amygdala, thus being rather restricted to the telencephalon (Mansour et al., 1988). In the spinal cord, δ receptors are present in the dorsal horn. The δ receptor is also present in peripheral organs, including the gastrointestinal system, sympathetic ganglia, and blood vessels (Hedner & Cassuto, 1987).

κ **Receptor**   The endogenous ligands for this receptor are preferentially dynorphins, and κ receptors are involved in mediation of spinal analgesia, cardiovascular effects, and sedation (Jaffe & Martin, 1985). A subclassification of this receptor has also been suggested. Within the CNS, κ-receptor binding occurs in the thalamus, hypothalamus, median eminence, caudate-putamen, amygdala, periaqueductal gray, raphe nuclei, locus coeruleus, nucleus tractus solitarius, and dorsal horn of the spinal cord (Mansour et al., 1988). This receptor is also widely distributed in the periphery, including sympathetic ganglia, the adrenal medulla, the heart and arteries, and the gut (Hedner & Cassuto, 1987).

Synthetic Opioid Receptor Agonists and Antagonists

The problem of opiates giving rise to addiction has prompted a search for analgesic drugs devoid of this side effect. Research has resulted in relatively pure antagonists like naloxone, antagonizing all opioid-mediated effects of morphine. Subsequently, actions of different drugs were regarded as opiate-like if they were antagonized by naloxone or naltrexone, and researchers have also tried to synthesize "pure" or "selective" agonists and antagonists for the respective receptor subtypes.

The most widely used antagonist is naloxone, which has high affinity to μ receptors, although doses 10 to 20 times those required to block the μ receptor also block δ and κ opioid receptors (Paterson, Robson, & Kosterlitz, 1983). In addition, when administered peripherally, naloxone penetrates rapidly into the brain and has a fast onset as antagonist. Generally, in the literature, higher doses of naloxone are required to antagonize effects of endogenously released opioid peptides compared with exogenously administered agonists, possibly depending on more favorable affinity, concentration, or proximity. However, some responses to high doses of naloxone may not be opioid receptor–mediated. Thus, naloxone can influence pharmacological responses to some nonopioid drugs, including those interacting with dopaminergic and GABAergic systems.

Reversal of Physiological Adjustments
To Physical Activity by Opioid Receptor Antagonists

A commonly used experimental strategy to study the involvement of endogenous opioid systems in physical activity has been to determine whether the physiological adaptations to exercise are altered by administration of naloxone or other opioid receptor antagonists. The following presentation focuses mainly on the behavioral effects, but several other areas, such as the effects on cardiovascular and respiratory regulation, hormonal secretion, thermoregulation, pain perception, and appetite and thirst have also been studied. While many authors have found opioid-mediated effects, it must be remembered that many studies in both humans and animals indicate that metabolic, endocrine, and thermoregulatory adjustments to exercise are not influenced by naloxone treatment.

The failure of naloxone to alter the various physiological responses to muscle exercise consistently may depend on the use of different types of physical activity, different levels of VO_2max, different doses of naloxone, and the interaction with various types of opioid receptors. In general, the involvement of endogenous opioid peptides appears to increase with increasing intensities of physical activity.

OPIOID SYSTEMS AND BEHAVIOR

Morphine was named after the Greek god of dreams, Morpheus, and dreamlike changes in mood, euphoria, drowsiness, and mental clouding are among its most pronounced effects. Following the discovery of the endogenous opioids, attempts were made to find connections between several types of behavioral disorders and mental illnesses and endogenous opioid peptides. In alcoholism and drug addiction, the opioid involvement is relatively well established, while our knowledge of the relationship between other behavioral disorders and endogenous opioid peptides is still very limited. In addition, many ordinary behaviors seen in normal subjects or animals, such as drinking, eating and feeding, aggression or defeat, motor activity, grooming, and sniffing, have been coupled to endogenous opioids.

A certain tonic endogenous opioid influence on mood seems to be present, because naloxone and naltrexone induce dysphoria in normal subjects (Cohen, Cohen, Pickar, Weingartner, & Murphy, 1983; File & Silverstone, 1981; Grevert, Albert, Intarrisi, & Goldstein, 1983; Judd, Janowsky, Segal, & Huey, 1980), although Malcolm, Mahlen, O'Neil, Von, and Dickerson (1987) did not find any effects. Further, stress can influence behavioral parameters via the endogenous opioid systems (Katoh, Nabeshima, & Kameyama, 1990). When mobilized, endogenous opioids participate in the modulation of general and locomotor activity, although the reported effects vary depending on type and dose of the agonist, the species, and the type of test. The behaviors are often, but not always, mediated by a mesolimbic opioid-dopaminergic connection (Calenco-Choukroun, Dauge, Gacel, & Roques, 1991).

Thus, naloxone decreases or has no effect on general or exploratory activity in rats and mice (Benton, Brain, & Brain, 1984; Walker, Berntson, Paulucci, & Champney, 1981). Spontaneous locomotor activity is increased by morphine and β-endorphin in mice and rats (Spanagel, Herz, Bals-Kubik, & Shippenberg, 1991; Volterra, Brunello, Cagiano, Cuomo, & Racagni, 1984), while β-endorphin has been reported to decrease ambulation in an open-field test (Weisner & Moss, 1986). Increased enkephalin levels enhance different types of motor behaviors (Heidbreder, Gewiss, Lallemand, Rogues, & DeWitte, 1992; Michael-Titus et al., 1989). The κ agonists dynorphin and U-50,488 both either decrease or increase motor activity (Bot, Chahl, Brent, & Johnston, 1992; Kavaliers & Innes, 1987), and the suppression of motility after stress is potentiated by κ agonists and inhibited by MR 2266 BS (Nabeshima, Kamei, & Kameyama, 1988).

In rats and cats, experimentally elicited aggressive and defensive behaviors can be reduced by different μ agonists and induced again by subsequent naloxone treatment (Brutus, Zuabi, & Siegel, 1988; Giraud, Cervo, Grignaschi, & Samanin, 1989; Shaikh, Lu, & Siegel, 1991); and in mice, both naloxone and the δ antagonist ICI 154,129 increased the incidence of defensive postures (Brain, Brain, & Benton, 1985). In monkeys, grooming as a social contact and reward releases CNS opioids (Keverne, Martensz, & Tuite, 1989), while naloxone treatment decreases social interaction (Martel, Nevison, Rayment, Simpson, & Keverne, 1993).

ACTIVATION OF ENDOGENOUS OPIOID SYSTEMS BY PHYSICAL ACTIVITY

Is there any evidence in support of the activation of endogenous opioid systems by physical activity? Many investigators have examined opioid concentrations in the plasma of both humans and animals before, during, and after exercise in an effort to answer this question. A few researchers have also attempted to measure levels of endogenous opioid peptides or receptor occupancy in the brain after physical activity in laboratory animals.

Concentrations of Opioid Peptides in Peripheral Blood After Physical Activity

The co-release of β-endorphin with the stress hormone ACTH from the anterior pituitary led early to the assumption that levels of circulating β-endorphin would increase in response to physical activity, and this has been confirmed in several human and animal studies. Forced prolonged swimming or acute running in trained or untrained rats increases plasma β-endorphin levels (Sforzo et al., 1986; Metzger & Stein, 1984), but plasma β-endorphin is also increased after voluntary running in wheels (Bittikofer-Griffin & Ely, 1987). In humans, mild or moderate aerobic exercise (<60% of VO_2max) only leads to minor changes in circulating β-endorphin (De Meirleir et al., 1986; Donevan & Andrew, 1987; Goldfarb, Hatfield, Armstrong, & Potts, 1990; Goldfarb, Hatfield, Potts, & Armstrong, 1991; Langenfeld, Hart, & Kao, 1987). After increased exercise intensity, regardless of the type of exercise performed, virtually all investigators report elevated plasma β-endorphin levels (De Meirleir et al., 1986; Donevan & Andrew, 1987; Goldfarb et al., 1990, 1991; Hatfield et al., 1987; Mougin et al., 1988; Olehansky, Zoltick, Herman, Mougey, & Meyerhoff, 1990). In most of these studies, peak values are reached within 15 min postexercise, and 1 hour after termination of exercise the β-endorphin levels have returned to preexercise control.

The response to exercise of circulating met- and leu-enkephalin, mainly released from the adrenals, has also been measured, but investigators have failed consistently to detect significant changes (Farrell et al., 1987; Kraemer, Armstrong, Marchitelli, Hubbard, & Leva, 1987; Mougin et al., 1987), although Jaskowski, Jackson, Raven, and Caffrey (1989) reported delayed disappearance of enkephalin *in vitro* in blood from trained subjects and after an exercise test.

Interestingly, long distance running has also been shown to increase plasma levels of immunoreactive hemorphin, and further, this increase was correlated to the increase in β-endorphin levels (Glämsta, Mθrkrid, Lantz, & Nyberg, 1993). Most of the β-endorphin measured in peripheral blood reflects a co-release with ACTH from the adenohypophysis rather than an increased hypothalamic-brainstem β-endorphin activity. In agreement with this finding, several investigators have reported a concomitant secretion of β-endorphin and ACTH after exercise (De Meirleir et al., 1986; Olehansky et al., 1990; Schwarz & Kindermann, 1990), and emotional stress may contribute to the rise in β-endorphin levels (Oltras, Mora, & Vives, 1987). Further doubt concerning the role of circulating opioids in CNS responses to physical activity is added by the lack of correlation between postexercise levels of endorphin and enkephalin and reported changes in mood, anxiety, and pain perception (Farrell et al., 1987; Hatfield et al., 1987; Heller et al., 1987), although Wildmann et al. (1986) found a correlation between changes in mood and plasma β-endorphin. Stress- or exercise-induced increases in plasma β-endorphin and ACTH are often not associated with increases in brain endorphin concentrations (Barta & Yashpal, 1981; Metzger & Stein, 1984; Sforzo et al., 1986). Additionally, the blood-brain barrier is fairly impermeable to circulating peptides, emphasizing the need for caution when attempting to assess central opioid activity from peripheral plasma opioid levels.

Central Endogenous Opioid Peptide Levels and Receptor Occupancy After Physical Activity

Few studies in experimental animals have, by direct measurement of endogenous opioid peptides or opioid receptor occupancy, addressed the question of whether or not central endogenous opioid systems are activated by physical activity. Unfortunately, most of these studies have used forced exercise, and some have even employed additional stressors such as ice water or extra weight attached to the rats during swimming.

Acute swimming (in warm water) has been reported to increase regional brain levels of immunoassayable β-endorphin, especially in the amygdala, nucleus interstitialis striae terminalis, nucleus raphe dorsalis, and nucleus paraventricularis, while hypophyseal β-endorphin levels were decreased (Barta & Yashpal, 1981). Similar results were reported by Blake et al. (1984), who found an increased content of β-endorphin in the nucleus accumbens and of leu-enkephalin in the ventral tegmentum after treadmill running for 2 hr. After chronic exposure to swimming or treadmill running, the levels were normalized, but they increased again immediately after a new bout of exercise (Barta & Yashpal, 1981; Blake et al., 1984). It has been suggested that during acute physical activity the activation of the opioid system is based mainly on the augmented release of β-endorphin, while in chronic exercise the production of β-endorphin is increased and exceeds the elevated release in hypophysis (Tendzegolskis, Viru, & Orlova, 1991). Acute sprinting for 5 min or chronic sprint training did not alter CNS β-endorphin levels (Metzger & Stein 1984). It has been reported by Radosevich et al. (1989) that CSF β-endorphin was increased during low-intensity exercise, whereas no increase was seen during high-intensity treadmill exercise in dogs.

After acute and chronic swimming, whether or not the mice were swum immediately before being killed, exogenous CNS leu-enkephalin binding was decreased, indicating an increased receptor occupancy by endogenous opioid peptides (Christie & Chesher, 1983; Christie, Chesher, & Bird, 1981). Sforzo et al. (1986) demonstrated, using an *in vivo* technique, decreased receptor binding by endogenous opioid peptides after 1 to 2 hr of weighted swimming in rats.

Taken together, these studies indicate an activation of CNS opioid systems after prolonged exercise but not after short-lasting, high-intensity running.

In our laboratory we have used a rat exercise model in which the running was completely voluntary. A wheel was attached to one side of each exercise group cage, to which the rat had free access. SHRs develop a completely voluntary running behavior during 3 to 5 weeks, reaching a maximum of about 5 km per 24 hr. The unique advantage of the model is that the running is spontaneous, therefore reducing any external influences and stress. Other exercise techniques (forced swimming, exercise on a treadmill or in electric wheels) will no doubt induce mental stress, which in turn may influence behavioral responses or endogenous opioid systems. After 5 to 6 weeks of voluntary exercise in SHRs, the immunoreactive β-endorphin CSF sampling concentration was significantly increased in runners compared with controls not given the opportunity to run (Hoffmann, Terenius, & Thoren, 1990). Interestingly, the cerebrospinal fluid β-endorphin concentration was still increased in SHRs that had their running wheel locked for 24 or 48 hr before CSF sampling, while 96 hr after the last exercise session, the β-endorphin concentration had returned to a level similar to that of the controls. This long-lasting increase in cerebrospinal fluid β-endorphin concentration is most interesting, because it has been suggested previously that altered opioid receptor occupancy in response to any type of experimental intervention is normalized within 60 to 120 min.

If the increased CSF concentration of immunoreactive β-endorphin reflects an elevation of opioid peptide release, this does not necessarily indicate an increased receptor activation. For instance, an opioid receptor desensitization and a reduction in receptor number after chronic agonist treatment has been shown. However, in rats exercised on a treadmill for 5 months, only a minor decrease in number of receptors and no change in affinity to β-endorphin were found (Houghten, Pratt, Young, Brown, & Spann, 1986). Thus, our findings probably reflect an increased receptor activation, especially because rats chronically exercised in the same model exhibit a naloxone-sensitive postexercise analgesia and a drop in blood pressure (Shyu, Andersson, & Thoren, 1982; Shyu & Thoren, 1986). The effect of running on CSF β-endorphin does not seem to be specific for the SHR strain. Thus, preliminary unpublished results indicate that a similar increase in CSF β-endorphin levels after voluntary exercise is also seen in normotensive rats (Daneryd & Hoffmann, unpublished observations).

In another exercise study using the same model we measured the activity of dynorphin-converting enzyme in CSF. Dynorphin-converting enzyme transforms the members of the dynorphin family of opioid peptides into leu-enkephalin-Arg[6]. The rats that were running had a dynorphin-converting enzyme activity in CSF that was 6 to 12 times higher than in sedentary control rats (Persson et al., 1993). Further, a significant correlation was found between running activity and dynorphin-converting enzyme activity. The increased dynorphin-converting enzyme activity in CSF most likely mirrors events taking place in the CNS. The increased dynorphin-converting enzyme activity would lead to increased formation of leu-enkephalin-Arg[6] and thus increased activation of δ receptors, and also reduced dynorphin concentration and reduced activation of κ receptors. An altered processing of prodynorphin-derived peptides could result in altered neurotransmission and thereby affect behavioral responses. Interestingly, δ receptors have been implicated in opioid reward mechanisms (Shippenberg, Bals-Kubik, & Herz, 1987).

ENDOGENOUS OPIOID SYSTEMS AND BEHAVIORAL EFFECTS OF EXERCISE

In general, exercise has three separate effects on mood and psychological tension. Thus, with increasing exercise intensity the well-known feelings of exhaustion and fatigue are experienced. This perceived exhaustion has been reported to be unaffected by naloxone (McMurray, Sheps, & Guinan, 1984), although Grossmann et al. (1984) reported a greater perceived effort during naloxone infusion. Grossman et al. (1984) observed a significant increase in ventilatory minute volume during the naloxone condition, and ventilation is known to influence effort sense.

In the immediate postexercise period, an increased sense of well-being, even joy and euphoria and decreased anxiety, has been reported (Dyer & Crouch, 1988; Farrell et al., 1986; Farrell et al., 1987; Janal et al., 1984; King et al., 1989; Moses et al., 1989; Nouri & Beer, 1989; Raglin & Morgan, 1987). Interestingly, somatic symptoms (e.g., EMG) of tension are also reduced after aerobic exercise (deVries, Wiswell, Bulbulian, & Moritani, 1981).

As mentioned previously, euphoric and tension-relieving effects of exercise have often been referred to as "endorphin calm" or "jogger's high." Although many investigators could show that with exercise, mood states became calmer, more relaxed, even tending away from depression and anger, they have often not been correlated to peripheral β-endorphin levels (Hatfield et al., 1987; Kraemer et al., 1990; McGowan et al., 1993), although Gerra et al. (1992) demonstrated higher basal β-endorphin levels and higher absolute postexercise β-endorphin levels in a group of subjects with evidence of anxiety compared with normal subjects. Wildmann et al. (1986) also showed that the increase in plasma β-endorphin level during long distance running was correlated to the change in feeling of pleasantness after running.

The positive mood changes after exercise have not always been naloxone- or naltrexone-reversible (Farrell et al., 1986). However, Janal et al. (1984) reported that naloxone attenuated the elevation in joy and euphoria but did not influence other psychological effects. Further, Allen and Coen (1987) and Daniel, Martin, and Carter (1992) demonstrated that positive mood shifts did not occur following physical activity in subjects pretreated with naltrexone or naloxone. Aerobic fitness and exercise are not only associated with positive psychological effects, but also with improved cardiovascular stress reactivity. Thus, McCubbin, Cheung, Montgomery, Bulbulian, and Wilson (1992) demonstrated that compared with subjects with low aerobic fitness, fit subjects showed lower heart rate reactivity during, and lower blood pressure after, psychological stress testing, and further, that these effects were eliminated by naltrexone.

Animal studies support the finding of decreased anxiety after a program of daily physical activity (Tharp & Carson, 1975). Voluntarily exercised rats, housed in population cages, have also been shown to exhibit less irritable aggression whereas defense against intruders was not decreased (Bittikofer-Griffin & Ely, 1987). Furthermore, habitual physical activity for weeks or months has been associated with improved psychological and mental health (Anthony, 1991; King et al., 1989; Stephens, 1988) and with improved coping ability and faster recovery from subjective anxiety (Brooke & Long, 1987; Moses et al., 1989). In addition, an aerobic exercise program resulted in improvements in depression, anxiety, hostility, and self-efficacy among psychiatrically institutionalized adolescents (Brown, Welsh, Labbé, Vitulli, & Kukarni, 1992). Interestingly, interruption of established exercise habits has negative effects on mood, and exercise may even become a compulsive behavior, leading to "dependence" (De Coverley Veale, 1987). However, there only appears to be one study that has examined the endogenous opioid peptide involvement in the chronic behavioral effects of exercise in humans. Thus, endurance training, consisting of jogging three times a week over 8 months, appeared to decrease resting plasma β-endorphin concentrations and depression scores in nonclinical depression in middle-aged men (Lobstein & Rasmussen, 1991). However, these investigators did not test the cause-and-effect relationship between the two variables.

Although not within the domain of this chapter, two hypothetically interesting points should be mentioned. First is the potential clinical implication of physical activity in the treatment of drug addiction and anorexia nervosa. That the endogenous opioids are linked to opiate addiction is rather obvious, but alcohol can also affect central endogenous opioid systems and neurotransmitters involved in morphine abstinence, and generally, opioid agonists increase and antagonists decrease experimental alcohol drinking. Clinically, naloxone can "awaken" patients who are somnolent due to alcohol intoxication (Lyon & Antony, 1982). This raises the interesting and clinically important question of whether or not a program of physical activity, together with other interventions, might facilitate the conversion of the addict from dependence on alcohol or exogenous opiates to an "endogenous endorphinist" (Thoren, Floras, Hoffmann, & Seals, 1990). Second, fasting in rats can induce changes in central opioid systems that result in an increased pain threshold and decreased blood pressure, and rat strains that normally do not exercise spontaneously will run up to 8 km per day when they are deprived of 10% of their normal food intake (Russell, Epling, Pierce, Amy, & Boer, 1987). Involvement of endogenous opioids in anorexia nervosa has been suggested by several investigators and excessive levels of opioids may be associated with several clinical symptoms of anorexia. However, clinical data are not straightforward because both increased and decreased opioid activity has been reported in patients with anorexia nervosa (Kaye et al., 1987), and opioid agonists stimulate while antagonists reduce food intake (Atkinson, 1987). Thus, physical activity might counter the effects of anorexia by restoring central opioid levels, or it could reinforce anorectic behavior by substituting exercise for fasting as a mechanism for opioid activation (Thoren et al. 1990).

In order to elucidate whether exercise could alter locomotor and aggressive behavior, we studied the effects of voluntary running in the SHR. In addition to being hypertensive, SHRs also provide a hyperactive as well as a hyperreactive animal model. Thus, several behavioral parameters were affected by physical activity, suggesting in general a reduction of the reported hyperactivity (Hoffmann, Thoren, & Ely, 1987). Exercise reduced the hyperactivity in the SHR almost to the level seen in the normotensive and normally active Wistar Kyoto rat. Parallel to the decreased exploratory activity, there was a tendency for decreased aggressive behavior in the runners. This was reversed when the running wheels were locked, after which the rats showed a pronounced increase in aggression. This hyperaggressiveness was not evident 2 days after the last night of exercise, but it was present 3 and 6 days postexercise, and then declined again to the level of the control SHR. The late onset and prolonged time course of the increased aggression after termination of exercise resembles an abstinence reaction to morphine withdrawal. Further, the delayed and protracted effect on aggression present in rats abstinent from running is consistent with the prolonged CNS β-endorphin activation previously described (Hoffmann, Terenius, & Thoren, 1990). Interestingly, the abstinence-like behavior was developed 4 days after termination of physical activity, simultaneously with the decline in central β-endorphin concentration. After termination of exercise, locomotor activity was also increased to the level of the control rats, although no further increase in any of the parameters measured was seen. However, the runners showed a type of displaced aggression, exhibited as digging, scratching, and biting in the home cage and open-field apparatus. This is in agreement with the results of Christie and Chesher (1982), who reported that naloxone elicited a withdrawal-like reaction in physically trained mice following exercise deprivation.

ARE OPIOID-MEDIATED EFFECTS OF EXERCISE ELICITED BY ACTIVATION OF AFFERENT NERVES FROM CONTRACTING MUSCLES?

The increase in blood pressure during static or dynamic muscle contraction has been called the *exercise pressor reflex*, which is only seen if Group III or Group IV muscle afferents are activated (Mitchell & Schmidt, 1983). These afferents respond to muscle stretch and contraction, and for this reason, Kniffki, Mense, and Schmidt (1981) termed the endings of these afferents "ergoreceptors." The *postexercise* cardiovascular effects can also be simulated by stimulation of afferent nerves. Prolonged, low-frequency stimulation of the intact sciatic nerve in conscious rats has been shown to result in a depressor response, bradycardia, and decreased splanchnic sympathetic activity lasting over 10 hours (Yao et al., 1982). The poststimulatory reduction in blood pressure was seen when stimulation intensities activating Group III afferents were used, and the drop in blood pressure after termination of nerve stimulation could be pretreated or reversed by a high dose of naloxone (Yao et al., 1982a, 1982b).

Generally, low-frequency peripheral transcutaneous or direct nerve stimulation is known to induce analgesia (Duranti, Pantaleo, & Bellini, 1988), and the analgesia to this type of peripheral nerve stimulation is considered to be mediated via Group III afferents (Kawakita & Funakoshi, 1982). Yao et al. (1982b) also reported a poststimulatory analgesia in response to stimulation of the sciatic nerve, using the same stimulation parameters as those that evoked the reduction in mean arterial pressure and heart rate. Interestingly, the poststimulatory analgesia lasted about 2 hours, and it was reversed by intravenous naloxone (1 mg/kg), as compared with the 10 hr and 15 mg/kg of naloxone required to reverse the cardiovascular depressor response, which suggests that different opioid systems are involved in the respective effects. Further, although it was not quantified, Yao et al. (1982a) also described a behavioral depression after the sciatic nerve stimulation.

In a set of experiments the effect of electrical muscle stimulation was studied in awake rats on behavior and also on blood pressure and pain threshold. The gastrocnemius muscles of one leg were stimulated for a total of 60 minutes. The intensity of the electric pulses was raised slowly to reach a maximum after 30 to 45 min of stimulation. Initially, the stimulation elicited only weak muscle twitches, while toward the end of stimulation powerful, dynamic muscle contractions were seen. In general, after cessation of the electrical stimulation of the gastrocnemius muscle a rapidly developing, long-lasting reduction in blood pressure was seen. The lowered blood pressure was accompanied by a behavioral calm with a markedly reduced spontaneous activity. An increase in pain threshold was also seen (Hoffmann, Carlsson, & Thoren, 1990). The effects are thus very similar to those seen after termination of exercise in humans or in laboratory animals.

The results show that electrically induced, rhythmic contractions of skeletal muscles induce a long-lasting, poststimulatory reduction in spontaneous activity and calm, and the time course of the behavioral calm seems to parallel the reduction in blood pressure. After termination of stimulation, sniffing, grooming, locomotor activity, and the total time the rats were active were all reduced compared with pre-stimulatory control levels, as well as with nonstimulated controls. Although the rats were calm, quiet, and rarely moved after the stimulation, they were easily and immediately aroused by any external stimulus. If they were left alone after such arousal, they slowly calmed down and returned to sleep. The poststimulatory sedation and decreased motor activity could also be influenced by opioid receptor antagonists. Thus, all behavioral effects studied were reversed toward pre-stimulatory control levels by high doses of naloxone, 15 mg/kg, while lower doses had no significant effect. When studying selective opioid receptor antagonists, the δ receptor antagonist ICI 154,129 did not significantly influence any of the behavioral parameters measured, whereas the κ receptor antagonist MR 2266 BS significantly increased the behavioral activity to almost pre-stimulatory levels. Pretreatment with the μ receptor antagonist β-Funaltrexamine did not significantly influence the poststimulatory depression in activity, further supporting the involvement of the κ receptor in the behavioral response to muscle stimulation (Hoffmann, Skarphedinsson, & Thoren, 1990). Interestingly, the poststimulatory reduction in blood pressure was also mediated by the κ receptor, while the analgesia was μ receptor mediated. The κ receptor is rather insensitive to naloxone, which may explain why several investigators have failed to influence the behavioral effects seen after termination of aerobic exercise, with low doses of naloxone.

CONCLUSION

The discovery of endogenous opioid peptides and their receptors 20 years ago gave rise to research on the role of these peptides in the autonomic and psychologic effects of physical activity. The animal and human experimental data reviewed in this chapter strongly indicate an activation of endogenous opioids by long-duration aerobic exercise and their involvement in the effects described.

It is suggested that some of the controversy in this area has arisen from the assumption that peripheral, plasma β-endorphin concentrations will reflect changes in CNS opioid activity. Indeed, because the blood-brain barrier is rather impermeable to circulating peptides, peripheral concentrations of β-endorphin would not be expected to modify CNS opioid activity. Although peripherally administered opioids can produce behavioral effects, these are seen when the opioid peptides are used in pharmacological doses.

Another commonly used experimental strategy has been to determine whether the physiological adjustments to physical activity are altered following administration of naloxone. The failure of naloxone to consistently alter the responses to exercise may be due to the use of low doses in some investigations. Thus, it can be hypothesized that higher doses of naloxone are required to antagonize the effects of endogenous opioid peptides than are required to antagonize the effects of exogenously administered opioid analogues. Further, higher doses are required to antagonize the effects mediated by the opioid δ and κ receptors, whereas the μ receptor is blocked effectively by lower doses.

Evidence is also presented in this chapter supporting the concept that the opioid-mediated effects of aerobic physical activity are elicited by an increased discharge from mechanosensitive nerve fibers arising from contracting skeletal muscles. It must be remembered that the postexercise "endorphin calm" is not an isolated phenomenon. The activation of "ergoreceptors" probably has functional significance in adapting the organism to both exercise and postexercise require-ments. Continued stimulation of ergoreceptors during prolonged aerobic exercise will thus lead to a release of endogenous opioids in the CNS. Increased opioid activation may exert a sympatho-inhibitory influence. With the cessation of exer-cise and its attendant excitatory inputs, the cardiovascular and behavioral effects of prolonged central opioid activation may become manifest, thus explaining the behavioral calm observed during recovery. Postexercise hormone secretion is also influenced, and this may be important in postexercise restoration of energy stores. In addition, the central opioid-mediated increase in pain threshold and sedation is presumably intended to reduce the physical discomfort associated with prolonged, fatiguing exercise. These mechanisms might therefore be of vital importance for improving endurance in the exercising animal and human.

Although the principal hypothesis of this review is that CNS opioid peptides are activated by prolonged exercise, it must be considered that several other transmitter systems such as catecholamines, serotonin, and other neuropeptides have been suggested to participate in the afferent, central, and efferent routes of the physiological adaptations to physical activity. It should also be noted that physiological responses to physical activity may be mediated by other pathways than afferent muscle nerves; i.e., central command and metabolic products, although these different systems probably work in concert to prepare the organ-ism for the demands of exercise.

Chapter 11

The Serotonin Hypothesis

Francis Chaouloff

There is substantial evidence that normal individuals who engage in physical activity experience positive health effects, including both psychological and physiological benefits (Bouchard et al., 1994). Interestingly, part of these positive effects on mood are observed after acute exercise, as is the case for anxiolysis (Morgan, 1987). In addition, physical exertion may also have positive effects in psychiatric patients, as illustrated by its antidepressive outcomes in mildly depressed subjects (chapter 6). Alternatively, excessive exercise (e.g., overtraining) or sudden disruption of a chronic training program may lead to mood disturbances (chapter 9). Taken together, these findings illustrate the tight, albeit complex relationships between exercise and mood. The neural bases for this interaction between exercise and mood are still unknown and only hypotheses can be advanced. Among these hypotheses, that related to a parallelism between the mechanisms underlying the antidepressant/anxiolytic effects of exercise and those involved in the therapeutic properties of "classical" antidepressant/anxiolytic drugs may prove fruitful (Ransford, 1982). In this context, the finding that central serotonergic systems are the targets for numerous antidepressant/anxiolytic compounds (Blier & De Montigny, 1994; Handley & McBlane, 1993) gives a new and promising insight into the relationships between physical activity and mood alterations. However, before assuming that central serotonergic systems play a key role (partly or totally) in the mood-improving effects of physical activity, it is necessary to show that physical activity is a paradigm that affects central serotonergic systems, and that the mood-elevating effects of physical activity can be diminished or prevented by treatments known to selectively affect central serotonergic tone. Actually, data derived from animal and human studies favor the hypothesis that central serotonergic systems are modified by physical activity (Chaouloff, 1989a), and this research literature serves as the

focus of this chapter. On the other hand, studies aimed at measuring the consequences of serotonergic manipulations on mood in exercising humans are still
lacking. Clearly, experiments devoted to this field of research should be encouraged because any conclusion regarding the involvement of serotonergic systems
in the mood-elevating effects of physical activity requires such an experimental
demonstration.

This chapter describes the different data supporting an interaction between
physical activity and central serotonin (5-hydroxytryptamine [5-HT]). To this
end, the first part of the chapter deals with the effects of physical exercise on
brain entry of tryptophan, the precursor in the 5-HT biosynthesis pathway. The
second part brings evidence for stimulatory effects of exercise on the synthesis
and metabolism of 5-HT. The third part of the chapter discusses, through 5-HT
receptor–related data and observations suggesting a stimulatory effect of exercise
on 5-HT release, more recent information related to putative changes in 5-HT
function during exercise. Most of the data provided in this chapter derive from
studies initially carried out with naive control animals (i.e., animals that are not
depressed or anxious) and forced exercise, and therefore, the validity and limitations of this work are discussed as well.

PHYSICAL ACTIVITY AND THE EXTRANEURONAL REGULATION OF 5-HYDROXYTRYPTAMINE SYNTHESIS

Peripheral Determinants of Tryptophan Supply to the Brain

In keeping with the early observations that the synthesis rate of 5-HT is dependent on both the levels of its first precursor, the amino acid tryptophan, and
tryptophan hydroxylase activity (the rate-limiting enzyme in 5-HT biosynthesis), and that tryptophan hydroxylase is not saturated under physiological
situations, it is not surprising that treatments (either physiological or pharmacological) that alter neuronal tryptophan concentration have consequences on
5-HT synthesis (Carlsson & Lindqvist, 1972) (Figure 1). However, because
tryptophan is an essential amino acid and brain proteolysis is of weak importance, brain tryptophan levels are strictly dependent upon the supply of tryptophan from the blood compartment. On that basis, one may assume that
alterations in blood tryptophan levels elicit parallel alterations in brain tryptophan supply, and then in 5-HT synthesis. However, the situation is complicated
by the respective influences of numerous variables (Figure 1). In blood, 9 molecules of tryptophan over 10 are bound to albumin (the remaining tryptophan
fraction being under a "free" form), and this equilibrium between tryptophan
and albumin-bound tryptophan molecules is displaced by circulating FFAs.
Thus, FFAs compete with tryptophan for its binding to albumin (McMenamy,

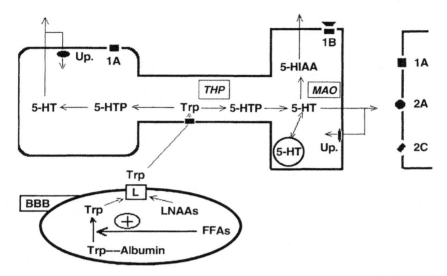

Figure 1 Schematic summary of the different extra- and intraneuronal mechanisms that regulate 5-hydroxytryptamine (HT) biosynthesis, release and/or metabolism. For clarity, only those 5-HT receptors mentioned in the text are indicated. With the exceptions of TPH (tryptophan hydroxylase), Up (5-HT uptake system), and BBB (blood-brain barrier), all abbreviations are defined in the text.

1965). Lipolysis will thereby increase the circulating level of the free form of tryptophan. Beside the impact of lipolysis and albumin on the circulating forms of tryptophan, there is another key determinant in the control of tryptophan supply to the brain, namely large neutral amino acids (LNAAs). These chiefly include the branched-chain amino acids (BCAAs; e.g. valine, leucine) and the aromatic amino acids (e.g., phenylalanine, tyrosine). Because all LNAAs, including tryptophan, compete for their respective entries into the brain at the level of a transporter (namely, the L system) located on the blood-brain barrier, the competition between tryptophan and the other LNAAs has direct influences on brain tryptophan entry, and then 5-HT synthesis (Fernstrom & Wurtman, 1972a). Thus, carbohydrate ingestion (or insulin administration) increases and protein ingestion decreases the supply of tryptophan to the brain by decreasing and increasing, respectively, the competition between tryptophan and the other LNAAs (Fernstrom & Wurtman, 1972b). One additional factor that is to be considered is a general change in blood-brain barrier permeability (via an alteration of the contraction of cerebral microvessels). Although not specific to tryptophan (changes in blood-brain barrier permeability affect brain entry of all LNAAs), this alteration has consequences on 5-HT synthesis. As an illustration, this mechanism partly underlies the enhancement in brain tryptophan supply consecutive to increased sympathetic activity (Chaouloff, 1993). Lastly, another key determinant of tryptophan supply to the brain is the intrinsic concentration of tryptophan (and albumin-bound tryptophan), which is controlled by the activity of tryptophan pyrrolase (Badawy, 1977). This hepatic enzyme, by metabolizing tryptophan in the kynurenine pathway, diminishes blood and tissue levels of tryptophan, which at high concentrations may be toxic. Interestingly, the activity of this enzyme is under the tight positive control of glucocorticoids, which thereby exert a buffering role.

The aforementioned data show that brain tryptophan supply depends on circulating tryptophan levels, circulating levels of competing LNAAs, and the intrinsic properties of both the L system and the blood-brain barrier. The key question is the following: Is it free tryptophan or total (free and albumin-bound) tryptophan that controls brain tryptophan levels? This question is still a matter of debate, and it is pertinent to answer that the identity of the substrate depends on the experimental conditions. For example, stress-induced elevation in brain tryptophan levels following immobilization is due to an increased entry of total tryptophan, whereas starvation-induced increases in brain tryptophan depend on lipolysis, and in turn, increased availability of free tryptophan for its transporter (Chaouloff, 1993).

Physical Activity Increases Tryptophan Supply to the Brain

There is a growing body of evidence in animal and human studies that physical activity affects blood tryptophan disposition. Thus, short-term physical activity increases the blood concentration of free tryptophan both in trained animals (Blomstrand, Perrett, Parry-Billings & Newsholme, 1989; Chaouloff, Elghozi, Guezennec, & Laude, 1985; Chaouloff, Kennett, Serrurier, Merino, & Curzon, 1986) and in humans (Blomstrand, Hassmen, & Newsholme, 1991; Davis et al., 1992; Fischer, Hollmann, & De Meirleir, 1991). Because circulating total tryptophan either slightly decreases or remains stable in these experiments, it is likely that increases in free tryptophan are due solely to lipolysis. Interestingly, the aforementioned selective increases in free, but not total, tryptophan extend to long-term physical activity (e.g., running a marathon) (Blomstrand, Celsing, & Newsholme, 1988; Blomstrand, Hassmen, Ekblom, & Newsholme, 1991; Conlay et al., 1989; Decombaz, Reinhardt, Anantharaman, von Glutz, & Poortmans, 1979). As noted previously, competition for entry into the brain between tryptophan and other LNAAs, especially BCAAs, is a key determinant. Actually, data regarding this subject are contradictory, and animal and human studies have reported *decreased* (Blomstrand et al., 1988; Blomstrand, Hassmen, Ekblom, & Newsholme, 1991; Blomstrand, Hassmen, & Newsholme, 1991; Decombaz et al., 1979), *increased* (Ahlborg, Felig, Hagenfeldt, Hendler, & Wahren, 1974; Blomstrand et al., 1989; Felig & Wahren, 1971; Ji, Miller, Nagle, Lardy, & Stratman, 1987), or *unchanged* BCAAs (Chaouloff et al., 1986; Conlay et al., 1989; Davis et al., 1992). However, in most cases, the ratio of free tryptophan over the sum of the other competing amino acids is increased by physical activity, thereby indicating that exercise increases the relative influx of tryptophan into the brain.

In keeping with the aforementioned acute exercise–induced changes in the blood compartment, it seems obvious that exercise should have a positive influence on brain tryptophan levels in rodents and possibly in humans. Indeed, analyses of whole brains (Chaouloff et al., 1985; Chaouloff et al., 1986), brain regions (Blomstrand et al., 1989; Chaouloff, Laude, & Elghozi, 1989), and CSF samples (Chaouloff, Laude, et al., 1986) from exercising rats confirm the above hypothesis. Nevertheless, one could argue that exercise-induced increases in blood free tryptophan and brain tryptophan are not causally related. For instance, if physical activity increases blood-brain barrier permeability or the intrinsic properties of the L system, brain levels of all amino acids (including tryptophan) are increased independently from exercise-elicited changes in the blood levels of these amino acids. Indeed, the examination of this hypothesis requires an analysis of both blood and brain levels of all LNAAs in exercising animals. This was actually achieved earlier in an investigation demonstrating that neither the blood levels nor the brain levels of most LNAAs (excluding tryptophan) were affected by acute treadmill exercise (Chaouloff, Kennett, et al., 1986). This research also confirmed that physical activity increases both circulating free tryptophan and brain tryptophan. Taken together, these data show that acute physical activity in trained animals does not affect the kinetics of the L system. In addition, because physical activity did not influence the brain influx of amino acids that enter the brain through different transporters, it was concluded that physical activity does not increase blood-brain barrier permeability (Chaouloff, Kennett, et al., 1986a). Clearly, exercise-induced increases in brain tryptophan are due solely to lipolysis and albumin-binding displacement. It now remains to be shown whether the latter evidence in animals applies to humans. Although difficult to confirm directly (for obvious ethical reasons), the fact that lipolysis is also a metabolic feature in exercising humans allows for a parallel between human and animal studies. Because CSF sampling is a technique routinely used by biological psychiatrists, it may be that in the near future some reports showing elevated CSF tryptophan levels following physical activity will be available. In this context, it is noteworthy that CSF sampling in depressed patients who have been exercised has revealed an increased 5-HT metabolism (as assessed by the measure of 5-hydroxyindoleacetic acid [5-HIAA]; Post, Kotin, Goodwin, & Gordon, 1973).

As mentioned earlier, acute running in trained rats does not affect blood-brain barrier permeability. However, it is noteworthy that such an indication applies to basal conditions only. Thus, it was found in one study that pretreatment of exercising rats (at the onset of acute exercise) with the noradrenaline uptake inhibitor desipramine (an antidepressant) markedly amplified running-induced elevations in brain tryptophan. Interestingly, however, this amplification could not be explained by the associated increase in blood free tryptophan (Chaouloff et al., 1985). Because the sympathetic nervous system controls both the blood level of most BCAAs and the permeability of the blood-brain barrier (Chaouloff, 1993), it is likely that in exercising rats displaying a high sympathetic tone, increased lipolysis, decreased competition between BCAAs and tryptophan for entry into the brain, and increased blood-brain barrier permeability account for the increase in brain tryptophan. In this context, it should be noted that we did use desipramine for a pharmacological property different from those mentioned earlier. Thus, it had been reported that desipramine is an inhibitor of tryptophan pyrrolase activity (Badawy & Evans, 1981), and thereby, desipramine-elicited increases in free and total tryptophan provide *in vivo* indices of tryptophan pyrrolase activity. These increases were more pronounced in exercising rats compared with sedentary controls, thus suggesting that exercise activates tryptophan pyrrolase. Such an activation may explain why total tryptophan is decreased in some studies but not in others.

There have been two animal studies designed to analyze whether training affects blood or brain tryptophan responses to an acute treadmill exercise. In the first study a comparison of responses in rats trained for 1 and 8 weeks for a 2-hr run revealed that plasma total tryptophan remained unaffected by training duration and acute exercise. Likewise, training duration did not affect brain tryptophan, but it did diminish the extent to which brain tryptophan rises during acute physical activity (Chaouloff, Laude, Serrurier, et al., 1987). In a second study, the impact of training intensity (duration of training was 11 weeks) on blood and brain tryptophan responses following acute running (to fatigue) was studied (Blomstrand et al., 1989). This investigation revealed that intense training increased both blood free tryptophan and brain tryptophan responses to fatigue, changes that were associated with a decrease in plasma total tryptophan and a marked increase in BCAAs. The apparent contradiction regarding the effects of training on brain tryptophan responses to acute physical activity between the two studies is likely due to differences in the protocols. Thus in the first study, acute exercise was similar in short- and long-term–trained rats, whereas in the second study acute exercise was of higher intensity and longer duration in highly trained rats.

PHYSICAL ACTIVITY AND 5-HYDROXYTRYPTAMINE SYNTHESIS AND METABOLISM

Acute Physical Activity Increases Brain 5-Hydroxytryptamine Synthesis and Metabolism

In keeping with the lack of saturation of tryptophan hydroxylase under physiological conditions, acute exercise-induced increases in brain tryptophan availability stimulate 5-HT synthesis and metabolism. Some investigators (Bailey, Davis & Ahlborn, 1993a; Barchas & Freedman, 1973; Blomstrand et al., 1989; Romanowski & Grabiec, 1974) have reported that acute treadmill exercise increases 5-HT levels either in whole brains or in selective brain regions, but this has not been confirmed by others (Chaouloff et al., 1985; Chaouloff, Laude, Serrurier, et al. 1987; Chaouloff et al., 1989; Heyes, Garnett, & Coates, 1988). Although contradictory at first glance, exercise-induced elevations in brain tryptophan but not in brain 5-HT levels does not exclude the hypothesis of increased 5-HT synthesis. Thus, 90% of assayed tissular 5-HT levels is constituted by neuronal 5-HT that is stored in vesicular stocks whereas the remaining 10% represents the sum of newly synthesized 5-HT molecules in the neurons and 5-HT released in the synaptic clefts. In keeping with the observation that newly synthesized 5-HT is readily metabolized in 5-HIAA, it is not surprising that increases in brain tryptophan that do not exceed 50% lead to marginal changes in tissue 5-HT levels. Conversely, because 5-HIAA molecules are not stocked in the neurons (and thus originate from newly synthesized 5-HT molecules), an analysis of tissue 5-HIAA levels gives a good index of 5-HT metabolism (Figure 1). If the activity of monoamine oxidase (the enzyme that transforms 5-HT into 5-HIAA) is not altered under the experimental conditions, then the analysis of tissue 5-HIAA levels provides also a good index of 5-HT synthesis. Actually, a great majority of animal studies have reported acute running-induced increases in 5-HIAA levels, whether the assays were performed in whole brains, in CSF, or in brain regions (e.g., Bailey et al., 1993a; Blomstrand et al., 1989; Chaouloff et al., 1985; Chaouloff, Laude, et al., 1986; Chaouloff et al., 1989; Heyes et al., 1988). It is interesting to note here that these regional increases in 5-HIAA extend to regions enriched in serotonergic nerve terminals (e.g., hippocampus, striatum, cortex, hypothalamus) as well as the midbrain (which contains the different raphe nuclei where all serotonergic cell bodies are localized). When viewed collectively, these data indicate that acute physical activity in trained animals promotes increases in tryptophan, and then in 5-HT synthesis and metabolism in most serotonergic neurons.

Because acute physical activity leads to the aforementioned changes, it is interesting to examine whether training has any influence per se, and whether training affects 5-HT response to acute exercise. In an early study, Brown et al., (1979) reported that an 8-week training program increased brain 5-HT levels, but such an effect of training was not observed in two subsequent studies (Blomstrand et al., 1989; Chaouloff, Laude, Serrurier, et al., 1987). As far as the relationships between chronic and acute physical activity are concerned, it was observed that acute exercise–elicited increases in brain 5-HIAA levels were less pronounced in rats trained for 8 weeks compared with rats trained for 1 week (Chaouloff, Laude, Serrurier, et al., 1987). Interestingly, acute exercise decreased 5-HT levels in rats trained for 8 weeks, but 5-HT did not change in the rats trained for 1 week (Chaouloff, Laude, Serrurier, et al., 1987). Indeed, this observation may bring a new insight into the relationships between physical activity and central serotonergic systems. In a second study, training intensity did not significantly affect 5-HT and 5-HIAA responses to exercise-elicited fatigue (Blomstrand et al., 1989).

Is There an Imbalance Between Tryptophan Availability and 5-Hydroxytryptamine Synthesis During Exercise?

An examination of the respective amplitudes of acute exercise–elicited increases in tryptophan, 5-HT and 5-HIAA (in studies in which both were measured) reveals that exercise has differential effects on these indoles. Thus, although tryptophan rises are large, those regarding 5-HT (if any) and 5-HIAA are relatively weak. This could suggest that beside the aforementioned effects of exercise on tryptophan, 5-HT, and 5-HIAA, one step in 5-HT biosynthesis is partly inhibited during physical activity. Actually, in one study in which control rats and acutely exercised rats (both being trained to run for the 4 preceding days) were either pretreated with different doses of tryptophan or were food-deprived (to increase tryptophan availability to the brain), it was found that tryptophan utilization toward synthesis of 5-HT and 5-HIAA was diminished by exercise (Chaouloff, Laude, Merino, et al., 1987). Indeed, double reciprocal plots of 5-HT synthesis and metabolism against brain tryptophan concentrations revealed that this effect of exercise was not due to an early saturation of tryptophan hydroxylase, but possibly to an inhibitory effect of exercise (partly through catecholaminergic systems) on the affinity of tryptophan hydroxylase (Chaouloff, Laude, Merina, et al., 1987). In another study, control and acutely exercised rats were pretreated with an inhibitor of 5-hydroxytryptophan (5-HTP) conversion into 5-HT. Under these experimental conditions, 5-HTP accumulates in a time-dependent manner, and this accumulation provides an *in vivo* index of tryptophan hydroxylase activity (Figure 1). Tryptophan hydroxylase activity was found to be diminished in the hippocampus and the striatum, but not in the midbrain of exercising rats (Chaouloff et al., 1989). This result was somewhat surprising because in vehicle-treated rats, hippocampal and striatal 5-HT and 5-HIAA levels were not diminished by exercise, as would be expected from a decrease in tryptophan hydroxylase activity. Conversely, administration of a high dose of tryptophan to control and running rats at the onset of exercise led to marked increases in 5-HT and 5-HIAA levels, the amplitudes of which were diminished in the hippocampus and the striatum of exercising rats (Chaouloff et al., 1989). The dose of tryptophan brought about huge but identical brain tryptophan levels in controls and runners.

These experiments suggest that the imbalance between marked brain tryptophan increases and weak increases in 5-HT synthesis and metabolism could be due to some inhibitory effects of exercise on tryptophan hydroxylase (through early 5-HT release, and in turn, autoreceptor-mediated feedback inhibition?). However, this is only one hypothesis that needs to be checked through appropriate *in vitro* techniques. Thus, all of these experiments rely on pharmacological approaches that suppose that the availability of the different drugs to their targets or that the pharmacokinetics of these are not different between control and exercising rats. The former hypothesis warrants more precise investigation because important variables such as the release of glucocorticoids, which affect drug metabolism and blood flow (which affects drug availability at its target), are affected by exercise. Furthermore, the observation that acute exercise to exhaustion increases plasma tetrahydrobiopterin (the cofactor for tryptophan hydroxylase) transiently in human subjects (Mizutani, Hashimoto, Ohta, Nakazawa, & Nagatsu, 1994) underlines the need for future investigation.

PHYSICAL ACTIVITY
AND 5-HYDROXYTRYPTAMINE RELEASE

As indicated in the previous section, there are numerous data in favor of an acute effect of exercise on 5-HT synthesis and metabolism. However, the most important matter concerns the functional relationships between exercise and 5-HT. Thus, if physical activity alters psychological or physiological functions, or both, through 5-HT–dependent mechanisms, it follows that exercise modifies 5-HT release in the synaptic cleft or in 5-HT receptor functions. As far as 5-HT release during physical activity is concerned, the aforementioned observation of exercise-elicited increases in 5-HT synthesis could indicate at first glance that physical activity actually increases 5-HT release. Unfortunately, the relationship between synthesis and release is not so straightforward, and past analyses of this relationship have led to controversy. Although available data suggest that reductions in synthesis lead to reductions in evoked release (Gartside, Cowen, & Sharp, 1992; Marsden, Conti, Strope, Curzon, & Adams, 1979), this relationship is not so clear-cut when synthesis of 5-HT is increased (see Kuhn, Wolf, & Youdim, 1986). Thus, some studies have reported increases in basal 5-HT release following tryptophan administration whereas other studies have shown that this happens only when the neuronal firing rate is increased (e.g. during particular stressful conditions), or when animals are pretreated with a monoamine oxidase inhibitor (to avoid intraneuronal metabolism of 5-HT into 5-HIAA; Figure 1). A good illustration of this uncertainty regarding synthesis-release relationships is provided by stress studies (Chaouloff, 1993). For instance, it has been claimed that some stressors (e.g., immobilization) promote increased 5-HT release through increases in synthesis. Conversely, other stressors (e.g. footshocks, insulin administration) have been claimed to enhance release independently from changes in tryptophan and synthesis. Indeed, it has been suggested that in these models stress increases tryptophan availability to the neurons (and then synthesis of 5-HT) to avoid release-induced depletion of 5-HT from serotonergic neurons. This view is confirmed by the observation that increases in 5-HT release happen within a few minutes after the onset of stress, whereas increases in tryptophan availability (and then synthesis of 5-HT) are not observed until 1 to 2 hours after stress onset (Chaouloff, 1993).

What about release of 5-HT during physical activity? While data related to the direct measurement of 5-HT release during physical activity are lacking, the following observations are worthy of mention. First, treadmill locomotion elevates 5-HT neuronal activity in the raphe obscurus of the trained cat (Jacobs & Fornal, 1993), thereby indicating that exercise increases neuronal activity in some serotonergic cell bodies. However, it remains to be shown whether this increase promotes 5-HT release from serotonergic cell bodies (and possibly, from some nerve terminals). This is important because acute administration of numerous serotonergic antidepressants has been shown to elicit a marked release of 5-HT from serotonergic cell bodies, as compared with that measured at nerve terminals (Artigas, 1993). Such a result would also support the hypothesis that besides catecholaminergic systems, 5-HT itself (through autoreceptor-mediated mechanisms) participates in the inhibition of tryptophan hydroxylase during physical activity. Second, an increase in extracellular 5-HT concentrations in the cerebral cortex of walking rats has been reported (Kurosawa, Okada, Sato, & Uchida, 1993). Nonetheless, it is important to note that the rats in this study were not trained prior to the exercise stressor, thereby rendering likely a stress effect due to novelty. Third, physical activity has been shown to increase extraneuronal 5-HIAA levels in the frontal cortex but not in the raphe dorsalis (Clement, Schäfer, Ruwe, Gemsa, & Wesemann, 1993), thereby suggesting that physical activity could have a differential influence on some serotonergic cell bodies (e.g., those located in the raphe obscurus), but not on others (e.g., those located in the raphe dorsalis). It is also important to note that the observation of exercise-elicited increases in extraneuronal 5-HIAA levels (such as those measured in the frontal cortex) does not mean that the exercise increases 5-HT release. It is possible that increases in extraneuronal 5-HIAA levels may simply indicate increased metabolism of 5-HT without prior release (Figure 1). Clearly, these series of observations suggest that acute physical activity may actually increase release of 5-HT, but further research is needed before a clear-cut conclusion can be reached. An identical statement applies to our knowledge of the relationships between physical activity and the synthesis and release of 5-HT. Thus, is exercise a model in which increased synthesis leads to increased release of 5-HT, or is it a model in which increased release of 5-HT (if any) is independent from increases in 5-HT synthesis? In this context, a partial answer is provided by the observation that acute physical activity in rats trained for 8 weeks slightly *increases* brain tryptophan and 5-HIAA levels, but actually *reduces* 5-HT levels, whereas exercise in rats trained for 1 week increases tryptophan and 5-HIAA but does not affect 5-HT (Chaouloff, Laude, Serrurier, et al., 1987). The most likely explanation for this effect of training duration is that when exercise-induced increases in tryptophan are not important (as seen in long-term trained rats), increases in 5-HT synthesis are not able to counteract 5-HT release or metabolism in 5-HIAA. If this explanation is correct, extension of past observations with different stress models (see Chaouloff, 1993) would suggest that exercise-induced increases in tryptophan and 5-HT synthesis serve to avoid an imbalance between synthesis of 5-HT and utilization (release or metabolism or both) of 5-HT. Hence, analyses of exercise-induced increases in 5-HT synthesis would not necessarily provide indices of 5-HT release. This is also true for the functional effects of tryptophan administration at the onset of exercise. In an investigation involving human subjects it was reported that such a treatment decreases the time to reach fatigue (Segura and Ventura, 1988). Assuming that exercise-elicited release of 5-HT (if any) should be amplified by tryptophan administration, this study suggests that 5-HT is endowed with a positive effect on exercise fatigue. However, this observation was not confirmed in a more recent investigation by Stensrud, Ingjer, Holm, and Stromme (1992). Besides the fact that this result contradicts earlier suggestions supporting a negative influence of 5-HT on endurance (Blomstrand et al., 1988; Chaouloff, 1989a), there is no indication that the functional consequences of tryptophan administration are partly or totally due to serotonergic systems. This analysis can be achieved solely by means of experiments including 5-HT receptor blockers. Thus tryptophan, which is involved in numerous metabolic pathways (e.g., synthesis of proteins, synthesis of nicotinamide dinucleotide), is able to have functional effects per se (e.g., on insulin release), including toxic ones (Chaouloff, 1989b).

As has been mentioned, there are some arguments favoring the hypothesis that decreases in 5-HT synthesis may have some functional effects on evoked release of 5-HT. However, because this possibility has never been investigated directly in exercising animals, its validity is still open to question. Despite this uncertainty, some investigators have assumed that an analysis of the consequences of prior blockade of tryptophan entry into the brain would provide information on the role of 5-HT during exercise. In human studies, for example, it has been reported that pretreatments with mixtures of BCAAs or treatments that decrease the ratio of free tryptophan to BCAAs reduce exercise fatigue (Blomstrand, Hassmen, Ekblom, & Newsholme, 1991; Blomstrand, Hassmen, & Newsholme, 1991; Davis et al., 1992). In keeping with the inhibitory effects of BCAAs on brain tryptophan availability, it has been suggested that the latter observation provides support for an inhibitory effect of central serotonergic systems on endurance. However, it should not be assumed that a treatment associated with prevention of exercise-elicited changes in serotonergic systems on the one hand, and reduction of fatigue on the other, represents a causal relationship. Although this BCAA–5-HT–fatigue relationship may prove to be correct in the future (thereby indicating that exercise elicits 5-HT release and in turn fatigue), the possibility that the positive effects of BCAAs are due to other systems (including metabolic ones) cannot be ignored at this time. In this context, it is noteworthy that pretreatment of trained rats with a dose of the BCAA valine, which has been shown to decrease evoked release of 5-HT (Gartside et al., 1992), did not diminish acute exercise-elicited corticosterone release (Chaouloff, unpublished data).

PHYSICAL ACTIVITY
AND 5-HYDROXYTRYPTAMINE RECEPTORS

As noted in the previous section, the suggestion that physical activity modifies central serotonergic function supposes that exercise alters 5-HT release and in turn 5-HT receptor–mediated functions. However, it is important to note here that 5-HT receptor–mediated functions may be altered independently from changes in 5-HT release. For example, glucocorticoids have both stimulatory and inhibitory (genomic) influences on some 5-HT receptors (Chaouloff, 1993). It is important to realize that exercise-elicited changes in 5-HT–mediated functions do not necessarily indicate that exercise alters 5-HT release. Furthermore, the uncertainty surrounding this issue can only be alleviated through pharmacological approaches (e.g., by means of inhibitors of 5-HT release, including 5-HT neurotoxins).

Central 5-HT$_{1A}$, 5-HT$_{2A}$, and 5-HT$_{2C}$ Receptors

Since the advent of gene cloning techniques, there have been rapid and extensive advances in the discovery of 5-HT receptor types. Beside confirming the existence of 5-HT receptor families, which were characterized in the 1980s through radioligand binding techniques, molecular biology has also helped to explain the respective localization of the mRNAs encoding for these receptors and how these receptors obey homologous or heterologous regulation (for a review, see Boess & Martin, 1994). The 5-HT$_1$ receptor family comprises the A, B, D (α,β), E, and F subtypes, with the B subtype being specific to rodents (the Dβ subtype being its human homologue). The 5-HT$_2$ receptor family comprises the A, B, and C subtypes (until recently, the 5-HT$_{2A}$ receptor and the 5-HT$_{2C}$ receptor were respectively termed 5-HT$_2$ and 5-HT$_{1C}$). In addition to these receptors, the 5-HT$_3$, 5-HT$_4$, 5-HT$_5$, 5-HT$_6$, and 5-HT$_7$ receptors have been characterized. Thus, 5-HT is endowed with a huge variety of functions that are mediated by more than a dozen receptors.

Although it is not the purpose of this section to describe the biochemical, pharmacological, and functional characteristics of these receptors (for a review, see Zifa & Fillion, 1992), some remarks related to central 5-HT$_{1A}$, 5-HT$_{2A}$, and 5-HT$_{2C}$ receptors must be mentioned because presently available data related to physical activity include only those three receptor types (Figure 1). Conversely, it is hoped that exercise data related to 5-HT$_{1B}$ autoreceptors (which are located on serotonergic nerve terminals where they negatively control 5-HT release; Figure 1), 5-HT$_3$ receptors (the stimulation of which promotes anxiety), and 5-HT$_6$ receptors (which bind numerous antidepressants) will be available in the near future.

5-HT$_{1A}$ receptors are located predominantly in brain regions concerned with mood and anxiety (e.g., the limbic system) (Zifa & Fillion, 1992). 5-HT$_{1A}$ receptors are located either at the postsynaptic level (e.g., in the limbic system) or at the presynaptic level (in the raphe nuclei of the midbrain where these receptors function as autoreceptors that negatively control the tone of serotonergic neurones; Figure 1). In both cases, 5-HT$_{1A}$ receptors mediate neuronal inhibition (hyperpolarization), and this property is thought to mediate the antidepressant and anxiolytic effects of commercially available 5-HT$_{1A}$ ligands (e.g., buspirone; Buspar). When injected in the rat, small doses of selective 5-HT$_{1A}$ receptor agonists such as 8-hydroxy-2-(di-n-propylamino)tetralin (8-OH-DPAT) promote feeding through the stimulation of 5-HT$_{1A}$ autoreceptors. At higher doses, these agonists stimulate postsynaptic receptors and thereby promote specific behaviors such as forepaw treading and flat body posture (components of the so-called 5-HT behavioral syndrome), but also neuroendocrine changes such as hyperglycemia and activation of the HPA. On repeated stimulation by synaptic 5-HT, presynaptic 5-HT$_{1A}$ receptors (like 5-HT$_{1B}$ autoreceptors) progressively desensitize, and such a time-dependent desensitization (which increases serotonergic tone) may explain why 2 to 3 weeks of medication are required for serotonergic antidepressants (especially selective 5-HT reuptake inhibitors: SSRIs) to express their therapeutic effects.

5-HT$_{2A}$ receptors, which are only postsynaptic, are found in numerous brain regions, but the highest concentrations can be measured in the frontal cortex (Zifa & Fillion, 1992). 5-HT$_{2A}$ receptors mediate neuronal excitation (depolarization) and are thought to be the targets of numerous hallucinogenic compounds. When injected in the rat, agonists such as 1-(4-iodo-2,5-dimethoxyphenyl)-2-aminopropane (DOI) promote specific changes such as head shaking and decreased slow-wave sleep, but also promote neuroendocrine changes such as hyperglycemia and activation of the HPA, as well as stimulation of the sympathetic nervous system. On repeated stimulation, 5-HT$_{2A}$ receptors rapidly desensitize, and such a change has often been observed with classical serotonergic antidepressants (although these compounds do not stimulate 5-HT$_{2A}$ receptors directly).

5-HT$_{2C}$ receptors are located postsynaptically and have a widespread distribution, with the highest concentrations being measured in the choroid plexus (Zifa & Fillion, 1992). Stimulation of 5-HT$_{2C}$ receptors by the nonselective agonist m-chlorophenylpiperazine (mCPP) elicits anxiety, hypophagia, hypolocomotion, and activation of the HPA. In humans, 5-HT$_{2C}$ receptors are thought to be additionally involved in 5-HT–elicited migraine. Interestingly, 5-HT$_{2C}$ receptors desensitize rapidly, and such a desensitization may be observed on repeated administration with some 5-HT–related antidepressants, such as the SSRIs. This finding actually reinforces the suggestion that SSRIs may possess therapeutic efficacy in the treatment of obsessive-compulsive disorders, panic disorders, and social phobia.

Physical Activity and Central 5-HT$_{1A}$, 5-HT$_{2A}$, and 5-HT$_{2C}$ Receptors

Data related to the putative effects of physical activity on radioligand binding at 5-HT receptors are lacking. Recently, Chauloff, Baudrie, and Coupry (unpublished data) have analyzed whether frontal cortex 5-HT$_{2A}$ receptor density (as measured by tritiated ketanserin binding) was affected by 4 days of treadmill training with or without 1 hour of acute exercise. These conditions have been shown to permit measurement of exercise-elicited increases in brain tryptophan and 5-HT synthesis. We were interested in frontal cortex 5-HT_{2A} receptors because, as mentioned earlier, this receptor subtype desensitizes rapidly on repeated stimulation (including the indirect one provided by numerous antidepressants), and extracellular 5-HIAA levels have been found to be increased in the frontal cortex of running rats. Surprisingly, neither training nor training plus acute exercise were found to affect the binding kinetics of cortical 5-HT_{2A} receptors (Table 1). In another study, rats were trained for 18 days on a treadmill according to a protocol that allowed the rats to run easily 1 hr/day at 20 m/min for the last 7 days. Twenty-four hours later, rats were injected acutely with the 5-HT_{2A} receptor agonist DOI and the number of head shakes elicited by this agonist were counted over 30 min. This paradigm was chosen on the basis of previous evidence indicating that the head shake response provides a good index of central 5-HT_{2A} receptor function and regulation. Moreover, trained rats were compared with both resting and immobilized rats (according to a time schedule analogous to that used for the runners) to examine whether the influence of physical activity on 5-HT_{2A} receptors (if any) was due to some nonspecific effect of repeated stress (and glucocorticoid release). Actually, it was found that none of the procedures affected the 5-HT_{2A} receptor–mediated head shake response (Figure 2). Interestingly, 18-day increases in body weights were diminished by immobilization but not by exercise, thereby suggesting adaptation to exercise but not to immobilization. Because 2 to 3 weeks (i.e., the period of time during which rats were trained to run) of antidepressant medication has often been shown to decrease this head shake response in control rats (Zifa & Fillion, 1992), this result shows that the mechanisms underlying the antidepressant effect of exercise (which still has to be demonstrated in rats) are not as simple to discover as one might anticipate. Aside from the aforementioned pilot data, other exercise studies have focused on 5-HT_{2A} receptors. In

Table 1 Effects of Physical Training With or Without Acute Exercise on Frontal Cortex 5-HT_{2A} Receptor Binding

Group	N	B_{max} (fmol/mg protein)	K_D (nM)
Rest	9	308 ± 24	0.55 ± 0.06
Trained	9	297 ± 19	0.48 ± 0.03
Trained + acute exercise	9	294 ± 43	0.50 ± 0.05

Note. Values are given as means $\pm$ SEM. Rats were trained for 4 days to run on a treadmill (maximal speed: 20 m/min); on the fifth day, rats were either kept in their home cages (trained) or exercised for 1 hr at a speed of 20 m/min (trained + acute exercise). This protocol is similar to that allowing the recognition of stimulatory effects of acute exercise on brain tryptophan availability and 5-HT synthesis (Chaouloff et al., 1985). Ninety minutes after the end of the fifth exercise session, all rats (including resting rats) were sacrificed and their frontal cortices dissected and stored at $-80°C$. Saturation binding curves with eight concentrations of [^{3}H]ketanserin were performed in duplicate from three cortices. Nonspecific binding was estimated by means of methysergide maleate. Note that resting rats were also placed on the treadmill according to the protocol used for 4-day trained rats (speed: 0 m/min).

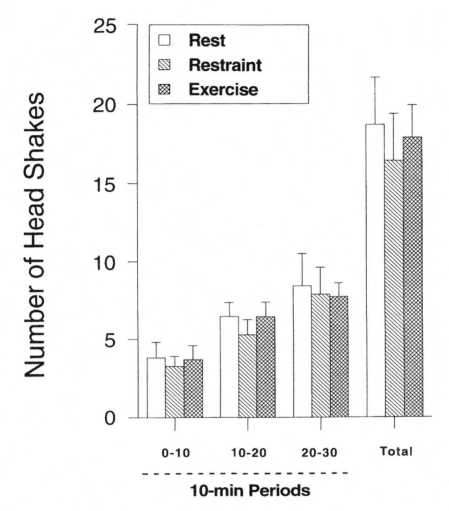

Figure 2 Head shake responses throughout the 30-min period that followed the acute administration of the 5-hydroxytryptamine (HT_{2A}) receptor agonist 1-(4-iodo-2,5-dimethoxyphenyl)-2-aminopropane (2 mg/kg subcutaneously) in rats that were either restrained or exercised on a treadmill. Values are given as mean ± SEM of 7 rats. Exercising rats were trained for 18 days (one daily session) so that they were able to run for 1 hr at a speed of 20 m/min for the last five training sessions. Rats from another group were immobilized for 18 days (one daily session) according to a time schedule identical to that of the exercising rats (i.e., rats were daily immobilized for 1 hr on the last 5 days). All rats, including the resting controls, were injected 24 hours after the end of their last exercise or restraint session. Note that the 18-day body weight increase was 106 ± 4 g in the resting rats (initial body weights: 200 to 210 g for all rats) whereas it was 81 ± 7 and 98 ± 4 g in the restrained rats and the exercising rats, respectively (at least $p < .05$ for the effect of restraint against rest or exercise).

humans, it has been reported that administration of the $5\text{-}HT_{2A}$ receptor antagonist ketanserin (see above) prevents exercise-elicited prolactin release (De Meirleir, L'Hermite-Baleriaux, L'Hermite, Rost, & Hollmann, 1985). This result suggests that exercise actually triggers 5-HT release, and in turn, stimulation of those $5\text{-}HT_{2A}$ receptors controlling prolactin release. Alternatively, because ketanserin is not selective for $5\text{-}HT_{2A}$ receptors at the dosage used (Leysen, 1989), it may be that the preventive effect of ketanserin is due to its effects on $5\text{-}HT_{2C}$ receptors or catecholaminergic receptors, or both.

Two animal studies have shown that pretreatment with LY 53857, a $5\text{-}HT_{2A}$ receptor-blocker endowed with $5\text{-}HT_{2C}$ receptor-blocker property (and catecholamine receptor-blocker properties when given at high dosage; Leysen, 1989), increases time to reach exhaustion (Bailey et al., 1993a; Bailey, Davis & Ahlborn, 1993b). Besides suggesting either that (a) exercise releases 5-HT, which in turn stimulates $5\text{-}HT_{2A}$ and/or $5\text{-}HT_{2C}$ receptors involved in the control of fatigue, or (b) 5-HT, under nonstimulated conditions, exerts a tonic control on these receptors (the blockade of which will diminish fatigue), these studies may bring evidence for a negative influence of 5-HT on exercise endurance. That administration of quipazine, a $5\text{-}HT_{2A}$ receptor agonist, or mCPP, a $5\text{-}HT_{2C}$ receptor agonist, increases treadmill fatigue (Bailey, Davis, & Ahlborn, 1992; Bailey et al., 1993b) supports the involvement of $5\text{-}HT_{2A}$ and $5\text{-}HT_{2C}$ receptors in the control of endurance. However, it has been pointed out previously that the effect of LY 53857 on endurance was neither dose-dependent nor observable at doses previously shown to be selective for $5\text{-}HT_{2A}$ and $5\text{-}HT_{2C}$ receptors, and that quipazine and mCPP elicit in control rats a set of behaviors (e.g., hypolocomotion, anxiety, head shakes, tremor) that may interact with the analysis of treadmill behavior (Chaouloff, 1994a). Hence, it would be premature to advance a conclusion at this time.

As far as $5\text{-}HT_{1A}$ receptors are concerned, a recent study conducted with resting rats, trained rats, and trained rats submitted to acute exercise (experimental conditions similar to those depicted in Table 1) examined whether training with or without acute exercise affects pre- (hyperphagia) and postsynaptic (forepaw treading, flat body posture) $5\text{-}HT_{1A}$ receptor–mediated behaviors (Chaouloff, 1994b). All behaviors were analyzed following administration of different doses of the selective $5\text{-}HT_{1A}$ receptor agonist 8-OH-DPAT (90 min after the end of acute exercise or 24 hr after the last training session). The results indicated clearly that neither hyperphagia nor components of the 5-HT behavioral syndrome were affected by training with or without acute exercise (Chaouloff, 1994b). In keeping with the observation that five immobilization sessions promote hypersensitivity of those $5\text{-}HT_{1A}$ receptors mediating forepaw treading and flat body posture (Kennett, Dickinson, & Curzon, 1985), this investigation confirms that different stressors (including exercise) have different and specific effects on serotonergic systems (Chaouloff, 1993). Furthermore, the lack of desensitization of 8-OH-DPAT–induced hyperphagia in repeatedly exercised animals is somewhat surprising in view of past evidence for increased 5-HT activity

in some cell bodies (such as those located in the raphe obscurus; Jacobs & Fornal, 1993) of acutely exercising animals. It could be that physical activity elicits
5-HT hyperactivity in some cell bodies (e.g., in the raphe obscurus), but not in
those involved with the control of food intake (e.g., in the raphe dorsalis and
medianus). It now remains to examine whether other 5-HT_{1A} receptor–mediated
functions are affected by exercise, and whether a longer training duration would
have some influence on 5-HT1A receptors (as underlined before, short-term
training or acute exercise protocols were chosen according to our previous data
related to the effects of short-term training or acute exercise on brain tryptophan
and 5-HT synthesis). As indicated above, it has been shown that 2 to 3 weeks of
antidepressant therapy desensitizes 5-HT_{1A} presynaptic receptors (autoreceptors).
Actually, this change in receptor sensitivity weakens the inhibitory feedback
effect of 5-HT on neuronal activity, thereby enhancing 5-HT release in the synaptic clefts. Whether a 2- or 3-week training duration would have similar effects is
a question that surely warrants future investigation.

PHYSICAL ACTIVITY, MOOD, AND
5-HYDROXYTRYPTAMINE: THE NEED FOR
A RELIABLE ANIMAL MODEL

The recent progress in 5-HT receptor pharmacology has helped to define part of
the mechanisms through which antidepressant therapies, especially those involving SSRIs such as fluoxetine, paroxetine, citalopram, and fluvoxamine, and anxiolytic therapies exert their positive effects. In keeping with this recent progress
and significant available information regarding dysfunctions of the serotonergic
system in psychiatric patients, it is likely that 5-HT plays a pivotal role in the etiology of some forms of depression and anxiety. As stated at the beginning of this
review, the hypothesis that 5-HT plays a key role in the positive effects of exercise on mood supposes that central serotonergic activity is affected by physical
activity. The different sets of data presented earlier offer strong support for the
validity of this hypothesis. It now remains to be shown whether 5-HT is involved
in the positive effects of exercise on mood. This open question will surely consti-
tute the most difficult but the most interesting issue to be investigated in the
future.

     As a prerequisite for such an investigation, it is important to know whether
currently available animal models are suitable, and if not, to develop more appropriate ones. Actually, this is the most important issue to solve at this point. Thus,
all animal studies have been carried out with prototypical "control" rats (Wistars,
Sprague-Dawleys) that were initially "trained" to run by means of aversive stimuli. Actually, the words "control" and "trained" perfectly define the possible pitfalls that may complicate the analysis of 5-HT–mood relationships during
physical activity. First, the use of control (i.e., naive) rats has proved efficient
enough to elucidate both the mechanisms by which antidepressants and anxiolytics affect central serotonergic systems, and some of the effects of physical activ-

ity on central serotonergic systems. Alternatively, one may underline the fact that exercise has positive mood effects in depressed and anxious human subjects, thereby indicating the need for exercise studies in animal models of depression and anxiety. For instance, it could be interesting to measure how central serotonergic systems are affected by exercise in animals previously submitted for several weeks to numerous unpredictable stressors, i.e., a model thought to parallel some traits of human anxiety and depression (Katz, 1981). Such an experiment could provide insight into some exercise–5-HT relationships that are hidden in control animals. Moreover, the use of control animals renders difficult any recognition of the positive mood effects of exercise because these animals already possess high and normal baseline scores, whereas exercise-induced reversal (if any) of low behavioral scores in stressed animals may be quantitated easily. An illustration of such a difficulty is provided in one recent study in which naive resting rats, trained rats, and trained rats undergoing acute exercise were compared in two animal models of anxiety, namely the elevated plus-maze and the social interaction test (Chaouloff, 1994b). At the opposite of what was observed in a previous study that used open-field and tunnel emergence measures (Tharp & Carson, 1975), neither training nor training plus acute exercise proved anxiolytic, although they both affected locomotion compared with the resting situation (Chaouloff, 1994b). On the other hand, it could be that chronic or acute physical activity would have proved anxiolytic in these tests if the resting animals had been stressed before the onset of the experiments.

Another experimental approach could rely on the use of rats from different strains. Thus, because genetic factors modulate behavioral and neuroendocrine responses to different stimuli (Figure 3), the study of 5-HT–mood relationships in exercising rodents from different strains (i.e., thus providing a huge array of behavioral responses to exercise) could prove fruitful. This kind of paradigm is actually the one our group has decided to develop. Second, the word "trained" is mentioned here to underline the fact that in most experiments, rats are forced initially to run on the treadmill through electric shock or air jet stimuli, thereby including a stress component that could interact with the exercise paradigm and its consequences. However, it is important to note here that although rats are forced to run on the first days of acclimation to the treadmill, this is not the case when training becomes effective. Actually, rats progressively and rapidly acquire running behavior and get conditioned to the exercise task with the result that aversive stimuli are no longer necessary. In addition, one may wonder whether depressed patients asked to exercise do not perceive the completion of this task as stressful initially. Lastly, that lipolysis, a metabolic change repeatedly observed in humans, is a key factor in exercise-elicited increases in 5-HT synthesis suggests that the aforementioned effects of exercise on central serotonergic systems are due mostly to exercise per se, rather than to some aversive components of stress.

To avoid this putative stress component, some investigators have used spontaneous wheel running behavior. These studies have led to the report that imme-

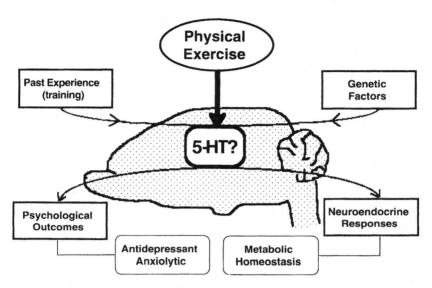

Figure 3 Schematic model integrating the mechanisms on which the positive effects of exercise on mood may rely. The psychological outcomes of exercise may depend (in a reciprocal manner) on adapted neuroendocrine responses to exercise because these neuroendocrine responses (corticotropic and sympathetic) permit a metabolic homeostasis. Both the psychological and neuroendocrine outputs are regulated by central systems (among which 5-hydroxytryptamine [HT]) may play a key role), the activity of which is dependent (a) on the past experience of the body with exercise (this training experience may generate a central print, probably through exercise-elicited release of glucocorticoids and then glucocorticoid-5-HT interactions), and (b) interindividual and genetic differences that may modulate positively or negatively this print.

diately after the last daily session of a 7-week exercise program neither brain tryptophan levels nor brain tryptophan hydroxylase activity were altered, whereas hippocampal 5-HT and 5-HIAA levels were decreased (Elam, Svensson, & Thoren, 1987; Hoffmann, Elam, Thoren, & Hjorth, 1994). In addition, the ratio of midbrain 5-HIAA to 5-HT levels was reported to be decreased in the study by Hoffmann et al. (1994). Taken together, these results suggest that spontaneous running does not affect brain tryptophan availability, but this form of physical activity possibly increases hippocampal 5-HT release. Although it is difficult to reconcile data from forced running and spontaneous running, the following observations are noteworthy. First, in the former model, rats were observed to run 1.2 to 1.5 km during a 1-hr period, but during spontaneous running rats averaged 4 km throughout the 12 hours of the dark cycle. Unlike humans, rats are active during their dark cycle. Thus, differences in exercise volume may explain the intermodel differences. Second, because rats consume most of their daily food requirements during the dark cycle, interactions between meal- and exercise-elicited changes in blood tryptophan disposition must be taken into account.

Third, humans who exercise (either the average jogger or the depressed patient) often run for a single bout (as in the forced exercise model) rather than for numerous short bouts (as in the spontaneous model). Clearly, both exercise models have positive and negative effects, and a model taking into account the qualities of both should be promising.

CONCLUSION

Data provided from both animal and human studies suggest that acute physical activity increases brain 5-HT synthesis and metabolism through lipolysis-elicited alterations in brain tryptophan availability. However, whether these changes promote increased release or are merely associated with it is a question that is yet to be answered. Such an uncertainty actually extends to release-dependent or -independent changes in 5-HT function(s). Clearly, future exercise experiments will need to rely on direct measurements of 5-HT release with the recognition of functional alterations in 5-HT receptors. Although there is evidence for central serotonergic systems playing a key role in the etiology of depression and anxiety, it remains to be shown whether such a contribution is significant in exercising subjects. The answer to this important question will only arise from studies employing both a suitable animal model and an integrative approach. In keeping with recent data, which indicate that glucocorticoids play a pivotal role in adaptive processes, partly through their actions on central serotonergic systems, it seems reasonable to propose that this approach should focus on the central effects of exercise-elicited release of glucocorticoids. Using this integrative approach will allow scientists to understand more about the role serotonin systems play in physical activity and mood elevation.

ADDENDUM

Since the completion of this chapter, four microdialysis studies have measured whether acute physical exercise affects 5-HT release. In one study, it was found that acute physical exercise did not affect extracellular 5-HT levels in the ventral horn of the spinal cord, thus reflecting combined increases in release and reuptake of 5-HT (Gerin, Becquet, & Privat, 1995). In two other studies, acute physical exercise was found to increase 5-HT release in the ventral funiculus of the spinal cord (Gerin, Legrand, & Privat, 1994) and in the hippocampus (Wilson & Marsden, 1996). However, the latter observation applied only to so-called "bad runners." Lastly, in food-deprived rats, acute physical exercise markedly increased 5-HT release in the ventral hippocampus (Meeusen, Thoren, Chaouloff, Sarre, DeMerleir, Ebinger, & Michotte, in press).

Chapter 12

The Norepinephrine Hypothesis

Rod K. Dishman

This chapter reexamines the norepinephrine hypothesis advanced as an explanation for the reductions in depression and anxiety reported by humans following physical activity (Morgan, 1985a; North et al., 1990; Petruzzello et al., 1991; Ransford, 1982). Previous discussions of the norepinephrine hypothesis have not provided sufficient detail about the role of norepinephrine in depression and anxiety. These reviews have also failed to provide biologically plausible explanations regarding the effects of physical activity on norepinephrine, or to provide direction for subsequent research.

The chapter is designed to (a) provide an overview of past and present views of how norepinephrine modulates brain-behavior relationships that are important for depression and anxiety; (b) summarize studies of the effects of exercise on norepinephrine within the context of brain-behavior integration; and (c) suggest some areas where research is especially needed. The conventional use of norepinephrine is adopted in this discussion rather than noradrenaline as the noun referring to the neuromodulator, and noradrenergic is adopted as the adjective referring to attributes or activity of the norepinephrine system. The terms physical activity, exercise, and physical fitness will be used consistent with conventional usage in public health (Pate et al., 1995).

THE NOREPINEPHRINE HYPOTHESIS: PAST AND PRESENT

Norepinephrine was the first substance identified as a mediator of peripheral nerve cell activity (Langley, 1901), but it wasn't until more than 50 years later

Thanks to Donna Smith for helping prepare this chapter.

that norepinephrine neurons were located in the brain (Dahlstrom & Fuxe, 1964; Vogt, 1954). Norepinephrine comprises only about 1% of the brain's neurotransmitters, and its actions are slower than those of classic neurotransmitters (seconds rather than milliseconds). Nonetheless, norepinephrine neurons are diffuse and topographically organized in the brain and peripheral nervous system, and norepinephrine is recognized as a major modulator of brain neural activity (Fillenz, 1990).

A norepinephrine hypothesis of human depression emerged from serendipitous findings in neurobiology and pharmacology (Maas, 1979; Whybrow, Akiskal, & McKinney, 1984). In the early 1950s the alkaloid reserpine, derived from *Rawolfia serpentina* (Indian snake root), was used to treat hypertension and was an alternative to phenothiazines in the treatment of mania and schizophrenia. About 15% of hypertensive patients receiving reserpine developed major depression. Because reserpine lowers presynaptic levels of norepinephrine by blocking norepinephrine uptake by vesicles within the cell body, a link between depressive illness and lowered synthesis of norepinephrine emerged (Goodwin & Bunney, 1971). About the same time, tuberculosis patients treated with iproniazid experienced euphoria. The subsequent clinical success of iproniazid in treating depression, coupled with its later identification as a monoamine oxidase inhibitor (Udenfriend, 1958) (thus promoting norepinephrine's availability at the synapse and its resynthesis) added to the credibility of the norepinephrine hypothesis. In addition, clinical tests of imipramine among psychiatric patients revealed its mood-elevating effects. Imipramine blocks the reuptake of monoamines, preferentially norepinephrine, by the presynaptic terminal (Strom-Olsen & Weil-Malherbe, 1958). Hence, monoamine oxidase inhibitors and tricyclic drugs (TCAs) were added to clinical treatment of depression, leading to the early hypothesis that depression resulted from low brain levels of norepinephrine (Bunney & Davis, 1965; Prange, 1964; Schildkraut, 1965).

Monoamine oxidase deaminates serotonin (5-hydroxytryptamine, 5-HT) as well as catecholamines, and imipramine blocks the reuptake of serotonin, although less specifically than for norepinephrine. Thus in Europe, an hypothesis similar to the norepinephrine hypothesis developed for serotonin (Coppen, 1969). The approaches taken to studying norepinephrine and serotonin in depression and anxiety have been similar. The serotonin hypothesis is addressed in chapter 12 by Chaouloff, and therefore, this discussion is restricted to norepinephrine, except where interactions between norepinephrine and serotonin are particularly informative. For example, an early interactionist view that is still relevant is the permissive biogenic amine hypothesis (Prange, 1964) that lowered serotonergic activity permits alterations in noradrenergic activity to cause depression, but that serotonergic dysregulation is not sufficient to cause depression.

The first clinical studies testing the norepinephrine hypothesis for depression and subsequent studies of norepinephrine after physical activity in depressed patients measured norepinephrine and its metabolites in urine and CSF. However, the precision of norepinephrine and metabolites in peripheral tissues for estimating brain noradrenergic levels or metabolic activity is inherently limited by the central and peripheral distribution of noradrenergic neurons in the body. Explaining the ways in which physical activity may alter norepinephrine to reduce depression or anxiety requires an understanding of how central and peripheral adaptations in the norepinephrine system may differ.

The cell bodies for synthesizing brain norepinephrine are located mainly centrally in brain neurons in the pons (locus coeruleus) and the ventral midbrain (the lateral tegmentum) and peripherally in postganglionic areas of the thoracic and upper lumbar spine and in chromaffin cells of the adrenal medulla (Feldman & Quenzer, 1984). In the brain, norepinephrine cell bodies represent two groups that innervate both dorsal and ventral ascending and descending structures. The major noradrenergic nucleus is the locus coeruleus (nucleus A6; Dahlstrom & Fuxe, 1964), which contains approximately half of all norepinephrine neurons in the brain. The locus coeruleus is located in the caudal pontine central gray. Fibers from the locus coeruleus form five major tracts that are mostly ipsilateral. Three of the tracts are ascending and innervate the periaqueductal gray, superior and inferior colliculi, thalamic nuclei, amygdala, hippocampus, and all of the frontal cortex. One other ascending tract innervates the cerebellum. The remaining descending tract innervates the mesencephalon and spinal cord (Cooper, Bloom, & Roth, 1991; Ungerstedt, 1971; Watson, Khachaturian, Lewis, Akil, 1986). A large number of brain norepinephrine neurons also lie outside the locus coeruleus and are located throughout the lateral ventral tegmental fields (nuclei A5 and A7; Dahlstrom & Fuxe, 1964). Fibers from these neurons intermingle with the locus coeruleus neurons, which contribute to the innervation of the mesencephalon and spinal cord as well as forebrain and diencephalon (Cooper et al., 1991).

Norepinephrine is synthesized in cell bodies from tyrosine taken up from blood. The rate of synthesis of norepinephrine varies with the degree of sympathetic nerve activity and its associated changes in tyrosine hydroxylase activity (Udenfriend & Dairman, 1971). Tyrosine hydroxylase is the rate-limiting enzyme in norepinephrine synthesis. If norepinephrine is not taken back up into the presynaptic neuron and bound in storage vesicles, it is metabolized by the enzymes monoamine oxidase and catechol-o-methyl transferase. The major metabolites of norepinephrine are 3,4 dihydroxy phenylglycol (DHPG) intraneuronally, and 3-methoxy-4-hydroxy phenylglycol (MHPG) extraneuronally.

The action of norepinephrine is mediated by two types of adrenergic receptors, α receptors and β receptors, which have been further subdivided into α-1 and α-2 and β-1 and β-2. When β-1 receptors bind with norepinephrine there is a stimulation of adenylate cyclase by the $G_{stimulatory}$ protein and a subsequent rise in the level of intracellular cAMP, which acts as a second messenger for neural transmission. α-2 receptor binding with norepinephrine is associated with an inhibition of noradrenergic activity. Presynaptic α-2 autoreceptors decrease norepinephrine neuron activity and the synthesis of norepinephrine by a G protein inhibition of tyrosine hydroxylase. When α-1 receptors are bound with norepinephrine, activity of the second-messenger phosphoinositide system is increased. Growing evidence indicates that the phosphorylation of regulatory proteins that control ion channels and neural conductance/resistance consequent to receptor–second messenger coupling plays the major role in brain noradrenergic activity. In the brain, β-2 receptors have the highest affinity for epinephrine and are associated primarily with glial cells rather than noradrenergic nerve transmission.

There is scientific consensus that noradrenergic neurons modulate a wide range of functions in the CNS, including behavior during threat, pituitary hormonal release, cardiovascular function, sleep, and analgesic responses (Cooper et al., 1991). In the following sections, norepinephrine in depression and anxiety is addressed with emphasis on the brain's locus coeruleus–norepinephrine system and the HPA.

Depression

Evidence for the involvement of brain noradrenergic systems in depression comes primarily from two sources. First, metabolites of norepinephrine in the CSF or urine of depressed patients have been sampled in some studies. This approach assumed that excretion of metabolites of norepinephrine such as MHPG reflects the activity of brain noradrenergic neurons. In general, the results of these studies demonstrated that in patients with bipolar depression, and some with unipolar depression, there were reduced levels of MHPG during depressive episodes and higher than normal levels during mania (Beckman & Goodwin, 1980; Schildkraut, 1975; Schildkraut, Orsulak, Schatzberg, & Rosenbaum, 1983). Lower than normal MHPG levels in CSF have not been substantiated (Hirschfeld & Goodwin, 1988). Urinary MHPG is generally collected over a 24-hour sampling period, while the lumbar puncture for CSF is acute. Therefore, samples of MHPG from CSF could exhibit a great deal of variability depending on the time of sampling.

The MHPG data are not fully consistent with the prediction by the original norepinephrine hypothesis of central depletion of norepinephrine. In some patients with unipolar depression, normal or higher than normal levels of MHPG were detected. Schildkraut et al. (1983) proposed that the differences in MHPG can discriminate three subtypes of unipolar depression. Patients in Subtype 1 present low levels of urinary MHPG prior to treatment. This low norepinephrine output may be due to a decrease in norepinephrine synthesis or decreased release from the norepinephrine neurons. Patients in Subtype 2 present intermediate levels of MHPG. These individuals may have normal norepinephrine metabolism but other neurochemical systems may be abnormal. Patients in Subtype 3 present with high MHPG levels prior to treatment, possibly due to less responsive noradrenergic receptors or increased cholinergic activity. Maas (1979) proposed that two subgroups of depression exist: patients presenting low MHPG and normal 5-hydroxy indoleacetic acid; 5 HIAA (the main metabolite of 5-HT), and patients presenting normal MHPG but low 5-HIAA. Although initial data from aggregated trials were consistent with these subtypes, subsequent findings were not (Davis et al., 1988).

Although these revised models are compatible with the norepinephrine hypothesis, each assumes that all of the MHPG in CSF, plasma, or urine is derived from the brain. Maas and Leckman (1983) estimated that 60% of MHPG is derived from the brain, while Blomberry, Kopin, Gordon, Markey, and Ebert (1980) estimated that only 20% is derived from brain. MHPG can be assayed as a free molecule or as conjugated MHPG in plasma and urine. In peripheral tissue, phenolsulfotransferase conjugates MHPG sulfate and glucuronyltransferase conjugates MHPG glucuronide. In the rat brain, and perhaps in primates (Fillenz, 1990), only MHPG sulfate is conjugated. Although the correlation between peripheral and central MHPG can be weak or high, recent consensus holds that urinary MHPG sulfate is a more reliable estimate of brain norepinephrine metabolism. In human plasma, total MHPG is comprised of about 30% free, 35% sulfate, and 35% glucuronide conjugates. In human urine less than 10% of total MHPG is free, with 40% sulfoconjugated and 50% in the glucuronide conjugate form. Based on these distributions, MHPG sulfate, rather than total MHPG or the glucuronide conjugate, appears the metabolite of choice for estimating central noradrenergic activity by assays of peripheral tissues (Peyrin, 1990).

A second line of evidence for a role of norepinephrine in depression comes from pharmacological studies examining the actions and effects of antidepressant drugs that are known to raise the levels of norepinephrine in the synapse. TCAs such as imipramine hydrochloride and desipramine hydrochloride block neuronal pumps and prevent norepinephrine from being taken back up into the presynaptic neuron. Thus, norepinephrine remains in the synaptic cleft longer for binding with receptors. Another class of antidepressants, monoamine oxidase inhibitors (e.g., phenelzine sulfate), prevent oxidative deamination, which also increases the availability of norepinephrine at postsynaptic receptor sites. New atypical drugs such as mianserin do not affect norepinephrine reuptake but presumably downregulate norepinephrine-producing cells by stimulating autoregulatory α-2 receptors that inhibit tyrosine hydroxylase. Other atypical drugs, such as venlafaxine hydrochloride, combine selective blockade of the reuptake of norepinephrine and 5-HT. They are designed to reduce anxiety and depression concomitantly with presumably fewer side effects of the less selective tricyclics. The efficacy of these antidepressant treatments is between 65% to 80%, while the placebo response rate is between 20% and 40% (Baldessarini, 1989). Although there is disagreement among clinicians over the relative effectiveness of tricyclics and the newer selective reuptake inhibitors, clinical trials indicate that the efficacy for reducing major depression in humans is similar for the two types of drugs (Workman & Short, 1993).

The aforementioned metabolic and pharmacologic studies reveal issues that are not easily resolved by the original hypothesis that reduced norepinephrine leads to depression. First, pharmacologic data reveal that both tricyclic antidepressants and monoamine oxidase inhibitors increase the availability of norepinephrine to the receptors. If depression is the result of low norepinephrine levels, then raising the levels should alleviate symptoms of depression in a matter of hours. However, clinical responses from antidepressant drugs generally are not observed for 10 to 20 days. In addition, some of the atypical antidepressants such as iprindole do not block the reuptake of norepinephrine, alter the metabolism of norepinephrine, or suppress the firing of norepinephrine cells in the locus coeruleus that commonly occurs after treatment with TCAs (Baldessarini, 1989; Sulser, Vetulani, Mobley, 1978). Because the therapeutic efficacy of antidepressant drugs does not appear dependent on acute levels of norepinephrine in the synapse (Maas, 1979), it is now accepted that the therapeutic effects of the drugs involve chronic adaptations in neural regulation (Siever & Davis, 1985).

Consensus effects of antidepressants on norepinephrine systems include acute and chronic outcomes (Baldessarini, 1989). First-line acute effects block the reuptake of monoamines. The reuptake of norepinephrine is blocked to a greater extent than is 5-HT, except in cases in which an atypical antidepressant is used such as fluoxetine, which selectively blocks the reuptake of 5-HT. A second acute effect is a reduction of firing rates for norepinephrine neurons in the brainstem. Third, there is a temporary reduction in the synthesis and turnover of norepinephrine. Fourth, receptors of the monoaminergic systems are blocked. α-1 Adrenergic receptors have a higher affinity for TCAs, while β receptors have the lowest affinity. The affinity of TCAs for the α-2 receptor is also low. Chronic effects of TCAs include continued blockade of reuptake; a temporary and reversible downregulation of presynaptic and postsynaptic α-2 receptors; a normalization of firing rates and turnover, which can lead to levels of monoamines that are above normal; increased release of norepinephrine; a downregulation of β receptors; and an increased affinity and sensitivity to α-1 agonists that may increase the number of α-1 receptors, and a possible upregulation of 5-HT receptors.

Contemporary views of the norepinephrine hypothesis focus on the regulation of noradrenergic neurons and their terminal fields. Such a focus is central for advances in understanding in what ways noradrenergic adaptations to exercise may account for reductions in depression and anxiety.

Locus Coeruleus–Norepinephrine System   There is an emerging consensus that the locus coeruleus–norepinephrine system integrates external and internal stimuli in order to regulate autonomic arousal, attention-vigilance, and neuroendocrine responses involved with behavioral responses to stress (Cooper et al., 1991; Fillenz, 1990). Most evidence indicates that norepinephrine hyperpolarizes neurons in the locus coeruleus terminal fields, thus enhancing their responsiveness to afferent signals from other neurons (Foote, Bloom, & Aston-Jones, 1983; Weiss & Simson, 1989). The locus coeruleus receives afferents from the central nucleus of the amygdala, from the CA1 region of the hippocampus, and from somatosensory afferents via the para-gigantocellular reticular nucleus with glutamate as a putative neurotransmitter (Fillenz, 1990). Activity in the locus coeruleus is inhibited presynaptically by norepinephrine, 5-HT, GABA, and opioid peptides including β-endorphin and met-enkephalin. Locus coeruleus activation can be regulated through distinct neurotransmitter pathways depending on the stressor (Weiss & Simson, 1989).

Experimental models of the locus coeruleus–norepinephrine system for anxiety and depression based on uncontrollable, inescapable stress have been developed in the rat using restraint and forced swimming (e.g., Porsolt, LePichon, & Jalfre, 1977), but escape from uncontrollable footshock is the most elaborated model. The hallmark response to uncontrollable, inescapable footshock is increased escape latency from controllable shock administered 24 to 72 hours later. The escape-deficit model after footshock was reported by McCulloch and Bruner (1939), and presumably results from motoric, emotive, or learning deficits consequent to depletion of norepinephrine in the locus coeruleus (Weiss et al., 1981). A single session of high-intensity uncontrollable footshock leads to a large decrease in brain norepinephrine (Bliss, Ailion, & Zwanziger, 1968; Maynert & Levi, 1964) with less reliable decreases in brain serotonin and dopamine levels perhaps due to slower resynthesis of norepinephrine. In addition to lowered brain norepinephrine in the locus coeruleus, hippocampus, hypothalamus, and frontal cortex (Weiss et al., 1981; Anisman & Zarcharko, 1986), uncontrollable footshock leads to behavior changes in the rat that mimic features of human depression or anxiety, or both, and are reversed by TCAs and other agonists and antagonists of noradrenergic (Sherman, Sacwuitne, & Petty, 1982) receptors. These features include altered sleep, weight loss, anhedonia, and reductions in physical activity, eating, and sexual behavior (Weiss & Simson, 1989).

Anxiety

Changes in brain monoamine activity and β-adrengergic receptors have been mentioned as possible mechanisms underlying reductions in anxiety following physical activity (e.g., Petruzello et al., 1991). However, norepinephrine has received little attention in the physical activity literature as a putative neuromodulator for anxiety. This is unfortunate because anxiety is a prominent feature of typical major depression and because there are both theoretical and clinical issues over whether anxiety and depression have independent etiologies. These issues emanate primarily from interpretations about the activation of the locus coeruleus–norepinephrine system under stressful conditions and are particularly relevant for future physical activity studies.

The aforementioned footshock escape-deficit model is largely isomorphic with shared features of human depression, but its construct validity for depression remains unclear because most of these features are also common to anxiety disorders. Early findings that the escape deficit was reversible by tricyclics, but not by anxiolytic drugs (Sherman & Petty, 1982), suggested predictive validity as a model of depression. Subsequent reports comparing anxiolytics and atypical antidepressants have not verified that the escape-deficit model has pharmacologic specificity for depression more so than for anxiety (Zarcharko & Anisman, 1989). Behavioral responses similar to those induced by inescapable footshock are seen after injection of the anxiety-inducing inverse benzodiazepine agonist β-carboline (Drugan et al., 1985), and the administration of the anxiolytic diazepam to rats prior to inescapable shock attenuates the escape-deficit 24 hours later (Drugan, et al., 1984).

Locus Coeruleus–Norepinephrine System   Redmond (1985) and Gray (1985) have argued that the locus coeruleus–norepinephrine depletion model conceptualizes the role of the dorsal ascending noradrenergic bundle for the regulation of depression in a way similar to its established role in inhibiting behavior under conditions of threat that is characteristic of anxiety. Prevailing animal models of anxiety and neurotic depression share similar neurobiological pathways consistent with their shared clinical symptoms of agitation, hypervigilance, decreased motor activity under threat, and HPA disruption (Redmond, 1985).

Other views (Panksepp, 1990) acknowledge that the locus coeruleus–norepinephrine system may be permissive or supportive of anxiety, but not causal. Increased neural activity in the locus coeruleus after injection of yohimbine (an α-2 antagonist) is associated with decreased open-field locomotion (a behavioral sign of anxiety or fear) (Weiss et al., 1986). This response is reversed by clonidine, which is an α-2 agonist. However, locus coeruleus–norepinephrine activity is increased by various changes in the environment that require behavioral adaptation and are not specific to anxiety or fear. Drugs that increase norepinephrine activity do not increase anxiety uniformly.

The norepinephrine model of arousal can, however, explain the absence of sedative effects for the 5-HT$_{1A}$ autoreceptor agonist buspirone, which is anxiolytic. Dorsal raphe (cell bodies for 5-HT in brain) activity is reduced, while dopamine and locus coeruleus cell body activity is increased. In contrast, benzodiazepines such as diazepam and alprazolam, the main anxiolytic drugs, decrease the neuron activity of norepinephrine, 5-HT, and dopamine cell bodies presumably via GABAergic inhibition (Laurent, Mangold, Humbel, & Haefely, 1983; Sanghera, McMillen, & German, 1983). One view (Eison & Temple, 1986) of the common anxiolytic effects of benzodiazapines and buspirone is that inhibition of the ascending norepinephrine system accounts for the sedating effects of benzodiazapines. Noradrenergic responses do not occur independently of serotonergic effects (Frazer, 1993; Shopsin, Gershon, Goldstein, Friedman, & Wilk, 1975). Serotonin can depolarize and increase membrane resistance via the excitatory amino acid glutamate in the locus coeruleus (Aston-Jones, Akaoka, Chariety, & Chouvet, 1991). Hence, 5-HT can both support and inhibit the actions of norepinephrine. Serotonin agonists such as clomipramine, which blocks the neuronal reuptake of 5-HT, are effective in treating some anxiety disorders, e.g., obsessive-compulsive disorder.

Norepinephrine and the
Hypothalamic-Pituitary-Adrenal Axis

Norepinephrine also is linked to the regulation of the HPA, which is dysregulated in major depression and certain anxiety disorders. In major depression (Gold, Goodwin, & Chrousos, 1988b) and panic disorder (Geracioti et al., 1990) the glucocorticoids and the brain monoaminergic systems apparently fail to restrain the

HPA response to stress. Activation of the brain noradrenergic and serotonergic systems during stress is believed to increase the secretion of ACTH by stimulating the secretion of corticotropin-releasing hormone (CRH) (Plotsky et al., 1989; Tuomisto & Mannisto, 1985). In turn, there is evidence that CRH feeds back to locus coeruleus cell bodies and increases locus coeruleus–norepinephrine activity (Menzaghi, Heinrichs, Pich, Weiss, & Koob, 1993; Valentino, 1988). Some evidence suggests that TCAs increase the sensitivity of glucocorticoid receptors, enhancing their autoregulatory inhibition of cortisol resulting in mood elevation (Barden, Reul, & Holsboer, 1995). Because depressed patients have higher free cortisol levels than normals, even though ACTH release is small during CRH stimulation, the adrenal cortex has apparently become hyperresponsive to ACTH. Indeed, patients diagnosed with major depression, including melancholia, often have an early escape from the normally suppressing effects on cortisol of the synthetic corticosteriod dexamethasone. There is evidence that the hippocampus downregulates the HPA in both rats and primates. Hypercortisolism can damage or destroy hippocampal cells containing glucocorticoid receptors that mediate the suppression of the CRH neuron (Sapolsky, Krey, & McEwen, 1984).

A model of depression based on dysregulation of the HPA is compatible with revisions of the norepinephrine hypothesis of depression. Excess norepinephrine could stimulate the overproduction of CRH. Conversely, Sachar (1985) has hypothesized that the functional depletion of norepinephrine in the hypothalamus leads to hypersecretion of cortisol. Another view is that the central action of norepinephrine on the HPA is inhibitory, thus reducing CRH and ACTH secretion. Central administration of catecholamine synthesis inhibitors such as reserpine and α-methyl-p-tyrosine leads to increased plasma corticosterone and ACTH (Tuomisto & Mannisto, 1985). The controversy over the stimulatory or inhibitory effects of norepinephrine on the HPA remains unresolved because norepinephrine apparently exerts different effects on ACTH at different levels of the HPA. In addition, norepinephrine actions are paradoxic at presynaptic and postsynaptic receptors. It has been hypothesized that norepinephrine reduces CRH and ACTH secretion through α-1 receptors and enhanced somatostatin release, while norepinephrine stimulation of α-2 receptors increases ACTH release (Plotsky et al., 1989; Tuomisto and Mannisto, 1985).

The inability to suppress plasma ACTH with cortisol infusion indicates a loss of sensitivity in steroid negative feedback mechanisms. A decreased resting ACTH and cortisol response to CRH among highly trained runners, despite expected increases in ACTH and cortisol during exercise has been interpreted as a hyposensitive HPA response (Luger, Deuster, Kyle, et al., 1987). In a study of trained middle-aged runners, however, Heuser, Wark, Keul, and Holsboer (1991) interpreted high resting ACTH and cortisol responses to CRH after dexamethasone as indicative of an attenuation of HPA negative feedback. ACTH during high-intensity exercise can increase despite infusion of CRH sufficient to saturate pituitary corticotrophs (Smoak, Deuster, Rabin, & Chrousos, 1991). Thus, releasing factors for ACTH other than CRH may be increased by exercise.

The pattern of HPA releasing factors appears stereotyped for different stressors (Antoni, 1986). Thus, it is important to determine whether chronic exercise elicits HPA hormonal responses similar to those observed for nonexercise stressors and whether brain norepinephrine regulates ACTH changes after chronic exercise. For example, the pituitary ACTH and β-endorphin responses to exercise appear to be dependent on sensory afference from muscle (Kjaer, Secher, Bach, Sheikh, & Galbo, 1989). Recent studies show that chronic treadmill training can lead to attenuated plasma corticosterone levels in response to acute treadmill running but elevated ACTH response to heterotypical (i.e., novel) immobilization (White-Welkley, Bunnell, Mougey, Meyerhoff, & Dishman, 1995) and elevated ACTH levels after heterotypical footshock (White-Welkley, Warren, Bunnell, Mougey, Meyerhoff, & Dishman, 1996). These findings indicate that treadmill exercise training leads to an increased potential for HPA responses to novel stressors. In contrast, we have reported that chronic voluntary running in an activity wheel does not moderate plasma levels of ACTH and corticosterone after footshock in male rats (Dishman et al., 1995) despite an elevation in norepinephrine levels in the locus coeruleus similar to that observed after treadmill training (Dishman et al., 1992, 1993). Studies are needed that examine noradrenergic responses to exercise in hypothalamic regions proximately involved with CRH release (e.g., paraventricular nucleus).

NOREPINEPHRINE AND PHYSICAL ACTIVITY: PERIPHERAL MEASURES

Revisions of the norepinephrine hypothesis more fully consider the chronic effects of antidepressant drugs on how noradrenergic neurons are regulated, rather than merely on levels of norepinephrine and its metabolites in brain and peripheral tissues (Maas, 1979; Siever & Davis, 1985; Whybrow et al., 1984). These revisions have received very little attention in the literature on physical activity and depression or anxiety (Dunn & Dishman, 1991).

In humans, changes in noradrenergic activity after acute physical activity typically have been estimated by measuring MHPG levels in urine, plasma, or CSF. Early studies examining the effects of acute physical activity on MHPG have been summarized and critiqued by Morgan and O'Connor (1988). Acute studies of urinary MHPG found increased MHPG excretion or no change after physical activity, but there were methodological problems with these studies. Sample sizes were small and different types of depression were present in the same treatment group. For example, unipolar and bipolar patients were assigned to the exercise condition. Also, exercise levels were not quantified, or very low levels of physical activity were used. Studies of acute physical activity and MHPG in nondepressed subjects have typically quantified the exercise stimulus, and some investigators have reported exercise intensity relative to maximal aerobic capacity. The findings have been mixed, and plasma MHPG typically was increased whereas urinary MHPG remained unchanged. The relative contributions of norepinephrine spillover from peripheral sympathetic nerves was not determined. Later studies reported increases in glucuronide and sulfated subfractions of MHPG (Peyrin 1990; Sothmann et al., 1990). However, the relevance of increased MHPG sulfate in plasma after acute exercise (Filser et al., 1988; Sothmann, et al., 1990) is unclear for the norepinephrine model of depression. There do not appear to be any chronic exercise studies that have examined changes in resting MHPG levels. Multivariate relationships among aerobic fitness and urinary norepinephrine metabolites with depression and anxiety have been reported for normal men following resting conditions (Sothmann & Ismail, 1985), but this research fails to demonstrate that the relationship is caused by physical activity.

Animal studies show increases in tyrosine hydoxylase activity in the adrenal gland and liver, but decreased tyrosine hydroxylase activity and decreased norepinephrine turnover in the heart, after exercise training (Mazzeo, 1991). Human studies indicate that exercise training usually does not alter plasma levels of norepinephrine (Cousineau et al., 1977; Peronnet et al., 1981; Winder, Hagberg, Hickson, Ehsani, & McLane, 1978) or muscle sympathetic nerve activity (MSNA) (Seals, 1991; Svedenhag, Wallin, Sundlof, & Henriksson, 1984) measured under resting conditions. After exercise training, plasma norepinephrine levels are lower at a given absolute exercise intensity but unchanged at the same intensity relative to maximal aerobic capacity (Cousineau et al., 1977; Peronnet et al., 1981; Winder et al., 1978; Winder, Hickson, Hagberg, Ehsani, & McLane, 1979). There also appears to be increased norepinephrine and epinephrine release at high exercise intensity (Kjaer & Galbo, 1988; Winder et al., 1978) among exercise-trained subjects. Plasma norepinephrine levels are imprecise estimates of sympathetic nerve activity (e.g., Chang, Kriek, van der Krogt, & van Brummelen, 1991), but studies show reduced MSNA during static handgrip exercise after exercise training (Somers, Leo, Shields, Clary, & Mark, 1992). These findings suggest that peripheral sympathetic nerve activity is reduced during standardized submaximal exercise following exercise training. However, there is an absence of evidence indicating that such effects of exercise training generalize to reduced responses during nonexercise stress relevant for depression or anxiety (Peronnet & Szabo, 1993; Sothmann, 1991).

Spontaneous and provoked cardiovascular hyperresponsiveness is a prominent feature of anxiety disorders including generalized anxiety and panic. Because chronic physical activity can lead to decreased cardiac sympathetic activity and increased cardiac vagal tone at rest (Cox, 1991; Smith, Hudson, Graitzer, & Raven, 1989), there is interest in the role of physical activity in altering autonomic balance during anxiety-provoking stress (Buckworth, Dishman, & Cureton, 1994). It has been hypothesized that decreases in self-reported anxiety and in heart rate and blood pressure responses to lab stressors after chronic physical activity are the result of *increased sensitivity* of β-adrenoreceptors (e.g., Crews & Landers, 1987; Petruzzello et al., 1991), but such hypotheses are not compatible with available evidence. For example, drugs that block β receptors (thus acutely downregulating the norepinephrine receptor-effector system) reduce both anxiety and heart rate responsiveness to psychosocial stressors (Mills & Dimsdale, 1991). In addition, the antidepressant tricyclic drugs lead to a downregulation of brain β receptors. Indeed, a downregulation of β receptors on the heart after chronic physical activity would better explain reduced heart rate and systolic blood pressure by attenuating the effect of norepinephrine on cardiac output.

Maki, Kontula, and Harkonen (1990) concluded that endurance-trained athletes have higher than normal β-adrenoreceptor density on lymphocytes and that acute, prolonged physical activity of high intensity is accompanied by increased β-adrenoreceptor binding on lymphocytes. In contrast, endurance training studies have reported decreased or unchanged β-adrenoreceptor density on lymphocytes. Lymphocyte adrenoreceptors are β-2 types with high affinity for epinephrine, like those found in skeletal and smooth muscle, the liver and peripheral sympathetic tissue. However, it is not known whether they provide a valid surrogate for peripheral sympathetic nervous system receptor populations, and they do not provide a measure of brain noradrenergic activity (Fillenz, 1990). Williams, Eden, Moll, Lester, and Wallace (1981) reported no effects of exercise training on β-receptor density or sensitivity in rat hearts. There is limited research showing increased α-2 adrenergic receptors on platelets (which mediate aggregation) in trained subjects (Lockette, McCurdy, Smith, & Carretero, 1987), but there is an absence of studies reporting the effects of physical activity on α-2 adrenoreceptors, which increase blood pressure.

Pharmacologic studies have shown that changes in receptor sensitivity can occur independently of changes in receptor density. Thus, exercise studies are needed of second-messenger systems including those linked to guanosine-dependent adenylate cyclase (5-HT$_{1A}$, α-2, and β receptors) and phosphoinositide (α-2, 5-HT$_2$) as well as intracellular transport of potassium and sodium. Plausible biological hypotheses explaining why the brain norepinephrine system is stimulated by exercise are needed. Sensory afference (such as Type Ib, III, and IV fibers from locomotory muscle) to the locus coeruleus, influences of locomotory muscle metabolism on central neurotransmitters, and motoric/limbic interactions (e.g., Mogenson, Brudzynski, Wu, Yang, & Yim, 1993) are plausible but untested at this time (Dunn & Dishman, 1991).

NOREPINEPHRINE AND PHYSICAL ACTIVITY: BRAIN

It is possible that chronic exercise, like other chronic stressors, affects the brain's noradrenergic system in ways qualitatively similar to the effects of pharmacologic interventions. Acute cold exposure, swimming, and treadmill running lead to decreased brain norepinephrine in locus coeruleus and its terminal areas (Barchas & Friedman, 1962; Stone, 1973). These findings suggest that the depletion of norepinephrine during acute stress is due to the inability of norepinephrine synthesis (beyond the rate-limiting step of tyrosine hydroxylation) to keep pace with release.

By contrast, chronic (14 to 30 days) intermittent stress by footshock or immobilization is accompanied by a decrease in cyclic-AMP accumulation to norepinephrine and reduced density of β-1 adrenoreceptors, indicating downreg-ulation. This has been seen in the hypothalamus, brainstem, and cortex, and has led to a postsynaptic subsensitivity theory of adaptation to stress (Stone & Platt, 1982). Other evidence suggests that chronic stress leads to enhanced presynaptic activity accompanied by a compensatory increase in norepinephrine storage (Fil-lenz, 1990). After chronic stress, increased activity of tyrosine hydroxylase has been observed in locus coeruleus–norepinephrine terminal areas in the hip-pocampus and frontal cortex, indicative of increased synthesis of dopamine and norepinephrine (Fillenz, 1990). Recent findings suggest that both treadmill exer-cise training and chronic activity wheel running lead to increasing norepineph-rine activity and storage (Dishman, Renner, et al., 1992; Dishman, Renner, Youngstedt, et al., 1993; Dunn, Reigle, Youngstedt, Armstrong, & Dishman, 1996). Exercise studies are needed to examine specific aspects of synthesis and metabolism of these neurotransmitters. Stone (1973) compared running stress with injections of reserpine or α methyl-p-tyrosine, which inhibit norepinephrine storage and synthesis, respectively. Running stress did not alter storage of nor-epinephrine, so it is likely that the norepinephrine depletion in the running condi-tion was derived from newly synthesized norepinephrine and not from reuptake mechanisms. Chronic stress (Stone & Platt, 1982) and tricyclics (Baldesserini, 1989) downregulate brain β adrenoreceptors, but the effects of physical activity on brain β (de Castro & Duncan, 1985) and α adrenoreceptors have not been examined using models of depression or anxiety.

Studies of noradrenergic responses to physical activity among animals (Chaouloff, 1989a; Dunn & Dishman, 1991) have not used an established experi-mental model of depression or anxiety to examine brain-behavior relationships. While positron emission imaging (Andreasen, 1988) could describe metabolism in brain regions implicated in anxiety and depression after acute and chronic exercise, this technology has not been employed in studies of physical activity with patients diagnosed as depressed or suffering from anxiety disorders.

Pharmacologic methods have been employed in a series of initial tests of established animal models of depression and anxiety, and results indicate that chronic activity wheel running attenuates the escape deficit induced by uncontrol-lable footshock (Dishman et al., 1993). This response was associated with higher concentrations of norepinephrine in the locus coeruleus and dorsal raphe for activ-ity wheel animals compared with sedentary animals, but higher concentrations of serotonin in the central amygdala and its metabolite 5-HIAA in the central amyg-dala and the CA1 area of the hippocampus for the sedentary animals. Lower 5-HT in the dorsal raphe for the sedentary animals is consistent with less locus coeruleus–norepinephrine inhibition of the dorsal raphe concomitant with locus coeruleus–norepinephrine depletion. Raphe cell bodies are densely innervated with noradrenergic cell terminals (Cooper et al., 1991), and it is believed that the locus coeruleus–norepinephrine and the dorsal raphe–serotonergic systems recip-rocally innervate each other (Frazer, 1993). These results suggest that chronic activity wheel running protects against the depletion of norepinephrine induced by uncontrollable footshock in sedentary animals. Higher norepinephrine in the locus coeruleus for the activity wheel group is consistent with past studies showing increased brain levels of norepinephrine after chronic treadmill running and activity wheel running (Chaouloff, 1989a; Dunn et al., 1996). Because various stressors that deplete norepinephrine acutely lead to increased synthesis and storage after chronic exposure (Fillenz, 1990), it is possible that activity wheel running also increases synthesis and storage, but the methods employed to date do not permit such an interpretation.

SUMMARY

Future studies examining the norepinephrine hypothesis as an explanation for reductions in self-rated depression and anxiety following physical activity must move beyond measuring levels of norepinephrine and its metabolites to consider the synthesis (e.g., enzyme activity or mRNA studies), release (e.g., using microdialysis), receptor-effector second messenger systems, and direct measures of neural activity (e.g., microneurography or positron emission imaging) in both brain and peripheral tissues. Beyond such technological advances, there is a great need for more sophisticated conceptualizations of brain-behavior regulation in physical activity studies. Even models of endogenous anxiety (e.g., panic disorder) and depression (e.g., major depression and melancholia) consider that stressful events precipitate, exacerbate, or manifest the symptoms of the disease. Hence, more attention is needed in physical activity studies on etiological models of depression and anxiety disorders. For example, the effects of physical activity may differ when depression has predominantly behavioral versus psychopharmacological origins. In addition, behavioral models of depression that are based on locus coeruleus–norepinephrine responses during aversive stress cannot be homologous to human depression if they do not address the anhedonia that is characteristic of decreased appetitive or reward-dependent behaviors. It appears that dopamine plays a more direct role in anhedonia than does norepinephrine (Koob, 1989). Future exercise studies should consider alternative models of depression that can address norepinephrine and 5-HT interactions (e.g., Vogel, Neill, Hagler, & Kors, 1990) and should examine how noradrenergic adaptations to physical activity interact with the GABA-benzadiazepine system in behavioral models of anxiety.

Finally, because behavioral and pharmacological models of depression and anxiety rely heavily on changes in brain-behavior relationships that follow the manipulation of selected brain neurotransmitter and neuromodulator systems in isolation of each other, views that a single neural system is responsible for each disease have been common. More recently, it has become clear that depression and anxiety each represent heterogenous illnesses in which signs and symptoms may vary (Zacharko & Anisman, 1989). Thus, the development of models of physical activity for depression and anxiety should consider noradrenergic, serotonergic, dopaminergic, GABAergic, or opiodergic neuron responses and their interactions to realize a truly enlightened and developed model.

Chapter 13

The Thermogenic Hypothesis

Kelli F. Koltyn

In addition to the endorphin (chapter 10) and monoamine (chapters 11 and 12) hypotheses advanced as the reasons for improved mood states associated with physical activity, there has been speculation about the role of other physiological factors in this process. One potential mechanism that has been studied involves the elevation in deep body temperature that occurs with physical activity. The hypothesis that increased core temperature may be responsible for the mediation of changes in mood following exercise does not rule out a potential role for endorphin and monoamine activity in this process. The thermogenic hypothesis of exercise-induced mood effects is reviewed in this chapter.

Elevation of body temperature has been used for centuries to produce a variety of therapeutic effects. During the Middle Ages and continuing through the early 1900s, it was common for aristocrats to travel to Baden and take the "cure," which consisted of soaking in the hot mineral-laden waters. The sauna bath has been used for centuries in Scandinavian countries to achieve alleged health benefits and the sensation of well-being. Kuusinen and Heinonen (1972), for example, reported that after a sauna bath subjects were more relaxed, less hostile, and less anxious than before the sauna. However, these investigators noted the same effects following a hot shower (Kuusinen & Heinonen, 1972). This finding has been replicated by Raglin and Morgan (1985), who reported that a 5-min shower, with water temperature maintained at 38.5°C, was associated with a significant decrease in state anxiety. It has also been reported that muscle tension levels are reduced following a sauna (deVries, Beckman, Huber, & Dieckmeir, 1968). The

The preparation of this chapter was supported in part by the University of Wisconsin Sea Grant Institute under grants from the National Sea Grant College Program, National Oceanic and Atmospheric Administration, U.S. Department of Commerce, and from the State of Wisconsin. Federal Grant NA90AA-D-56469, Project R/NI-18.

213

reduction in tonic muscle activity observed by deVries et al. (1968) was attributed to decreased muscle spindle fiber activity as opposed to a generalized decrease in cortical activity. This explanation was based in part on an earlier report by von Euler and Soderberg (1957), who found that gamma motor neuron activity was correlated with increased hypothalamic temperature and EEG recordings. These investigators employed whole-body warming as well as direct brain warming using a cat model, and this intervention was found to have a profound influence on central neuron activity.

Pyrogenic therapy, which consisted of injecting pyrogens into the patients, was used to treat individuals suffering from paresis during the 1930s and the early 1940s. This procedure resulted in elevated temperatures lasting for almost 2 weeks, and it was reported by Bennett, Cash, and Hockstra (1941) that EEG improvements were observed in patients undergoing this therapy. These investigators noted an increase in alpha wave frequency following treatment, and this normalized EEG was found to persist after 3 years of follow-up. This form of therapy was eventually discontinued in favor of simply heating patients, and hyperthermia therapy has continued to the present day. Whole-body hyperthermia, for example, is currently employed as a treatment modality for cancer patients. Robins, Kalin, Shelton, Schecterle, et al. (1987) have reported marked pain relief and a sense of well-being in patients undergoing this treatment, and these investigators postulated that whole-body hyperthermia might result in increases in the opiate peptide, β-endorphin. In a subsequent study, Robins, Kalin, Shelton, Martin, et al. (1987) measured β-endorphin levels during hyperthermia treatment. A linear relationship was observed between thermal stress and duration of hyperthermia, and the quantitative rise in plasma β-endorphin levels. β-endorphin levels increased significantly as core temperature increased during the hyperthermia treatment (Robins et al., 1987a).

Changes in mood state have been assessed in cancer patients before and after whole-body hyperthermia (Koltyn, Robins, Schmitt, Cohen, & Morgan, 1992). A radiant heat device was employed, and core temperature increased to 41.8°C in these patients. Changes in mood state were measured with the POMS (McNair et al., 1992), and a significant decrease in depression was observed following the hyperthermia treatment. This antidepressant effect persisted for 72 hours following the intervention. Scores on the POMS scales designed to measure vigor and fatigue decreased and increased, respectively, following whole-body hyperthermia, but these changes returned to baseline levels within 72 hours. This investigation supports the view that transient increases in core temperature are associated with improved mood.

There is also evidence that disturbances in temperature regulation are associated with affective disorders. Avery, Wildschiodtz, and Rafaelsen (1982), for example, compared 9 patients diagnosed with primary affective disorder with 12 normal control subjects. It was found that the depressed patients had higher nocturnal temperatures than the control subjects, and that these elevated nocturnal temperatures returned to normal with recovery in the depressed sample. It has been hypothesized by Avery, Wildschiodtz, Smallwood, Martin, and Rafaelson (1986) that a relationship exists between REM sleep and thermoregulation. These investigators studied the relationship between core temperature and REM sleep in 9 depressed patients and 11 nondepressed controls. It was found that REM latency was shorter in the depressed group, and furthermore, that REM latency lengthened with recovery in these depressed patients. Rectal and tympanic temperatures were also both found to be higher in the depressed group, and this elevated temperature decreased following recovery.

The effects of passive versus active (e.g., exercise) heating on sleep have been compared by Horne and Staff (1983). Eight trained subjects took part in an experiment consisting of: (a) two, 40-min treadmill runs at 80% of VO_2max; (b) two 80-min treadmill runs at 40% of VO_2max; and (c) two 40-min sessions that involved sitting in a hot bath. The water temperature was adjusted in order to elevate each subject's rectal temperature to the same level produced during the high-intensity exercise condition. The results indicated that similar increases in slow wave sleep resulted from high-intensity physical activity and passive heating.

In an investigation by Holland, Sayers, Keatinge, Davis, and Peswani (1985), mood state was assessed before and after subjects were immersed in warm or thermoneutral water and asked to perform memory and reasoning tasks. A significant increase in irritability was observed in the warm condition, but these results should be viewed with caution for two reasons. First, the validity of the instrument employed to measure mood has not been demonstrated, and second, it is possible that the memory and reasoning tasks may have influenced mood state.

Different conditions that elevate core temperature have been associated with changes in subjective, electrocortical (brain), and neuromuscular correlates of anxiety. This seems to be the case for both passive heating as well as physical activity, and there is extensive literature indicating that aerobic exercise is associated with reductions in state anxiety (see chapter 7). Exercise increases core temperature in direct proportion to the intensity of exercise (Davies, Brotherhood, & Ziedifard, 1976), and this has led deVries (1987) to propose that the anxiolytic effect of physical activity may be caused by elevations in body temperature. However, there has been very little research dealing with the relationship between emotions such as anxiety on the one hand, and core temperature during and following physical activity on the other. The principal research strategy up to this point has involved manipulation of the customary temperature response that occurs during exercise in order to quantify whether or not changes in anxiety are independent of core temperature. If anxiety were observed to decrease in the absence of a rise in core temperature, for example, this would serve to refute the hypothesis that exercise-induced anxiolytic effects are caused by increased body temperature. Conversely, if anxiolytic effects were not observed following physical activity that did not produce a rise in body temperature, this would offer evidence in support of the thermogenic hypothesis. A principal concern in this area has involved the question of how deep body temperature should be measured, and this issue is addressed in the following section.

MEASUREMENT OF BODY TEMPERATURE

Examination of various studies designed to test the thermogenic hypothesis leads to the conclusion that compelling evidence is lacking. However, there are a number of reasons why this hypothesis should not be discounted on the basis of existing research. Various methods have been employed to measure core temperature in studies involving the impact of exercise and temperature manipulation on anxiety. Furthermore, there is an absence of universal agreement regarding which site is the best for assessment of core body temperature in humans. Each of the temperature sites employed in human studies has advantages and disadvantages, and to the extent possible, selection of a site should be governed by the question being asked. A brief review of temperature assessment is presented in this section.

Rectal Temperature

Rectal temperature has been the most widely used approximation of deep body temperature because of its convenience and low error rate (Molnar & Read, 1974); it also has widespread clinical acceptance (Armstrong, Maresh, Crago, Adams, & Roberts, 1994). While rectal temperature has been found to be independent of ambient temperature (Nadel & Horvath, 1970), it exhibits an initial inertia. Furthermore, the reliability of rectal temperature has been questioned in cases of rapid changes in temperature. Esophageal temperature has been shown to be a more accurate measure when rapid changes in core temperature take place. For example, esophageal temperature response has been shown to respond faster to passive heating (Robins et al., 1985). Rectal temperature lagged approximately 15 min behind the response time noted for esophageal temperature in this study. However, after 15 min, rectal temperature and esophageal temperature did not differ significantly.

Esophageal Temperature

Esophageal temperature is measured by inserting a catheter or a thermistor through the nasal passage to the throat, and the subject then swallows the probe until it reaches a specific anatomical position. However, the measurement of esophageal temperature is repulsive to some individuals, and it has been estimated that 10% of the population cannot suppress the gag reflex during insertion of the probe (Brengelmann, Johnson, & Hong, 1979). This is an important consideration because measurement of esophageal temperature may induce anxiety in some subjects, and it may also suppress or dampen the anxiolytic effects normally observed following various interventions.

Tympanic Temperature

Tympanic membrane temperature has also been used as a measure of deep body temperature, and it has been proposed that tympanic temperature actually reflects the temperature of the hypothalamus (Benzinger, 1959). This is important because the hypothalamus is thought to be the brain center responsible for temperature regulation. Benzinger (1959) was the first to propose the tympanic membrane as a possible site for accurate recording of hypothalamic temperature. Because it is usually not possible to measure brain temperature in humans, most of the research in this area has been conducted using animal models. Tympanic and hypothalamic temperatures have been compared in experiments using different animal species. Randall, Rawson, McCook, and Peiss (1963), for example, reported opposite shifts of tympanic temperature and hypothalamic temperature after occlusion of the common carotid artery in anesthetized cats, and concluded that the two were not closely related. However, Baker, Stocking, and Meehan (1972) reached the opposite conclusion on the basis of research using unanesthetized cats. They reported parallel changes of tympanic and hypothalamic temperature during feeding, sleeping, and arousal at different ambient temperatures. Tanabe and Takauri (1964) found that tympanic and hypothalamic temperature underwent parallel shifts during carotid heating or cooling in rabbits, whereas changes in rectal temperature were delayed if they occurred at all. In anesthetized pigs submitted to whole-body hyperthermia, mean tympanic temperature has been reported to remain within a range of $\pm 0.2°C$ of brain temperature (Dickson, MacKenzie, & McLeod, 1979). Research conducted with monkeys has also revealed that tympanic temperature parallels hypothalamic temperature (Baker et al., 1972; Rawson & Hammell, 1963). There is very little direct information regarding the relationship between hypothalamic and tympanic temperature in humans (Brinnel & Cabanac, 1989); and most of what has been written about the relationship in humans has been generalized from animal research. This could be problematic because of the differences in temperature regulation between species. However, there is limited research of both a direct and an indirect nature that has been conducted with humans.

Inferred Brain Temperature in Humans

Cabanac (1986) has proposed that a "selective cooling of the brain" occurs in humans during hyperthermic states such as those known to occur with exercise. This view is based on a study by Cabanac and Caputa (1979) in which the occurrence and magnitude of natural selective cooling of the human brain were investigated. In this study, subjects were immersed in a warm water ($38.6°C$ to $38.7°C$) bath and exposed to different conditions. One condition consisted of exposing the face to a fan that produced a wind at 6 m/s for 30 to 40 min. The other condition consisted of having subjects lift their left arms out of the water and expose them to the same wind while insulating their heads against the wind. Inferred brain temperature (i.e., tympanic), core temperature (i.e., esophageal) and perceptual ratings (pleasure and displeasure) were assessed in the different conditions. Fanning of the face resulted in a decrease in tympanic temperature, an increase in esophageal temperature, and an increase in perceptual ratings. In comparison, fanning of the arm resulted in a decrease in esophageal temperature, no change in tympanic temperature and no change in perceptual ratings. Cabanac and Caputa (1979) concluded that brain temperature could be affected independent of body temperature, and that such cooling had significant psychological and physiological effects.

Nielsen and Jessen (1992) have argued that brainstem cooling does not occur during face fanning. These investigators measured the speed of conduction of auditory evoked potentials to explore brainstem temperature changes, and found it to be accelerated during hyperthermia. In this study, subjects exercised in a hot environment while wearing an impermeable garment. In one condition the head was covered with a hood to hinder heat loss. In another condition the head was bare and the face was fanned. These two hyperthemic conditions were compared with a control condition. Results indicated that speed of conduction was increased significantly in the control condition compared with the hyperthermic conditions. However, the hyperthermic condition with the head covered did not differ from the hyperthermic condition with the head uncovered and the face fanned. Nielsen and Jessen (1992) concluded that no selective brain cooling occurred in this experiment. Cabanac (1993) has disagreed with the conclusion drawn by Nielsen and Jessen on the grounds that during face fanning tympanic temperature decreased significantly, but the magnitude of the decrease was only 0.15°C. This small change in tympanic temperature may explain why there was no significant change in the auditory evoked potentials. The limit of detection for a change of brainstem temperature by the auditory evoked potentials method is 0.39°C. Cabanac (1993) also pointed out that although small, some cooling nevertheless took place on the skin. There was a small decrease in heart rate, as well as a small but significant decrease of forearm skin blood flow. These decreases indicate that heat stress was diminished by face fanning even with esophageal temperature staying constant in the two hyperthermic conditions. Thus, Cabanac (1993) hypothesizes that brain temperature (i.e., tympanic temperature) was lowered enough by face fanning to diminish heat stress.

Direct Measurement
of Brain Temperature in Humans

There is very little research available involving the direct measurement of human brain temperature. However, there are several reports involving brain temperature in seriously injured and critically ill patients (Mellergard & Nordstrom, 1990; Whitby & Dunkin, 1971). Intraventricular and epidural temperatures were measured along with tympanic and rectal temperature in 7 neurosurgical patients in a study by Mellergard and Nordsrom (1990). Rectal temperature was reported to "reflect the epidural temperature adequately in most of the patients" (p. 33). There was a mean difference of 0.48°C between rectal and epidural temperature. Tympanic temperature was lower (0.3 to 0.5) than the epidural temperature in approximately 90% of the observations. The temperature of the air in the external ear canal was reported to possibly be a factor of major importance in measuring tympanic temperature. However, sealing the external ear canal from ambient air by means of insulation material did not significantly alter the recorded temperatures of the patients in this study. It was also found that tympanic temperature followed variations in epidural temperature more closely than did rectal temperature. It was concluded that tympanic temperature appears to be more reliable than rectal temperature as an index of epidural temperature. However, it was also reported that measurement of tympanic temperature was a difficult and tedious procedure. There were often difficulties getting the thermocouple in the proper position to measure tympanic temperature, and it was reported that even comatose patients showed signs of discomfort during the slightest manipulation of the temperature probe. However, advances in the instrumentation employed to measure tympanic temperature have eliminated many of these problems, and tympanic temperature is now employed routinely in exercise research (Trine, 1994).

Summary   Rectal temperature has been the basis for measurement of deep body or core temperature in most investigations dealing with evaluation of the thermogenic hypothesis of exercise-induced anxiolytic effects (Koltyn & Morgan, 1990, 1992a; Koltyn, Shake, & Morgan, 1993; Petruzello, Landers, & Salazar, 1993). Tympanic temperature has been employed in two studies dealing with this question (Reeves, Levison, Justesen, & Lubin, 1985; Trine, 1994), and esophageal temperature has been employed in one study (Youngstedt, Dishman, Cureton, & Peacock, 1993). While the question being asked should ultimately govern the choice of site, there are other considerations that must be made as well. Tympanic temperature would seem to be the most attractive option at this time for studies concerned with the relationship between deep body temperature and anxiety. First of all, there is evidence suggesting that tympanic temperature is associated with hypothalamic temperature. Second, measurements of esophageal temperature can be sufficiently aversive to render it impractical in studies involving dependent variables such as anxiety. Third, rectal temperature not only lags behind other measures of core temperature, but it is also associated with concerns from the standpoint of disease transmission and personal modesty in the case of research with humans. In addition, when rectal temperature is employed, it would seem prudent to employ disposable probes. While this approach is more expensive, and potentially prohibitive in studies involving large samples, it minimizes concerns about disease transmission.

TEMPERATURE MANIPULATION

Investigations designed to test the thermogenic hypothesis of exercise-induced anxiolytic effects by manipulating deep body temperature are reviewed in this section. While this design strategy is attractive from an experimental standpoint, it has proven to be problematic for two reasons. First, investigators have experienced difficulty in blocking the normal rise in deep body temperature associated with vigorous physical activity. Second, effective temperature-blocking paradigms, because of potential stress, can actually result in elevated anxiety. A chronological summary of research using this experimental paradigm follows.

Study I

The first experiment in this area was conducted by Reeves et al. (1985), who assessed core temperature and affective changes in 20 male subjects before and after 20 min of calisthenics. The test subjects were assigned randomly to a control condition that consisted of exercise while wearing shorts, T-shirt, socks, and shoes. The participants in the experimental group wore insulated clothing (including a hood and gloves) while performing the same set of calisthenics for 20 min. In addition, the subjects in the experimental group were covered with two blankets and a surgical mask following exercise. Anxiety and tympanic temperature were assessed before and after exercise. The experimental manipulation resulted in the desired temperature response in that the control group did not experience a change, but tympanic temperature increased significantly ($\pm 1.2°C$) in the experimental group. The subjects in the experimental group experienced a significant elevation in anxiety, but there was no change in anxiety observed for the control group.

This study (Reeves et al., 1985) seems to refute the hypothesis that physical activity reduces anxiety, and suggests that the absence of such an anxiolytic effect is independent of increased core temperature. It is possible that increased anxiety with elevated body temperature resulted from discomfort associated with the wear of excessive and restrictive clothing in this study. Likewise, while the two conditions resulted in the desired change in body temperature for the experimental group, the intensity and duration of the physical activity were not sufficient to provoke the customary rise in core temperature observed with vigorous physical activity. In other words, this study did not involve a direct test of the thermogenic hypothesis advanced to explain exercise-induced anxiolytic effects.

Study II

In an attempt to block the normal temperature rise associated with physical activity, Koltyn and Morgan (1990) employed whole-body cooling prior to exercise in a pilot study. Six male subjects walked at 70% of VO_2max for 30 min following a period of either whole-body cooling, or quiet rest in a sound-dampened chamber (control). Whole-body cooling consisted of immersion (head out) in a bath maintained at 25°C for 30 min whereas the control condition consisted of resting quietly in a chamber with a noise level of 8 dB. The two conditions (whole-body cooling/control) were counterbalanced and randomly assigned to subjects. Exercise performed following whole-body cooling resulted in a mean rectal temperature of 37.8°C compared with 38.5°C in the control group, and this difference of 0.7°C was statistically significant. State anxiety decreased significantly under the control condition when a customary rise in core temperature occurred, but it was not reduced following physical activity that was preceded by whole-body cooling. This pilot study offered preliminary support for the view that reduced anxiety following exercise may be governed, in part, by increased body temperature.

Study III

It has been shown that core temperature does not rise during physical activity performed underwater at temperatures of 18°C to 29°C, and underwater exercise was employed in the next experiment (Koltyn & Morgan, 1992a). Fifteen male certified scuba divers completed 20 min of underwater exercise at a pace of 0.52 m/s in 25°C water. State anxiety and rectal temperature were measured simultaneously before divers entered the water; before exercise in the water; immediately after exercise; and 15 min after exercise. The results indicated that core temperature did not change significantly following underwater exercise. The mean core temperature response of the divers before entering the water was 37.1°C ($SD = 0.3$), and following 20 min of underwater exercise the mean temperature was 37.0°C ($SD = 0.2$). This exercise protocol was effective in eliminating the customary rise in core temperature following exercise, and state anxiety was observed to decrease significantly at 15 min postexercise. This finding serves to refute the thermogenic hypothesis, and it was concluded that the anxiolytic effect of underwater exercise is not dependent on increases in core temperature (Koltyn & Morgan, 1992a).

Study IV

The finding that anxiety can be reduced following physical activity even though core temperature does not rise offers good evidence that the anxiolytic effect of exercise is not dependent on increased body temperature (Koltyn & Morgan, 1992a). However, a more compelling refutation of the thermogenic hypothesis would be the demonstration that anxiolytic effects occur with and without increased core temperature following the same exercise stimulus. For this reason, the same underwater protocol was employed in a subsequent study, but another condition was included in order to make a direct comparison between exercise with and without increased core temperature (Koltyn & Morgan, 1993). This was achieved by having subjects complete an additional trial while wearing a 1/4-inch-thick neoprene wetsuit. Thirteen male scuba divers completed 20 min of underwater exercise at a pace of 0.52 m/s in 24°C water with and without a wetsuit. The order of conditions was counterbalanced, randomly assigned, and performed on separate days. In this study (Koltyn & Morgan, 1993), state anxiety and core temperature were assessed as previously described (Koltyn & Morgan, 1992a). Core temperature increased significantly following underwater exercise in the wetsuit condition, but temperature did not change following exercise in the control condition. Results for state anxiety revealed different responses for the two conditions. State anxiety actually increased following exercise when subjects wore a wetsuit and experienced an increase in core temperature. In contrast, there was a significant decrease in state anxiety when subjects performed underwater exercise without a wetsuit and did not have an increase in core temperature. A basic premise of this study was that a decrease in anxiety in the absence of a rise in core temperature would offer evidence to refute the thermogenic hypothesis suggested to explain exercise-induced anxiolytic effects. These results provide further evidence that the anxiolytic effect of underwater exercise occurs in the absence of an increase in core temperature (Koltyn & Morgan, 1993).

Study V

It has also been shown that state anxiety increases following exercise in which core temperature falls (Koltyn et al., 1993). Ten male divers were evaluated before and after 30 min of underwater physical activity in 18°C or 29°C water. The physical activity was performed both with and without a wetsuit in the two conditions. Core temperature did not change significantly following 30 min of underwater exercise in 18°C water while wearing a wetsuit, or in 29°C water with or without a wetsuit. However, core temperature decreased significantly following underwater exercise in 18°C water without a wetsuit. Thus, the customary rise in core temperature following exercise on land was not evident following exercise underwater. An increase in state anxiety was observed following underwater exercise performed in 18°C water without a wetsuit. There was also an increase in state anxiety following underwater exercise performed in 29°C water without wearing a wetsuit even though core temperature did not change significantly. These results offer further refutation of the temperature hypothesis.

Study VI

Other investigators have attempted to study this problem by having subjects exercise in shoulder-deep water at different temperatures (Youngstedt et al., 1993). Eleven male subjects were assigned randomly to four 20-min conditions consisting of cycling at 70% of VO_2peak in thermoneutral water (32°C to 35°C); cycling at 70% of VO_2peak in cold water (18°C to 23°C); passive warm water exposure (39°C to 41°C); and quiet rest. Esophageal temperature increased equally during thermoneutral cycling ($+1.45°C \pm 0.05°C$) and passive heating ($+1.51°C \pm 0.06°C$), was blunted during cold cycling ($+0.40°C \pm 0.12°C$), and was unchanged at rest. State anxiety, mean radial arterial pressure, and brain electrocortical activity were assessed before and after each of the four conditions. Results revealed a significant reduction in mean arterial pressure following cycling in the thermoneutral condition and after passive heating. However, the reduction in blood pressure was not accompanied by concomitant changes in brain electrocortical activity or self-reported state anxiety. Conversely, blood pressure can be operationalized as an anxiety measure. In agreement with earlier research (Bahrke

& Morgan, 1978; Raglin & Morgan, 1987), state anxiety was reduced following quiet rest. The results for state anxiety in the thermoneutral condition are not in agreement with most published studies because it has generally been reported that a decrease in self-reported state anxiety follows acute physical activity (chapter 7). Youngstedt et al. (1993) acknowledged that the novelty of their experimental conditions may have prevented an anxiolytic effect, and it is possible that measurement of esophageal temperature is sufficiently aversive that commonly observed changes in anxiety are suppressed or dampened.

Study VII

Another approach to this problem has involved the comparison of subjects who exercised in warmer and cooler conditions in comparison with a control condition (Petruzello et al., 1993). In the control condition, subjects ran at 75% of VO_2max for 30 min in regular running clothing (i.e., T-shirt, shorts, socks, and shoes). In the warmer condition, subjects ran at 75% of VO_2max for 30 min with full-leg lycra tights, nylon running pants, long sleeve T-shirt, a nylon sweat jacket, and a terry cloth neck wrap. In the cooler condition, subjects exercised as described in the normal condition, but had their shirts and shorts dampened with cold water prior to exercise. Subjects also wore a terrycloth neck wrap filled with ice. Core temperature was assessed with a rectal probe before, during, and after exercise in all three conditions, and state anxiety was assessed prior to exercise, as well as 5, 10, 20, and 30 min postexercise. Results indicated that rectal temperature increased significantly in all three conditions following exercise, with the highest increase being observed for the warmer condition. State anxiety decreased significantly in all three conditions, but it should be kept in mind that core temperature was not blocked in this study. That is, exercise in the experimental conditions resulted in temperature values that differed, but all conditions were characterized by elevated rectal temperature. These results can be viewed as providing limited support for the temperature hypothesis because anxiety fell at a point following increases in core temperature.

Study VIII

Tympanic temperature was employed in the most recent research conducted in this area (Trine, 1994). This research differed from the related research involving physical activity, deep body temperature, and anxiety in three important respects. First, individuals who regularly exercised in the morning, at noon, or in the evening completed three sessions of running exercise from 6 a.m. to 8 a.m., 11 a.m. to 1:30 p.m., and 6 p.m. to 8 p.m. Second, each individual exercised at an intensity that was based on his or her "preferred exertion" (Morgan, 1994a). In other words, unlike prior research in which subjects exercised at the same relative or absolute intensity selected by the investigator(s), each participant ran at his or her customary or preferred pace. Third, the participants consisted of 15 women and 15 men, whereas the earlier research has been based almost entirely on male test subjects. State anxiety and tympanic temperature were assessed before and after each of the runs. A significant decrease in state anxiety was observed following exercise for both women and men, and this effect was independent of time of day for both groups. The reduced anxiety was associated with increased tympanic temperature in the men but not the women, and this difference reflects the higher exercise intensity selected by the male participants in this study.

Summary

Some of the research reviewed in this section suggests that reduced anxiety following acute physical activity is associated with elevated core temperature, while other studies fail to demonstrate that such a relationship exists. Even where an association between anxiety and core temperature has been demonstrated, there is an absence of compelling data in support of a causal link. Furthermore, efforts to test the thermogenic hypothesis by blocking the customary rise in core temperature associated with vigorous physical activity have failed to yield consistent findings. Investigators in this area of inquiry have employed different: methods of measuring core temperature; different modes and intensities of physical activity; and different measures of anxiety. Therefore, the inconsistency of research findings may be due to the use of different independent and dependent variables by investigators. At any rate, it seems reasonable to conclude that the temperature hypothesis remains tenable. It appears that one of the most attractive experimental strategies at this point involves the manipulation of core temperature, but it is imperative that investigators who elect to employ "blocking" paradigms consider two issues. First, the procedure should be effective in preventing an increase in core temperature; that is, merely blunting the customary rise in temperature is not sufficient. Second, blocking procedures should not be so stressful that anxiety is actually provoked. It should be understood, of course, that methods of measuring core temperature should not be anxiety-provoking either.

FUTURE DIRECTIONS

The thermogenic hypothesis of exercise-induced anxiolytic effects remains tenable, and additional research is needed before this explanation can be discounted. If tympanic temperature is a measure of brain temperature, and if it is selectively cooled during exercise, it may have differential effects on affective states independent of body warming as reflected by increases in rectal temperature. With the advent of new technology such as infrared tympanic temperature scanners, it may be possible in future research to examine the thermogenic hypothesis in a less distressing and more accurate manner.

Most of the research in this area has been restricted to the study of anxiety, and there is a need to investigate the relationship between physical activity, temperature, and changes in other mood states such as depression. In a recent study by Nelson and Morgan (1994), for example, it was reported that acute physical activity resulted in an antidepressant effect in depressed college students, and this improvement in mood was independent of exercise intensity. Furthermore, all but one of the investigations published thus far in this area have employed college-age men, and there is a need to investigate the relationship between temperature and affective changes in women, as well as women and men from additional age groups.

Another consideration to be made before discounting the thermogenic hypothesis involves the possibility that various hypothesized mechanisms (e.g., endorphin, norepinephrine, serotonin, temperature) may operate in an interactive or redundant manner. It is possible, for example, that each of the hypothesized mechanisms, including core temperature, influences anxiety in a redundant manner. If this were the case, one could theoretically eliminate a selected mechanism (e.g., temperature), but owing to the inherent redundancy and interaction, an axiolytic effect might still occur. For example, changes in body temperature affect cellular structures, enzyme systems, and numerous temperature-dependent chemical reactions that take place in the body. It has been shown that thermal stress causes increases in some hormonal responses, such as catecholamines, glucagon, growth hormone, and cortisol during prolonged exercise (Dulac et al., 1987; Galbo et al., 1979; Hartley et al., 1972; Viti, Lupo, & Lodi, Bonifazi, & Martelli, 1989).

The effect of water temperature on the hormonal response to prolonged swimming has been studied by Galbo et al. (1979). Six male subjects swam for 60 min at approximately 68% of VO_2max in water at 21°C, 27°C, and 33°C. Significant increases were observed in plasma noradrenaline at all three water temperatures. Thus, with both increases and decreases in core temperature, there was a significant change in noradrenaline level. Furthermore, Barchas and Freedman (1962) demonstrated that manipulation of temperature in rats will alter the rate and extent of change in brain levels of serotonin and norepinephrine. The significance of this observation is addressed thoroughly in chapters 11 (Chaouloff) and 12 (Dishman) of this book. It has also been demonstrated that injection of norepinephrine into the anterior hypothalamus of rats just before exercise not only attenuated the rise in core temperature, but produced hypothermia (Gisolfi & Christman, 1980). It appears that there is an interaction between temperature and catecholamine response in both humans and animals. Thus, further research is needed to investigate the interaction between changes in temperature (i.e., with exercise) and changes in brain levels of monoamines.

The interaction between temperature and changes in β-endorphins needs further study as well. The results of pharmacological studies (Clark, 1979; Olson, Olson, Kastin, & Coy, 1982; Rezvani, Gordon, & Heath, 1982) in which endogenous opioid peptides were administered have indicated that the thermoregulatory effects of opioid peptides are variable and numerous. In animal studies, exogenous β-endorphin administration causes alterations in thermoregulatory control that are dependent on ambient temperature, dosage, and route of administration (Bloom & Tseng, 1981; Clark, 1979; Yehuda & Kastin, 1980). Research in humans by Kelso, Herbert, Gwazdauskas, Goss, and Hess (1984) has indicated that the β-endorphin and β-lipotropin response pattern closely parallels changes in rectal temperature during physical activity. The endorphin hypothesis is reviewed in detail by Hoffmann in chapter 10. It is possible that several of the hypothesized mechanisms (e.g., temperature, monoamines, endorphins) influence anxiety or other affective states in an interactive (or redundant) manner, but this possibility has not been addressed systematically.

SUMMARY

There appears to be limited indirect evidence supporting a potential role for temperature in the mediation of exercise-induced anxiolytic effects. Different conditions that elevate core temperature have been associated with changes in subjective, biochemical, electrocortical, cardiovascular, and neuromuscular correlates of anxiety. However, efforts to perform direct tests of the thermogenic hypothesis have not yielded compelling evidence in support of this hypothesis. Indeed, there is some evidence refuting the thermogenic hypothesis. Our knowledge in this area will not advance until study of the anxiolytic and mood enhancing correlates of physical activity are approached from a multidisciplinary perspective. It is important that future efforts to identify the contribution of core temperature in the mediation of improved affective states include biochemical, cardiovascular and neurophysiological parameterization. In the meantime it is important to recognize that passive warming of the human body by means of common interventions (e.g., warm baths, showers, sauna) leads to an improved sense of well-being and mood. Furthermore, whole-body heating (hyperthermia therapy) is directly correlated with a rise in plasma β-endorphin levels and improved mood. Because vigorous physical activity can also lead to an increase in core temperature, it has been logical to assume that a causal link exists. However, anxiety has been shown to decrease following exercise performed at an intensity or under environmental conditions in which body temperature does not rise. This is a very important finding because it offers additional support (see chapter 3) for the view that physical activity does not need to be performed at a high intensity in order for selected physical and mental benefits to occur.

Chapter 14

Conclusion: State of the Field and Future Research

William P. Morgan

It has been reported by the National Institute of Mental Health (NIMH) that 22% of the population is affected by mental disorders each year. It has also been estimated that 5 million American adults experience the most severe of these illnesses, including major depression, manic-depressive disorder, schizophrenia, panic disorder, and obsessive-compulsive disorder. However, these severe illnesses represent only a small portion of a much broader problem, and a large number of individuals are affected by various mental and behavioral disorders that occur independent of age, gender, race, and socioeconomic status. These mental disorders result in a cost of $148 billion each year for treatment and indirect costs, and the cost of depression alone is estimated at $53 billion a year in the United States (NIMH, 1995). Serious depression affects approximately 15% of the U.S. population at least once in a lifetime, but it is estimated that only 1 person in 10 with such disorders gets adequate treatment. The solution to this pandemic public health problem is prevention, and a theoretical rationale for prevention has been addressed in chapter 2. One concern is that two thirds of the people suffering from depression never get treated for this disorder, and half of this group never even seeks treatment. Furthermore, a national advisory panel on depression has reported that even when patients seek treatment insurance and managed care companies actively discourage them from seeking mental health care services (Hirschfeld, 1996).

There are many psychological and medical procedures such as psychotherapy and drug therapy that are used effectively to treat various mental problems such as anxiety and depression, but these interventions can be costly and time-consuming. Treatment for depression, for example, may require months and years of therapy or long-term treatment with antidepressive drugs. It has been reported that many insurance plans are motivated to contain costs, and this can lead to caps on the number of therapy visits and limits on the type and length of time drugs may be prescribed (Hirschfeld, 1996). Furthermore, while drug therapy is often effective in the treatment of severe depression, it can lead to undesired side effects in the case of mild or moderate depression. This has led to a search for nonpharmacologic therapies, and physical activity, the focus of this book, has proven to be associated with desirable psychological outcomes in individuals with mild to moderate levels of mood disturbance. This book represents an effort to evaluate the efficacy of physical activity in the prevention and treatment of mental disorders such as depression (chapter 6), anxiety (chapter 7), and low self-esteem (chapter 8).

This book represents the most current review of physical activity and mental health, and it differs from earlier volumes of a related nature in several respects. First, a multidisciplinary approach has been employed, and the contributors include scientists with specialization in various fields such as behavioral medicine, epidemiology, experimental psychology, clinical psychology, psychiatry, physiology, physical education, endocrinology, kinesiology, and exercise science. Second, the book includes a discussion of selected mechanisms underlying the psychological changes accompanying physical activity. One of the most exciting and promising avenues of research in the area of physical activity and mental health involves the influence of exercise on brain monoamine levels. While research involving the influence of exercise on brain chemistry and behavior has only been pursued systematically in recent years, it is noteworthy that William James (1899) stated almost a century ago that:

> The nervous system and the muscles need exercise in order that their vital metamorphoses shall contribute to the normal chemical composition of the blood that bathes the brain. (p. 221)

Potential mechanisms examined in this book include the endorphin (chapter 10), serotonin (chapter 11), norepinephrine (chapter 12), and thermogenic (chapter 13) hypotheses. While none of these hypotheses can be viewed as providing proof of a causal link between physical activity and improved psychological well-being, each can be regarded as tenable. Further research will be necessary in order to establish evidence of biological plausibility. It is also possible that dopaminergic mechanisms play an important role in this process, but there is not sufficient research of a systematic nature to warrant such an explanation at this time. There is also limited research literature suggesting that a correlation may exist between electrocortical and affective changes during and after physical activity. However, it would be premature to suggest that indirect measures (e.g., EEG) of this nature play a causal role in exercise-induced anxiolysis until alternative hypotheses can be ruled out. At any rate, there are numerous biochemical changes that have been shown to occur in the CNS during and after physical activity. While this work has relied almost entirely on animal models, the observations have direct relevance for, and parallel, hypothesized changes in the human.

There is considerable evidence supporting the view that physical activity is associated with improved physical health and increased longevity, but there is less support for the view that physical activity can serve to develop and maintain mental health (Bouchard et al., 1994). This book represents an effort to summarize the existing research dealing with the influence of physical activity on mental health, as well as the potential mechanisms underlying psychological outcomes. An effort has been made throughout the book to not only synthesize existing knowledge in this area, but emphasis is also place on the creation of a research agenda for the future. It is hoped that this feature of the book will be attractive to beginning students, established investigators, and applied health professionals alike.

There has been a general tendency in related volumes, as well as in quantitative and qualitative review articles and chapters, to ignore crucial methodological issues that are known to influence psychological outcomes in efficacy research. This book begins with a chapter dealing with methodological considerations, and it is now apparent that much of the outcome or efficacy research in this area of inquiry has been influenced by various behavioral artifacts such as the halo and Hawthorne effects, as well as expectancies, demand characteristics, lack of blind paradigms, inadequate control or placebo groups, failure to control for response distortion, inappropriate sample size, and so on. In addition to discussing these issues at some length in chapter 1, contributors have made an effort to comment on methodological issues germane to the focus of each chapter.

An effort has been made in this book to address the circumstances under which physical activity is appropriate as a treatment strategy, as well as the conditions that serve to maximize psychological outcomes. The prescription of exercise is addressed in chapter 3, and the approach taken in this chapter differs substantially from conventional treatments of the subject. The authors introduce the concept of "lifestyle" exercise, and this may prove to represent a major advance in health promotion efforts. It is also known that over half of all individuals who adopt exercise programs quit within 6 to 8 weeks, and further attrition occurs with the passage of time. Prevention of sedentary lifestyles is discussed in chapter 2, and the related problem of adherence to physical activity programs is addressed in chapter 4. While the problem of exercise adherence remains a puzzle and a challenge, consideration of the principles presented in chapter 2 (prevention) and chapter 3 (prescription) should prove to be useful to therapists and researchers alike.

Despite the absence of evidence that physical activity actually *causes* the improved psychological states observed following exercise, there is overwhelming evidence that both acute and chronic physical activity are accompanied by improved psychological well-being. However, there is an exception to this generalization, and it involves the case in which an individual exercises to the point that "overtraining" occurs. Individuals who fall into this category may experience psychological distress characterized by elevated levels of anxiety and depression, as well as endocrine and cardiovascular dysregulation, and this clinical syndrome has been labeled "staleness" in the exercise science literature. This complex, psychobiological problem is addressed in chapter 9, and it needs to be considered within the context of exercise prescription (chapter 3) and adherence (chapter 4). In other words, an ideal exercise prescription should theoretically lead to enhanced adherence, but the adherence (self-imposed or otherwise) should not lead to overtraining and staleness. This important paradoxical aspect of physical activity should not be ignored because it can lead to the very problems (e.g., anxiety, depression) one hopes to prevent or treat.

It is not uncommon for individuals with various forms of depression and anxiety disorders to receive various drugs in the treatment process. These may include neuroleptics, antidepressants, lithium, minor tranquilizers, and β-adrenergic blocking agents. Therefore, while physical activity is sometimes promoted as a nondrug intervention in the management of depression and anxiety disorders, it is not uncommon for clients in physical activity programs to receive drugs concurrently for various physical and mental disorders. For this reason, the issue of drug therapy and physical activity is addressed in chapter 5, and there is good evidence that patients who are receiving psychopharmacological agents can exercise safely if monitored by a physician.

FUTURE RESEARCH

There is no need for further research or reviews dealing with the question of whether or not physical activity results in improved mood. There is compelling evidence supporting the efficacy of physical activity in the prevention and treatment of both physical and mental disorders (Bouchard et al., 1995; Morgan & Goldston, 1987; Nicoloff & Schwenk, 1995). There are, however, many questions that remain unanswered, and these questions will hopefully be addressed in the decade ahead.

It is unclear whether a threshold or optimal exercise dose exists, and there is some evidence that low intensity physical activity that fails to produce physiological changes results in improved psychological states. In this respect, it has been shown that individuals experience a comparable anxiolytic effect following vigorous physical activity and quiet rest (Bahrke & Morgan, 1978; Raglin & Morgan, 1987), and this observation has led to formulation of the "distraction" hypothesis, which proposes that the exercise-induced anxiolysis may be due to distraction from the cares and worries of the day (Morgan, 1985a). It has also been reported by Nolen-Hoeksema and Morrow (1993) that mildly to moderately depressed individuals became significantly less depressed following 8 min of focusing their attention on descriptions of geographic locations and objects (i.e., distraction). Conversely, a depressed group that focused their attention on current feeling states and personal characteristics (i.e., rumination) became significantly more depressed. Rather than hypothesizing that improved mood following exercise is due to alterations in brain levels of neurotransmitters or endorphins, one could hypothesize that observed psychological changes are caused by the distraction afforded by exercise. It is customary when conducting scientific inquiry not only to test one's hypothesis (e.g., monoamine hypothesis), but there is also a need to rule out alternative hypotheses.

Future research in this area will also need to address the related issues of *exercise mode* (e.g., running, walking); *intensity* (e.g., low, moderate, high); *duration* (e.g., 15, 30, 45 min); *frequency* (e.g., 1, 3, 5 days per week); *preferred versus prescribed* exertion levels; *personalized prescription* (e.g., based on personality structure); and *lifestyle versus traditional exercise prescription* (see chapter 3).

There are many other factors that will need to be addressed in future work. For example, there has been a tendency to conceptualize mood in exercise science research as a unitary rather than a two-dimensional construct (Clark, Watson, & Leeka, 1993). As a consequence, investigators have examined either negative or positive affect. The decision to study one or both of these dimensions of mood should be based on the question being asked, and this needs to be taken into account in future research. Other factors such as the circadian rhythm that are known to occur for various affective measures (Clark et al., 1993) warrant attention as well, but this issue has been largely ignored by investigators interested in the psychological effects of physical activity (Trine & Morgan, 1995). Finally, individuals with certain psychological characteristics (e.g., high trait anxiety) appear to experience more injuries and fatalities when pursuing certain high-risk recreational activities such as scuba diving (Morgan, 1995). This phenomenon needs to be addressed for other high-risk activities (e.g., rock climbing, sport parachuting).

SUMMARY

The relationship between regular physical activity and psychological well-being has been very well established. Indeed, Nicoloff and Schwenk (1995) have reported that exercise is just as effective as psychotherapy and antidepressant therapy in the treatment of mild to moderate depression. Furthermore, a much earlier report by Franz and Hamilton (1905) suggests that exercise can also be effective as an adjunct in the treatment of major depression. Beginning with the early narrative reviews by Layman (1960) and Cureton (1963), there have been a number of qualitative and quantitative meta-analyses of acute and chronic experiments that support the view that physical activity is associated with an improvement in psychological well-being. However, there is an absence of compelling evidence in support of the view that physical activity *causes* the anxiolytic or antidepressant effects that occur, and the search for underlying mechanisms that can be used to explain these outcomes has only begun. This book not only summarizes what is currently known about the effects of physical activity on various affective measures, but an effort is also made to address the important issue of the potential mechanisms responsible for mediation of such effects. In other words, an attempt has been made to generate a research agenda, as well as to present a state-of-the-art summary for use by health care providers concerned with both the prevention and treatment of mental health problems. A lifestyle that includes regular physical activity is clearly associated with psychological well-being.

References

Ahlborg, G., Felig, P., Hagenfeldt, L., Hendler, R., & Wahren, J. (1974). Substrate turnover during prolonged exercise in man. *Journal of Clinical Investigation, 53,* 1080–1090.

Ainsworth, B.E., Montoye, H.J., & Leon, A.S. (1994). Methods of assessing physical activity during leisure and work. In C. Bouchard, R.J. Shephard, & T. Stephens (Eds.), *Physical activity, fitness, and health: International proceedings and consensus statement* (pp. 146–159). Champaign, IL: Human Kinetics Publishers.

Akil, H., Watson, S.J., Young, E., Lewis, M.E., Khachaturian, H., & Walker, J.M. (1984). Endogenous opioids: Biology and function. *Annual Review of Neuroscience, 7,* 223–255.

Aksnes, E.G. (1977). Beta-blockers: Dangerous for skiers? *Journal of the Norwegian Medical Association, 12,* 576.

Albanes, D., Blair, A., & Taylor, P.R. (1989). Physical activity and risk of cancer in the NHANES I popoulation. *American Journal of Public Health, 79,* 744–750.

Allen, M.E., & Coen, D. (1987). Naloxone blocking of running-induced mood changes. *Annals of Sports Medicine, 3,* 190–195.

American College of Sports Medicine (1978). The recommended quantity and quality of exercise for developing and maintaining fitness in healthy adults. *Medicine and Science in Sports, 10,* vii–x.

American College of Sports Medicine (1990). The recommended quality and quantity of exercise for developing and maintaing fitness in healthy adults. *Medicine and Science in Sports and Exercise, 22,* 265–274.

American College of Sports Medicine (1995). *Guidelines for exercise testing and prescription* (5th ed.). Baltimore, MD: Williams & Wilkins.

American College of Sports Medicine (1993). Physical activity, physical fitness, and hypertension: Position stand. *Medicine and Science in Sports and Exercise, 25,* i–x.

American Medical Association (1966). *Standard nomenclature of athletic injuries.* Chicago: Author.

American Psychiatric Association. (1980). *Diagnostic and statistical manual of mental disorders* (3rd ed.). Washington, DC: Author.

American Psychiatric Association (1994). *Diagnostic and statistical manual of mental disorders* (4th ed.). Washington, DC: Author.

Andersen, S.D., Bye, P.T.P., Perry, C.P., Hamor, G.P., Theobald, G., & Nyberg, G. (1979). Limitations in work performance in normal adult males in the presence of beta-adrenergic blocade. *Australian and New Zealand Journal of Medicine, 9,* 515–520.

Andreasen, N.C. (1988). Brain imaging: Applications in psychiatry. *Science, 239,* 1381–1385.

Anisman, H., & Zacharko, R.M. (1986). Behavioral and neurochemical consequences of stressors. In D.D. Kelly (Ed.), *Stress-induced analgesia* (pp. 205–225). New York: Academy of Science.

Anthony, J. (1991). Psychologic aspects of exercise. *Clinics in Sports Medicine, 10,* 171–180.

Antoni, F.A. (1986). Hypothalamic control of adrenocorticotropin secretion: Advances since the discovery of 41-residue corticotropin releasing factor. *Endocrine Reviews, 7*, 351–378.

Aref, M.A., El-Badramany, M., Hannora, N. et al. (1982). Lithium loss in sweat. *Psychosomatics, 23*, 407.

Arlin, M. (1976). Causal priority of social desirability over self-concept: A cross-lagged correlation analysis. *Journal of Personality and Social Psychology, 33*, 267–272.

Armstrong, C.A., Sallis, J.F., Hovell, M.F., & Hofstetter, C.R. (1993). Stages of change, self-efficacy, and the adoption of vigorous exercise: A prospective analysis. *Journal of Sport and Exercise Psychology, 15*, 190–402.

Armstrong, L.E., Maresh, C.M., Crago, A.E., Adams, R., & Roberts, W.O. (1994). Interpretation of aural temperatures during exercise, hyperthermia, and cooling therapy. *Medicine, Exercise, Nutrition and Health, 3*, 9–16.

Artigas, F. (1993). 5-HT and antidepressants: New views from microdialysis studies. *Trends in Pharmacological Sciences, 14*, 262–263.

Åsberg, M., Perris, C., Schalling, D., & Sedvall, G. (1978). The CPRS-development and applications of a psychiatric rating scale. *Acta Psychiatrica Scandinavica, Suppl 271*, 1–27.

Aston-Jones, G., Akaoka, H., Chariety, P., & Chouvet, G. (1991). Serotonin selectively attenuates glutamate-evoked activation of noradrenergic locus coeruleus neurons. *Journal of Neuroscience, 11*, 760–769.

Åstrand, P.O., & Saltin, B. (1961). Maximum oxygen uptake and heart rate in various types of muscular activity. *Journal of Applied Physiology, 16*, 977–981.

Atkinson, R.L. (1987). Opioid regulation of food intake and body weight in humans. *Federation Proceedings, 46*, 178–182.

Avery, D.H., Wildschiodtz, G., & Rafaelsen, O.J. (1982). Nocturnal temperature in affective disorders. *Journal of Affective Disorders, 4*, 61–71.

Avery, D.H., Wildschiodtz, G., Smallwood, R.G., Martin, D., & Rafaelsen, O.J. (1986). REM latency and core temperature relationships in primary depression. *Acta Psychiatrica Scandinavica, 74*, 269–280.

Baandrup, U., Christensen, S., & Bagger, S.P. (1987). Muscle. In F.N. Johnson (Ed.), *Depression and mania: Modern lithium therapy* (pp. 236–239). Washington, DC: IRL Press.

Badawy, A.A.B. (1977). The functions and regulation of tryptophan pyrrolase. *Life Sciences, 21*, 755–768.

Badawy, A.A.B., & Evans, M. (1981). Inhibition of rat liver tryptophan pyrrolase activity and elevation of brain tryptophan concentration by administration of antidepressants. *Biochemical Pharmacology, 30*, 1211–1216.

Baekeland, F. (1970). Exercise deprivation: Sleep and psychological reactions. *Archives of General Psychiatry, 22*, 365–369.

Bahrke, M.S., & Morgan, W.P. (1978). Anxiety reduction following exercise and meditation. *Cognitive Therapy and Research, 2*, 323–334.

Bailey, S.P., Davis, J.M., & Ahlborn, E.N. (1992). Effect of increased brain serotonergic (5-HT$_{1C}$) activity on endurance performance in the rat. *Acta Physiologica Scandinavica, 146*, 76–77.

Bailey, S.P., Davis, J.M., & Ahlborn, E.N. (1993a). Neuroendocrine and substrate responses to altered brain 5-HT activity during prolonged exercise to fatigue. *Journal of Applied Physiology, 74*, 3006–3012.

Bailey, S.P., Davis, J.M., & Ahlborn, E.N. (1993b). Serotonergic agonists and antagonists affect endurance performance. *International Journal of Sports Medicine, 14*, 330–333.

Baker, M.A., Stocking, R.A., & Meehan, J.P. (1972). Thermal relationship between tympanic membrane and hypothalamus in conscious cat and monkey. *Journal of Applied Physiology, 32*, 739–742.

Baldessarini, R.J. (1989). Current status of antidepressants: Clinical pharmacology and therapy. *Journal of Clinical Psychiatry, 50*, 117–126.

Bandura, A. (1977). Self-efficacy: Toward a unifying theory of behavior change. *Psychological Review, 84*, 191–215.

Barchas, J.D., & Friedman, D.X. (1962). Brain amines: Response to physiological stress. *Biochemistry and Pharmacology, 12*, 1232–1235.

Barchas, J.D., & Freedman, D. (1973). Brain amines: Response to physiological stress. *Biochemistry and Pharmacology, 30*, 1211–1216.

Barden, N., Reul, J.M.H.M., & Holsboer, F. (1995). Do antidepressants stabilize mood through actions on the hypothalamic-pituitary-adrenocortical system? *Trends in Neurosciences, 18*, 6–10.

Barron, J.L., Noakes, T.D., Levy, W., Smith, C., & Millar, R.P. (1985). Hypothalamic dysfunction in overtrained athletes. *Journal of Clinical Endocrinology and Metabolism, 60*, 803–806.

Barta, A., & Yashpal, K. (1981). Regional redistribution of β-endorphin in the rat brain: The effect of stress. *Progress in Neuropsychopharmacology, 5*, 595–598.

Beck, A.T., Ward, C.H., Mendelsohn, M., Mock, J., & Erbaugh, H. (1961). An inventory for measuring depression. *Archives of General Psychiatry, 4*, 561–571.

Beckmann, H., & Goodwin, F.K. (1980). Urinary MHPG in subgroups of depressed patients and normal controls. *Neuropsychobiology, 6*, 91–100.

Beecher, H.K. (1958). *Experimentation in man.* Springfield, IL: Charles C Thomas.

Belisle, M., Roskies, E., & Levesque, J.M. (1987). Improving adherence to physical activity. *Health Psychology, 6*, 159–172.

Ben-Shlomo, L.S., & Short, M.A. (1986). The effects of physical conditioning on selected dimensions of self-concept in sedentary females. *Occupational Therapy in Mental Health, 5*, 27–46.

Bennett, A.E., Cash, P.T., & Hockstra, C.S. (1941). Artificial fever therapy in general paresis with electroencephalographic studies. *Psychiatric Quarterly, 15*, 750–771.

Benson, H. (1975). *The relaxation response.* New York: William Morrow & Company.

Benton, D., Brain, S., & Brain, P.F. (1984). Comparison of the influence of the opiate delta receptor antagonist, ICI 154,129, and naloxone on social interaction and behaviour in an open field. *Neuropharmacology, 23*, 13–17.

Benzinger, T.H. (1959). On physical heat regulation and the sense of temperature in man. *Proceedings of the National Academy of Sciences USA, 45*: 645–659.

Berger, B., & Owen, D.R. (1983). Mood alteration with swimming: Swimmers really do "feel better." *Psychosomatic Medicine, 45*, 425–433.

Berger, B.G., & Owen, D.R. (1988). Stress reduction and mood enhancement in four exercise modes: Swimming, body conditioning, hatha yoga and fencing. *Research Quarterly for Exercise and Sport, 59*, 148–159.

Berger, B.G., & Owen, D.R. (1992). Preliminary analysis of a causal relationship between swimming and stress reduction: Intense exercise may negate the effects. *International Journal of Sport Psychology, 23*, 70–85.

Berglund, B., & Säfström, H. (1994). Psychological monitoring and modulation of training load of world-class canoeists. *Medicine and Science in Sports and Exercise, 26*, 1036–1040.

Bernstein, L., Henderson, B.F., Hanisch,R., Sullivan-Halley, J., & Ross, R.K. (1994). Physical exercise and reduced risk of breast cancer in young women. *Journal of the National Cancer Institute, 86*, 1403–1408.

Bewsher, P.D. (1967). Pranolol, blood-sugar and exercise. *Lancet, 289*, 104.

Bittikofer-Griffin, E., & Ely, D. (1987). Decrease in irritable aggression due to long-term voluntary aerobic exercise in spontaneously hypertensive rats. *Federation Proceedings, 46*, 952.

Blair, S.N. (1993). 1993 C.H. McCloy Research Lecture: Physical activity, physical fitness and health. *Research Quarterly for Exercise and Sport, 64*, 365–376.

Blair, S.N. (1994). Physical activity, fitness, and coronary heart disease. In C. Bouchard, R.J. Shephard, & T. Stephens (Eds.), *Physical activity, fitness, and health: International proceedings and consensus statement* (pp. 579–590). Champaign, IL: Human Kinetics Publishers.

Blair, S.N., Jacobs, D.R., Jr., & Powell, K.E. (1985). Relationships between exercise or physical activity and other health behaviors. *Public Health Reports, 100*, 172–180.

Blair, S.N., Kohl, H.W., & Gordon, N.F., Paffenbarger, R.S. (1992). Physical activity and health: A lifestyle approach. *Medicine, Exercise, Nutrition and Health, 1*, 54–57.

Blair, S.N., Kohl, H.W., Paffenberger, R.S., Clark, K., Cooper, H., & Gibbons, L.W. (1989). Physical fitness and all-cause mortality: A prospective study of health men and women. *Journal of the American Medical Association, 262,* 2395–2401.

Blair, S.N., Piserchia, P.V., Wilbur, C.S., & Crowder, J.H. (1986). A public health intervention model for worksite health promotion: Impact on exercise and physical fitness in a health promotion plan after 24 months. *Journal of the American Medical Association, 255,* 921–926.

Blake, M.J., Stein, E.A., & Vomachka, A.J. (1984). Effects of exercise training on brain opioid peptides and serum LH in female rats. *Peptides, 5,* 953–958.

Blier, P., & De Montigny, C. (1994). Current advances and trends in the treatment of depression. *Trends in Pharmacological Sciences, 15,* 220–226.

Bliss, E.L., Ailion, J., & Zwanziger, J. (1968). Metabolism of norepinephrine, serotonin, and dopamine in rat brain with stress. *Journal of Pharmacology and Experimental Therapy, 164,* 122–133.

Blomberry, P.A., Kopin, I.J., Gordon, E.K., Markey, S.P., & Ebert, M.H. (1980). Conversion of MHPG to vanillylmandelic acid. *Archives of General Psychiatry, 37,* 1095–1098.

Blomstrand, E., Celsing, F., & Newsholme, E.A. (1988). Changes in plasma concentrations of aromatic and branched-chain amino acids during sustained exercise in man and their possible role in fatigue. *Acta Physiologica Scandinavica, 133,* 115–121.

Blomstrand, E., Hassmen, P., Ekblom, B., & Newsholme, E.A. (1991). Administration of branched-chain amino acids during sustained exercise: Effects on performance and on plasma concentration of some amino acids. *European Journal of Applied Physiology, 63,* 83–88.

Blomstrand, E., Hassmen, P., & Newsholme, E.A. (1991). Effect of branched-chain amino acid supplementation on mental performance. *Acta Physiologica Scandinavica, 143,* 225–226.

Blomstrand, E., Perrett, D., Parry-Billings, M., & Newsholme, E.A. (1989). Effect of sustained exercise on plasma amino acid concentrations and on 5-hydroxytryptamine metabolism in six different regions of the rat. *Acta Physiologica Scandinavica, 136,* 473–481.

Bloom, A.S., & Tseng, L.F. (1981). Effect of β-endorphin on body temperature in mice at different ambient temperatures. *Peptides, 2,* 293–297.

Bloom, B.L. (1984). *Community mental health: A general introduction* (2nd ed.). Belmont, CA: Brooks/Cole Publishing Company.

Bloom, B.L. (1985). Focal issues in the prevention of mental disorders. In H.H. Goldman & S.E. Goldston (Eds.), *Preventing stress-related psychiatric disorders.* (DHHS Publication No. ADM 85–1366). Washington, DC: U.S. Government Printing Office.

Blumenthal, J.A. (1989). Response to Abbot and Peters. *Psychosomatic Medicine, 51,* 218–221.

Blumenthal, J.A., Emery, C.F., Madden, D.J., George, L.K., Coleman, R.E., Riddle, M.W., McKee, D.C., Reasoner, J., & Williams, R.S. (1989). Cardiovascular and behavioral effects of aerobic exercise training in healthy older men and women. *Journal of Gerontology, 44,* 147–157.

Boess, F.G., & Martin, I.L. (1994). Molecular biology of 5-HT receptors. *Neuropharmacology, 33,* 275–318.

Borg, G.A.V. (1973). Perceived exertion: A note on "history" and methods. *Medicine and Science in Sports, 5,* 90–93.

Boshes, B. (1960). The status of tranquilizing drugs—1959. *Annals of Internal Medicine, 52,* 182–194.

Bot, G., Chahl, L.A., Brent, P.J., & Johnston, P.A. (1992). Effects of intracerebroventricularly administered mu-, delta- and kappa-opioid agonists on locomotor activity of the guinea pig and the pharmacology of the locomotor response to U50,488H. *Neuropharmacology, 31,* 825–833.

Bouchard, C., Shephard, R.J., & Stephens, T. (Eds.). (1994). *Physical activity, fitness and health.* Champaign, IL: Human Kinetics Publishers.

Bouchard, C., Shephard, R.J., Stephens, T., Sutton, J.R., & McPherson, B.D. (1990). Exercise, fitness, and health: The concensus statement. In C. Bouchard, R.J. Shephard, T. Stephens, J.R. Sutton, & B.D. McPherson (Eds.), *Exercise, fitness, and health: A concensus of current knowledge.* Champaign, IL: Human Kinetics Publishers.

Boutcher, S.H., & Landers, D.M. (1988). The effects of vigorous exercise on anxiety, heart rate, and alpha activity of runners and nonrunners. *Psychophysiology, 23*, 696–702.

Bowman, W.C. (1980). Effects of adrenergic activators and inhibitors on the skeletal muscles. In L. Szekeres (Ed.), *Adrenergic activators and inhibitors*. Berlin: Springer-Verlag.

Brain, P.F., Brain, S., & Benton, D. (1985). Ethological analyses of the effects of naloxone and the opiate antagonist ICI 154,129 on social interactions in male house mice. *Behavioral Process, 10*, 341–354.

Breckenridge, A. (1982). Jogger's blocade. *British Medical Journal, 284*, 532–533.

Brengelmann, G.L., Johnson, J.M., & Hong, P. (1979). Electrocardiographic verification of esophageal temperature probe position. *Journal of Applied Physiology, 47*, 638–642.

Brinnell, H., & Cabanac, M. (1989). Tympanic temperature is a core temperature in humans. *Journal of Thermal Biology, 14*, 47–53.

Brooke, S.T., & Long, B.C. (1987). Efficiency of coping with a real-life stressor: A multimodal comparison of aerobic fitness. *Psychophysiology, 24*, 173–180.

Brown, B.S., Payne, T., Kim, C., Moore, G., Krebs, P., & Martin, W. (1979). Chronic response of rat brain norepinephrine and serotonin levels to endurance training. *Journal of Applied Physiology, 46*, 19–23.

Brown, D.R. (1992). Physical activity, ageing, and psychological well-being: An overview of the research. *Canadian Journal of Sport Sciences, 17*, 185–193.

Brown, D.R., Morgan, W.P., & Raglin, J.S. (1993). Effects of exercise and rest on the state anxiety and blood pressure of physically challenged college students. *Journal of Sports Medicine and Physical Fitness, 33*, 300–305.

Brown, R.D., & Harrison, J.M. (1986). The effects of a strength training program on the strength and self-concept of two female age groups. *Research Quarterly for Exercise and Sport, 57*, 315–320.

Brown, S.W., Welsh, M.C., Labbé, E.E., Vitulli, W.F., & Kulkarni, P. (1992). Aerobic exercise in the physiological treament of adolescents. *Perceptual and Motor Skills, 74*, 555–560.

Brown, W.A., Johnson, M.F., & Chen, M.G. (1992). Clinical features of depressed patients who do and do not improve with placebo. *Psychiatry Research, 41*, 203–214.

Brownell, K.D., Stunkard, A.J., & Albaum, J.M. (1980). Evaluation and modification of exercise patterns in the natural environment. *American Journal of Psychiatry, 137*, 1540–1545.

Bruin, G., Kuipers, H., Keizer, H.A., & Vander Vusse, G.J. (1994). Adaptations and overtraining in horses subjected to increased training loads. *Journal of Applied Physiology, 76*, 1908–1913.

Brutus, M., Zuabi, S., & Siegel, A. (1988). Effects of D-ALA^2-Met^5-enkephalinamide micro injections placed into the bed nucleus of the stria terminalis upon affective defense behavior in the cat. *Brain Research, 473*, 147–152.

Buckworth, J.B., Dishman, R.K., & Cureton, K.J. (1994). Autonomic responses of women with parental hypertension: Effects of VO_2max and physical activity. *Hypertension, 24*, 576–584.

Budgett, R. (1990). Overtraining syndrome. *British Journal of Sports Medicine, 24*, 231–236.

Budgett, R. (1994). ABC of sports medicine: The overtraining syndrome. *British Medical Journal, 309*, 465–468.

Bunney, W.E., Jr., & Davis, J.M. (1965). Norepinephrine in depressive reactions: A review. *Archives of General Psychiatry, 13*, 483–494.

Burd, S. (1993, March 10). U.S. judge's ruling sets up new battle over care of lab animals. *The Chronicle of Higher Education*, 30.

Burfoot, A. (1994). The brain connection. *Runner's World, 29*, 70–75.

Burke, E.J., & Franks, B.D. (1975). Changes in VO_2max resulting from bicycle training at different intensities holding total mechanical work constant. *The Research Quarterly, 46*, 31–37.

Byrne, A., & Byrne, D.G. (1993). The effect of exercise on depression, anxiety, and other mood states: A review. *Journal of Psychosomatic Research, 37*, 565–574.

Cabanac, M. (1986). Keeping a cool head. *News in Physiological Sciences, 1*, 41–44.

Cabanac, M. (1993). Brain-stem cooling by face fanning severely hyperthermic humans. *Pflugers Archives, 424*, 367.

Cabanac, M., & Caputa, M. (1979). Natural selective cooling of the human brain: Evidence of its occurrence and magnitude. *Journal of Physiology, 286,* 255–264.

Calenco-Choukroun, G., Dauge, V., Gacel, G., & Roques, B.P. (1991). Lesion of dopamine mesolimbic neurons blocks behavioral effects induced by the endogenous enkephalins but not by a μ-opioid receptor agonist. *European Journal of Pharmacology, 209,* 267–271.

Califano, J.A., Jr. (1979). *Healthy people: The surgeon general's report on health promotion and disease prevention.* Washington, DC: U.S. Government Printing Office.

Callister, R., Callister, R.J., Fleck, S.J., & Dudley, G.A. (1990). Physiological and performance responses to overtraining in judo athletes. *Medicine and Science in Sports and Exercise, 22,* 816–824.

Camacho, T.C., Roberts, R.E., Lazarus, N.B., Kaplan, G.A., & Cohen, R.D. (1991). Physical activity and depression: Evidence from the Alameda County Study. *American Journal of Epidemiology, 134,* 220–231.

Campbell, D.T., & Stanley, J.C. (1966). *Experimental and quasi-experimental designs for research.* Chicago: Rand McNally.

Caplan, G. (1964). *Principles of preventative psychiatry.* New York: Basic Books.

Carlsson, C., Dencker, S.J., Grimby, G., & Heggendal, J. (1967). Noradrenaline in human blood plasma and urine during exercise in patients receiving large doses of chlorpromazine. *Acta Pharmacology et Toxicology, 25,* 97–106.

Carlsson, C., Dencker, S.J., Grimby, G., & Heggendal, J. (1968a). Circulatory studies during physical exercise in mentally disordered patients. I. Effects of large doses of chlorpromazine. *Acta Medica Scandinavica, 184,* 499–509.

Carlsson, C., Dencker, S.J., Grimby, G., & Heggendal, J. (1968b). Circulatory studies during physical exercise in mentally disordered patients. II. Effects of physical training with and without administration of chlorpromazine. *Acta Medica Scandinavica, 184,* 511–516.

Carlsson, E., Fellenius, E., Lundborg, P., & Svensson, L. (1978). Beta-adrenoreceptor blockers, plasma potassium, and exercise. *Lancet, ii,* 425–426.

Carlsson, A., & Lindqvist, M. (1972). The effect of L-tryptophan and psychotropic drugs on the formation of 5-hydroxytryptophan in the mouse brain in vivo. *Journal of Neural Transmission, 34,* 23–43.

Carver, C.S. (1979). A cybernatic model of self-attention process. *Journal of Personality and Social Psychology, 37,* 1251–1281.

Caspersen, C.J., Merritt, R.K., & Stephens, T. (1994). International physical activity patterns: A methodological perspective. In R.K. Dishman (Ed.), *Advances in exercise adherence* (pp. 73–110). Champaign, IL: Human Kinetics Publishers.

Cauley, J.A., LaPorte, R.E., Sandler, R.B., Orchard, T.J., Slemenda, C.W., & Petrini, A.M. (1986). The relationship of physical activity to high density lipoprotein cholesterol in postmenopausal women. *Journal of Chronic Diseases, 39,* 687–697.

Centers for Disease Control (1990). CDC surveillance summaries, June. *Morbidity and Mortality Weekly Report, 39* (No. SS-2), 8.

Centers for Disease Control and American College of Sports Medicine (1993). Summary statement: Workshop on physical activity and public health. *Sports Medicine Bulletin, 28,* 7.

Chang, P.C., Kreik, E., van der Krogt, J., & van Brummelen, P. (1991). Does regional norepinephrine spillover represent local sympathetic activity? *Hypertension, 18,* 56–66.

Chaouloff, F. (1989a). Physical exercise and brain monoamines: A review. *Acta Physiologica Scandinavica, 137,* 1–13.

Chaouloff, F. (1989b). About the effect of L-tryptophan on exercise performance: Lacunae and pitfalls. *International Journal of Sports Medicine, 10,* 383.

Chaouloff, F. (1993). Physiopharmacological interactions between stress hormones and central serotonergic systems. *Brain Research Reviews, 18,* 1–32.

Chaouloff, F. (1994a). Serotonin$_{1C,2}$ receptors and endurance performance: An illustration of the limits of pharmacological tools in exercise science. *International Journal of Sports Medicine, 5,* 339.

Chaouloff, F. (1994b). Influence of physical exercise on 5-HT$_{1A}$ receptor- and anxiety-related behaviours. *Neuroscience Letters, 76,* 226–230.

Chaouloff, F., Elghozi, J.L., Guezennec, Y., & Laude, D. (1985). Effects of conditioned running on plasma, liver and brain tryptophan and on brain 5-hydroxytryptamine metabolism of the rat. *British Journal of Pharmacology*, *86*, 33–41.

Chaouloff, F., Kennett, G.A., Serrurier, B., Merino, D., & Curzon, G. (1986). Amino acid analysis demonstrates that increased plasma free tryptophan causes the increase of brain tryptophan during exercise in the rat. *Journal of Neurochemistry*, *46*, 1647–1650.

Chaouloff, F., Laude, D., & Elghozi, J.L. (1989). Physical exercise: Evidence for differential consequences of tryptophan on 5-HT synthesis and metabolism in central serotonergic cell bodies and terminals. *Journal of Neural Transmission*, *78*, 121–130.

Chaouloff, F., Laude, D., Guezennec, Y., & Elghozi, J.L. (1986). Motor activity increases tryptophan, 5-hydroxyindoleacetic acid, and homovanillic acid in ventricular cerebrospinal fluid of the conscious rat. *Journal of Neurochemistry*, *46*, 1313–1316.

Chaouloff, F., Laude, D., Merino, D., Serrurier, B., Guezennec, Y., & Elghozi, J.L. (1987). Amphetamine and α-methyl-p-tyrosine affect the exercise-induced imbalance between the availability of tryptophan and synthesis of serotonin in the brain of the rat. *Neuropharmacology*, *26*, 1099–1106.

Chaouloff, F., Laude, D., Serrurier, B., Merino, D., Guezennec, Y., & Elghozi, J.L. (1987). Brain serotonin response to exercise in the rat: The influence of training duration. *Biogenic Amines*, *4*, 99–106.

Charles, R.B., Kirkham, A.J.T., Guyatt, A.R., & Parker, S.P. (1987). Psychomotor, pulmonary and exercise responses to sleep medication. *British Journal of Clinical Pharmacology*, *24*, 191–197.

Christie, M.J., & Chesher, G.B. (1982). Physical dependence on physiologically released endogenous opiates. *Life Sciences*, *30*, 1173–1177.

Christie, M.J., & Chesher, G.B. (1983). [^{3}H] leu-enkephalin binding following chronic swim-stress in mice. *Neuroscience Letters*, *36*, 323–328.

Christie, M.J., Chesher, G.B., & Bird, K.D. (1981). The correlation between swim-stress induced antinociception and [^{3}H] leu-enkephalin binding to brain homogenates in mice. *Pharmacology, Biochemistry, and Behavior*, *15*, 853–857.

Clark, W.G. (1979). Influence of opioids on central thermo-regulatory mechanisms. *Pharmacology, Biochemistry, and Behavior*, *10*, 609–613.

Clark, L.A., Watson, D., & Leeks, J. (1993). Diurnal variation in the positive affects. *Motivation and Emotion*, *13*, 205–234.

Clement, H.W., Schäfer, F., Ruwe, C., Gemsa, D., & Wesemann, W. (1993). Stress-induced changes of extracellular 5-hydroxyindoleacetic acid concentrations followed in the nucleus raphe dorsalis and the frontal cortex of the rat. *Brain Research*, *614*, 117–124.

Cobb, L.A., Thomas, G.I., Dillard, D.H, Merendino, K.A., & Bruce, R.A. (1959). An evaluation of internal-mammary-artery ligation by a double-blind technic. *New England Journal of Medicine*, *260*, 1115–1118.

Cockerill, I.M., Nevill, A.M., & Byrne, B.A. (1992). Mood, mileage and the menstrual cycle. *British Journal of Sports Medicine*, *26*, 145–150.

Cogan, K.D., Highlen, P.S., Petrie, T.A., Sherman, W.M., & Simonsen, J. (1991). Psychological and physiological effects of controlled intensive training and diet on collegiate rowers. *International Journal of Sport Psychology*, *22*, 165–180.

Cohen, J. (1988). *Statistical power analysis for the behavioral sciences* (2nd ed.), Hillsdale, NJ: Lawrence Erlbaum Associates.

Cohen, J. (1992). A power primer. *Psychological Bulletin*, *112*, 155–159.

Cohen, J. (1994). The earth is round (p < .05). *American Psychologist*, *49*, 997–1003.

Cohen, M.R., Cohen, R.M., Pickar, D., Weingartner, H., & Murphy, D.L. (1983). High-dose naloxone infusions in normals. *Archives of General Psychiatry*, *40*, 613–619.

Cohen, S., Tyrell, D.A.J., & Smith, A.P. (1991). Psychological stress and susceptibility to the common cold. *New England Journal of Medicine*, *325*, 606–612.

Collomp, K.R., Ahmaid, S.B., Cailland, C.F., Audran, M.A., Chanal, J.L., & Préfaut, C.G. (1993). Effects of benzodiazepine during a Wingate test: Interaction with caffeine. *Medicine and Science in Sports and Exercise*, *25*, 1375–1380.

Conlay, L.A., Wurtman, R.J., Lopez-Coviella, I., Blusztajn, J.K., Vacanti, C.A., Logue, M., During, M., Caballero, B., Maher, T.J., & Evoniuk, G. (1989). Effects of running the Boston marathon on plasma concentrations of large neutral amino acids. *Journal of Neural Transmission, 76,* 65–71.

Cooper, J.R., Bloom, F.E., & Roth, R.H. (1991). *The biochemical basis of neuropharmacology* (6th ed.). New York: Oxford University Press.

Coppen, A. (1969). Defects in monoamine metabolism and their possible importance in the pathogenesis of depressive symptoms. *Psychiatrica, Neurologia, Neurochirurgia, 72,* 173–180.

Costill, D.L., Flynn, M.G., Kirwan, J.P., Houmard, J.A., Mitchell, J.B., Thomas, R., & Park, S.H. (1988). Effects of repeated days of intensified training on muscle glycogen and swimming performance. *Medicine and Science in Sports and Exercise, 20,* 249–254.

Costill, D.L., King, D.S., Thomas, R., & Hargreaves, H. (1985). Effects of reduced training on muscular power in swimmers. *The Physician and Sportsmedicine, 13,* 94–101.

Counsilman, J.E. (1955). Fatigue and staleness. *The Athletic Journal, 15,* 16–44.

Cousineau, D., Ferguson, R.J., de Champlain, J., Gauthier, P., Cote, P., & Bourassa, M. (1977). Catecholamines in coronary sinus during exercise in man before and after training. *Journal of Applied Physiology, 43,* 801–806.

Cowen, E.L. (1980). The wooing of primary prevention. *American Journal of Community Psychology, 8,* 258–284.

Cox, R.H. (1991). Exercise training and response to stress: Insights from an animal model. *Medicine and Science in Sports and Exercise, 23,* 853–859.

Cramer, S.R., Nieman, D.C., & Lee, J.W. (1991). The effects of moderate exercise training on psychological well-being and mood state in women. *Journal of Psychosomatic Research, 35,* 437–449.

Crauford, D.I., Creed, F., & Jayson, M.I. (1990). Life events and psychological disturbance in patients with low-back pain. *Spine, 15,* 490–494.

Crews, D.J., & Landers, D.M. (1987). A meta-analytic review of aerobic fitness and reactivity to psychosocial stressors. *Medicine and Science in Sports and Exercise, 19* (Suppl.), S114–S120.

Crocker, P.R., & Grozelle, C. (1991). Reducing induced state anxiety: Effects of acute aerobic exercise and autogenic relaxation. *Journal of Sports Medicine and Physical Fitness, 31,* 277–282.

Cureton, T.K. (1963). Improvement of psychological states by means of exercise-fitness programs. *Journal of the Association for Physical and Mental Rehabilitation, 17,* 14–25.

Dahlstrom, A., & Fuxe, K.I. (1964). Evidence for the existence of monoamine-containing neurons in the central nervous system. I. Demonstration of monoamines in the cell bodies of brainstem neurons. *Acta Physiologica Scandinavica, 62* (Suppl. 232), 1–55.

Dalsky, G.P., Stocke, K.S., Ehsani, A.A., Slatoplsky, E., Lee, W.C., & Birge, S.J. (1988). Weight-bearing exercise training and lumbar bone mineral content in post menopausal women. *Annals of Internal Medicine, 108,* 824–828.

Daniel, M., Martin, A.D., & Carter, J. (1992). Opiate receptor blockade by naltrexone and mood state after acute physical activity. *British Journal of Sports Medicine, 26,* 111–115.

Davidson, J.R.T. (1992). Monoamine oxidase inhibitors. In E.S. Paykel (Ed.), *Handbook of affective disorders* (pp. 345–358). Edinburgh: Churchill Livingstone.

Davidson, R.J. (1994). Asymmetric brain function, affective style, and psychopathology: The role of early experience and plasticity. *Development and Psychopathology, 6,* 741–758.

Davidson, R.J., & Sutton, S.K. (1995). Affective neuroscience: The emergence of a discipline. *Current Opinion in Neurobiology, 5,* 217–224.

Davies, C.T., Brotherhood, J.R., & Ziedifard, E. (1976). Temperature regulation during severe exercise with some observations on effects of skin wetting. *Journal of Applied Physiology, 41,* 772–776.

Davis, J.M., Bailey, S.P., Woods, J.A., Galiano, F.J., Hamilton, M.T., & Bartoli, W.P. (1992). Effects of carbohydrate feedings on plasma free tryptophan and branched-chain amino acids during prolonged cycling. *European Journal of Applied Physiology, 65,* 513–519.

Davis, J.M. Koslow, S.H., & Gibbons, R.D. (1988). Cerebrospinal fluid and urinary biogenic amines in depressed patients and healthy control. *Archives of General Psychiatry, 45,* 705–717.

DeBusk, R.F., Hakansson, U., Sheehan, M., & Haskell, W.L. (1990). Training effects of long versus short bouts of exercise in health subjects. *American Journal of Cardiology, 65,* 1010–1013.

deCastro, J.M., & Duncan, G. (1985). Operantly conditioned running effects on brain catecholamine concentrations and receptor densities in the rat. *Pharmacology, Biochemistry, and Behavior, 23,* 494–500.

Dechant, K.L., & Clissold, S.P. (1991). Paroxetine. A review of its pharmacodynamic and pharmacocinetic properties, and therapeutic potential in depressive illness. *Drugs, 41,* 225–253.

Decombaz, J., Reinhardt, P., Anantharaman, K., von Glutz, G., & Poortmans, J.R. (1979). Biochemical changes in a 100 km run: Free amino acids, urea, and creatinine. *European Journal of Applied Physiology, 41,* 61–72.

De Coverley Veale, D.M.W. (1987). Exercise dependence. *British Journal of Addiction, 82,* 735–740.

De Geus, E.J.C., Van Doornen, L.J.P., & Orlebeke, J.F. (1993). Regular exercise and aerobic fitness in relation to psychological make-up and physiological stress reactivity. *Psychosomatic Medicine, 55,* 347–363.

De Meirleir, K., L'Hermite-Baleriaux, M., L'Hermite, M., Rost, R., & Hollmann, W. (1985). Evidence for serotoninergic control of exercise-induced prolactin release. *Hormone and Metabolic Research, 17,* 380–381.

De Meirleir, K., Naaktgeboren, N., Van Steirteghem, A., Gorus, F., Olbrecht, J., and Block, P. (1986). Beta-endorphin and ACTH levels in peripheral blood during and after aerobic and anaerobic exercise. *European Journal of Applied Physiology, 55,* 5–8.

Dennison, B.A., Straus, J.H., Mellits, E.D., & Charney, E. (1988). Childhood physical fitness tests: Predictor of adult physical activity levels? *Pediatrics, 82,* 324–330.

Department of Health and Human Services (1990). *Healthy people 2000: National health promotion and disease prevention objectives* (DDHS(PHS) 91–50212, p. 107). Washington, DC: U.S. Government Printing Office.

Department of Health and Human Services (1993). *Midcourse review. Healthy People 2000: National health promotion and disease prevention objectives* (DHHS(PHS) Publication No. 93–50212). Washington, DC: U.S. Government Printing Office.

Depression Guideline Panel. (1993). Depression in primary care: Vol. 1. Diagnosis and detection. (Clinical Practice Guidelines No. 5, AHCPR Pub. No. 93-0550). Rockville, MD: U.S. Dept. of Health and Human Services, Public Health Service, Agency for Health Care Policy and Research.

Desharnais, R., Jobin, J., Coté, C., Lévesque, L., & Godin, G. (1993). Aerobic exercise and the placebo effect: A controlled study. *Psychosomatic Medicine, 55,* 149–154.

deVries, H.A. (1987). Tension reduction with exercise. In W.P. Morgan & S.E. Goldston (Eds.), *Exercise and Mental Health* (pp. 99–104). Washington, DC: Hemisphere.

deVries, H.A., & Adams, G.M. (1972). Electromyographic comparison of single doses of exercise and meprobamate as to effects on muscular relaxation. *American Journal of Physical Medicine, 51,* 130–141.

deVries, H.A., Beckman, P. Huber, H., & Dieckmeir, L. (1968). Electromyographic evaluation of the effects of sauna on the neuromuscular system. *Journal of Sports Medicine and Physical Fitness, 8,* 1–11.

deVries, H.A., Wiswell, R.A., Bulbulian, R., & Moritani, T. (1981). Tranquilizer effect of exercise. *American Journal of Physical Medicine, 60,* 57–66.

DiBianco, R., Shoomaker, F.W., Sigh, J.B., Awan, N.A., Bennett, T., Canosa, F.L., Kawanishi, D.T., Bamrah, V.S., Glasser, S.P., & Barey, W. (1992). Amlodipine combined with beta blocade for chronic angina: Results of a multicenter, placebo-controlled, randomized double-blind study. *Clinical Cardiology, 15,* 519–524.

Dickson, J.A., MacKenzie, A., & McLeod, K. (1979). Temperature gradients in pigs during whole-body hyperthermia at 42°C. *Journal of Applied Physiology, 47,* 712–717.

Dishman, R.K. (1981). Biologic influences on exercise adherence. *Research Quarterly for Exercise and Sport, 52,* 143–159.

Dishman, R.K. (1982). Compliance/adherence in health-related exercise. *Health Psychology, 1,* 237–267.

Dishman, R.K. (1984). Motivation and exercise adherence. In J.M. Silva III & R.S. Weinberg (Eds.), *Psychological Foundations of Sport*. Champaign, IL: Human Kinetics Publishers.

Dishman, R.K. (1987). Exercise adherence and habitual physical activity. In W.P. Morgan & S.E. Goldston (Eds.), *Exercise and Mental Health* (pp. 57–82). Washington, DC: Hemisphere.

Dishman, R.K. (Ed.). (1988a) *Exercise adherence: Its impact on public health*. Champaign, IL: Human Kinetics Publishers.

Dishman, R.K. (1988b). Supervised and free-living physical activity: No differences in former athletes and nonathletes. *American Journal of Preventive Medicine, 4*, 153–160.

Dishman, R.K. (1990). Determinants of participation in physical activity. In C. Bouchard, R.J. Shephard, T. Stephens, J.R. Sutton, B.D. McPherson (Eds.), *Exercise, fitness and health* (pp. 75–102). Champaign, IL: Human Kinetics Publishers.

Dishman, R.K. (1991). Increasing and maintaining exercise and physical activity. *Behavior Therapy, 22*, 345–378.

Dishman, R.K. (1992). Physiological and psychological effects of overtraining. In K.D. Brownell, J. Rodin & J.H. Whilmore (Eds.), *Eating, body weight, and performance in athletes. Disorders of modern society* (pp. 248–272). Philadelphia: Lea & Febiger.

Dishman, R.K. (1994a). Biological psychology, exercise and stress. *Quest, 64*, 28–59.

Dishman, R.K. (Ed.). (1994b). *Advances in exercise adherence*. Champaign, IL: Human Kinetics Publishers.

Dishman, R.K. (1994c). Prescribing exercise intensity for health adults using perceived exertion. *Medicine and Science in Sports and Exercise, 26*, 1087–1094.

Dishman, R.K., & Buckworth, J. (1996). Increasing physical activity: A quantitative synthesis. *Medicine and Science in Sports and Exercise, 28*, 706–719.

Dishman, R.K., Darracott, C., & Lambert, L. (1992). Failure to generalize determinants of self-reported physical activity to a motion sensor. *Medicine and Science in Sports and Exercise, 24*, 904–910.

Dishman, R.K., Farquhar, R.P., & Cureton, K.J. (1994). Responses to preferred intensities of exertion in men differing in activity levels. *Medicine and Science in Sports and Exercise, 26*, 783–790.

Dishman, R.K., & Ickes, W. (1981). Self-motivation and adherence to therapeutic exercise. *Journal of Behavioral Medicine, 4*, 421–438.

Dishman, R.K., Ickes, W., & Morgan, W.P. (1980). Self-motivation and adherence to habitual physical activity. *Journal of Applied Social Psychology, 10*, 115–132.

Dishman, R.K., Renner, K.J., White, J.E., Bunnell, B.N., Youngstedt, S.D., & Armstrong, R.B. (1992). Effects of treadmill training on locus coeruleus monoamines following running and immobilization. *Medicine and Science in Sports and Exercise, 24* (Suppl.), S25.

Dishman, R.K., Renner, K.J., Youngstedt, S.D., Reigle, T., Kedzie, K.A., Bunnell, B.N., & Yoo, H. (1993). Spontaneous physical activity moderates escape latency and brain monoamines after uncontrollable footshock. *Medicine and Science in Sports and Exercise, 25* (Suppl.), S90.

Dishman, R.K., & Sallis, J. (1994). Determinants and interventions for physical activity and exercise. In C. Bouchard, R.J. Shephard, T. Stephens, J.R. Sutton, & B.D. McPherson (Eds.), *Exercise, fitness and health*. Champaign, IL: Human Kinetics Publishers.

Dishman, R.K., Warren, J.M., Youngstedt, S.D., Yoo, H., Bunnell, B.N., Mougey, E.H., Meyerhoff, J.L., Jaso-Friedmann, L., & Evans, D.L. (1995). Activity-wheel running attenuates suppression of natural killer cell activity after footshock. *Journal of Applied Physiology, 78*, 1547–1554.

Donahoe, C.P., Lin, D.H., Kirschenbaum, D.S., & Kesey, R.E. (1984). Metabolic consequences of dieting and exercise in the treatment of obesity. *Journal of Consulting and Clinical Psychology, 52*, 827–836.

Donevan, R.H., & Andrew, G.M. (1987). Plasma β-endorphin immunoreactivity during graded cycle ergometry. *Medicine and Science in Sports and Exercise, 19*, 229–233.

Donovan, R.J., & Owen, N. (1994). Social marketing and population-level intervention. In Dishman, R.K., (Ed.), *Advances in exercise adherence* (pp. 249–290). Champaign, IL: Human Kinetics Publishers.

Doyne, E.J., Chambless, D.L., & Beutler, L.E. (1983). Aerobic exercise as a treatment for depression in women. *Behavioral Therapy, 14,* 434–440

Doyne, E.J., Ossip-Klein, D.G, Bowman, E.D., Osborn, K.M., McDougall-Wilson, I.B., & Neimayer, R.A. (1987). Running versus weightlifting in the treatment of depression. *Journal of Consulting and Clinical Psychology, 5,* 748–754.

Dressendorfer, R.H., & Wade, C.E. (1983). The muscular overuse syndrome in long-distance runners. *The Physician and Sportsmedicine, 11,* 116–126.

Dressendorfer, R.H., & Wade, C.E. (1991). Effects of a 15-d race on plasma steroid levels and leg muscle fitness in runners. *Medicine and Science in Sports and Exercise, 23,* 954–958.

Dressendorfer, R.H., Wade, C.E., & Scaff, J.H. (1985). Increased morning heart rate in runners: A valid sign of overtraining? *The Physician and Sportsmedicine, 13,* 77–86.

Drugan, R.C. (1984). Librium prevents the analgesia and shuttlebox escape deficit typically observed following inescapable shock. *Pharmacology of Biochemistry Behavior, 21,* 749–754.

Drugan, R.C., Maier, S.F., & Skolnick, P. (1985). An anxiogenic benzodiazepine receptor ligand induces learned helplessness. *European Journal of Pharmacology, 113,* 453–457.

Duffy, E. (1962). *Activation and behavior.* New York: Wiley.

Dulac, S., Quiron, A., DeCarufel, D., LeBlanc, J., Jobin, M., Cote, J., Brisson, G.R., LaVoie, J.M., & Diamond, P. (1987). Metabolic and hormonal responses to long-distance swimming in cold water. *International Journal of Sports Medicine, 8,* 352–356.

Duncan, J.J., Gordon, N.F., & Scott, C.B. (1991). Women walking for health and fitness: How much is enough?. *Journal of the American Medical Association, 266,* 3295–3299.

Duncan, T.E., & McAuley, E. (1993). Social support and efficacy cognitions in exercise adherence: A latent growth curve analysis. *Journal of Behavioral Medicine, 16,* 199–218.

Dunn, A.L., & Dishman, R.K. (1991). Exercise and the neurobiology of depression. *Exercise and Sport Sciences Reviews, 19,* 41–98.

Dunn, A.L., Reigle, T.G., Youngstedt, S.D., Armstrong, R.B., & Dishman, R.K. (1996). Brain norepinephrine and metabolites after treadwell training and wheel running in rats. *Medicine and Science in Sports and Exercise, 28,* 204–209.

Duranti, R., Pantaleo, T., & Bellini, F. (1988). Increase in muscular pain threshold following low frequency-high intensity peripheral conditioning stimulation in humans. *Brain Research, 452,* 66–72.

Durnin, J.V.G.A. (1990). Assessment of physical activity during leisure and work. In C. Bouchard, R.J. Shephard, T. Stephens, J.R. Sutton, & B.D. McPherson (Eds.), *Exercise, fitness and health: A consensus of current knowledge* (pp. 63–70). Champaign, IL: Human Kinetics Publishers.

Dyer, J.B., III, & Crouch, J.G. (1988). Effects of running and other activities on moods. *Perceptual and Motor Skills, 67,* 43–50.

Ebbesen, B.L., Prkachin, K.M., Mills, D.E., & Green, H.J. (1992). Effects of acute exercise on cardiovascular reactivity. *Journal of Behavioral Medicine, 15,* 489–507.

Ebisu, T. (1985). Splitting the distance of endurance running: On cardiovascular endurance and blood lipids. *Japanese Journal of Physical Education, 30,* 37–43.

Egleston, S.A., & Sonstroem, R.J. (1993). Life adjustment correlates of perceived physical competencies [abstract]. *Medicine and Science in Sports and Exercise, 25,* 761.

Eichner, E.R. (1989). Chronic fatigue syndrome: How vulnerable are athletes? *The Physician and Sportsmedicine, 17,* 157–160.

Eimer, M., Cable, T., Gal, P., Rothenberger, L.A., & McCue, J.D. (1985). The effect of clorazepate on breathlessness and exercise tolerance in patients with chronic airflow obstruction. *Journal of Family Practice, 21,* 359–362.

Eison, A.S., & Temple, D.L. (1986). Buspirone: Review of its pharmacology and current perspectives on its mechanism of action. *American Journal of Medicine, 80* (Suppl 3B), 1–11.

Ekelund, L.G., Haskell, W.L., Johnson, J.L., Whaley, F.S., Criqui, M.H., & Sheps, D.S. (1988). Physical fitness as predictor of cardiovascular mortality in asymptomatic North American men: The Lipid Research Clinics Mortality Follow-up Study. *New England Journal of Medicine, 319,* 1379–1384.

Elam, M., Svensson, T.H., & Thoren, P. (1987). Brain monoamine metabolism is altered in rats following spontaneous, long-distance running. *Acta Physiologica Scandinavica, 130*, 313–316.

Epstein, L.H., Koeske, R., & Wing, R.R. (1984). Adherence to exercise in obese children. *Journal of Cardiac Rehabilitation, 4*, 185–195.

Epstein, L.H., Wing, R.R., Koeske, R., Ossip, D., & Beck, S. (1983). A comparison of lifestyle change and programmed aerobic exercise on weight and fitness changes in children. *Behavior Therapy, 13*, 651–665.

Epstein, S.E., Robinson, B.F., Kahler, R.L., & Braunwald, E. (1965). Effects of beta adrenergic blockade and the cardiac response to maximal and submaximal exercise in man. *Journal of Clinical Investigation, 44*, 1745–1753.

Erling, J., & Oldridge, N.B. (1985). Effect of a spousal-support program on compliance with cardiac rehabilitation. *Medicine and Science in Sports and Exercise, 17*, 284.

Evans, F.J. (1968). Critique and comment: Recent trends in experimental hypnosis. *Behavioral Science, 13*, 477–487.

Ewart, C.K., Stewart, K.J., & Gillilan, R.E. (1986). Usefulness of self-efficacy in predicting overexertion during programmed exercise in coronary artery disease. *American Journal of Cardiology, 57*, 557–561.

Ewart, C.K., Taylor, C.B., Reese, L.B., & DeBusk, R.F. (1983). Effects of early postmyocardial infarction exercise testing on self-perception and subsequent physical activity. *American Journal of Cardiology, 51*, 1076–1080.

Eysenck, H.J. (1952). The effects of psychotherapy: An evaluation. *Journal of Consulting Psychology, 16*, 319–324.

Eysenck, H.J. (1994). Meta-analysis and its problems. *British Medical Journal, 309*, 789–792.

Eysenck, H.J., & Eysenck, S.B.G. (1975). *Manual for the Eysenck Personality Questionnaire.* San Diego: Educational and Industrial Testing Service.

Faria, I.E. (1970). Cardiovascular response to exercise as influenced by training of various intensities. *Research Quarterly, 41*, 44–50.

Farina, A., Fisher, J.D., Getter, H., & Fischer, E.H. (1978). Some consequences of changing people's views regarding the nature of mental illness. *Journal of Abnormal Psychology, 87*, 272–279.

Farmer, M.E., Locke, B.Z., Moscicki, E.K., Dannenberg, A.L., Larson, D.B., & Radloff, L.S. (1988). Physical activity and depressive symptoms: The NHANES I Epidemiologic Follow-Up Study. *American Journal of Epidemiology, 128*, 1340–1351.

Farrell, P.A., Gustafson, A.B., Garthwaite, T.L., Kalhoff, R.K., Cowley, A.W., & Morgan, W.P. (1986). Influence of endogenous opioids on the response of selected hormones to exercise in man. *Journal of Applied Physiology, 61*, 1051–1057.

Farrell, P.A., Gustafson, A.B., Morgan, W.P., & Pert, C.B. (1987). Enkephalins, catecholamines, and psychological mood alterations: Effects of prolonged exercise. *Medicine and Science in Sports and Exercise, 19*, 347–353.

Feldman, R.S., & Quenzer, L.F. (1984). *Fundamentals of Neuro-psychopharmacology.* Sunderland, MA: Sinauer Associates, Inc.

Felig, P., & Wahren, J. (1971). Amino acid metabolism in exercising man. *Journal of Clinical Investigation, 50*, 2703–2714.

Fernstrom, J.D., & Wurtman, R.J. (1972a). Brain serotonin content: Physiological regulation by plasma neutral amino acids. *Science, 178*, 414–416.

Fernstrom, J.D., & Wurtman, R.J. (1972b). Elevation of plasma tryptophan by insulin in rat. *Metabolism, 21*, 337–342.

File, S.E., & Silverstone, T. (1981). Naloxone changes self-ratings but not performance in normal subjects. *Psychopharmacology, 74*, 353–354.

Fillenz, M. (1990). *Noradrenergic neurons.* New York: Cambridge University Press.

Filser, J.G., Spira, J., & Fischer, M. (1988). The evaluation of 4-hydroxy-3-methoxyphenylglycol sulfate as a possible marker of central norepinephrine turnover: Studies in healthy volunteers and depressed patients. *Journal of Psychiatric Research, 22*, 171–181.

Fischer, H.G., Hollmann, W., & De Meirleir, K. (1991). Exercise changes in plasma tryptophan fractions and relationship with prolactin. *International Journal of Sports Medicine, 12*, 487–489.

Fitts, W.H. (1965). *Manual: Tennessee self-concept scale*. Nashville, TN: Counselor Recordings and Tests.

Fitzgerald, L. (1991). Overtraining increases the susceptibility to infection. *International Journal of Sports Medicine, 12*(Suppl. 1), 5–8.

Fletcher, G.F., Blair, S.N., Blumenthal, J., Caspersen, C., Chaitman, B., Epstein, S., Falls, H., Froelicher, E.S.S., Froelicher, V.F., & Piña, I.L. (1992). Position statement. Statement on exercise: Benefits and recommendations for physical activity programs for all Americans. A statement for health professionals by the Committee on Exercise and Cardiac Rehabilitation of the Council on Clinical Cardiology, American Heart Association. *Circulation, 86*, 340–344.

Flynn, M.G., Pizza, F.X., Boone, J.B., Andres, F.F., Michaud, T.A., & Rodriguez-Zayas, J.R. (1994). Indices of training stress during competitive running and swimming seasons. *International Journal of Sports Medicine, 15*, 21–26.

Folkins, C.H., & Sime, W.E. (1981). Physical fitness and mental health. *American Psychologist, 36*, 373–389.

Foote, S.L., Bloom, F.E., & Aston-Jones, G. (1983). Nucleus locus ceruleus: New evidence of anatomical and physiological specificity. *Physiological Reviews, 63*, 844–914.

Ford, H.T., Puckett, J.R., Blessing, D.L., & Tucker, L.A. (1989). Effects of selected physical activities on health-related fitness and psychological well-being. *Psychological Reports, 64*, 203–208.

Forgays, D.G. (1991). Primary prevention of psychopathology. In M. Hersin, A.P. Kazdin, & A.S. Bellack (Eds.), *The clinical psychology handbook* (2nd ed., pp. 743–761). New York: Pergamon Press.

Foster, V.L., Hume, G.J.E., Byrnes, W.C., Dickinson, A.L., & Chatfield, S.J. (1989). Endurance training for elderly women: Moderate vs low intensity. *Journal of Gerontology, 44*, M184–M188.

Fox, K.H. (1990). *The physical self-perception profile manual*. DeKalb, IL: Northern Illinois University, Office for Health Promotion.

Fox, K.H., & Corbin, C.B. (1989). The physical self-perception profile: Development and preliminary validation. *Journal of Sport and Exercise Psychology, 11*, 408–430.

Franz, S.I., & Hamilton, G.V. (1905). The effects of exercise upon the retardation in conditions in depression. *American Journal of Insanity, 62*, 239–256.

Frazer, A. (1993). Regionally selective effects in brain of typical and atypical antidepressants. *Neurobiology of affective disorders* (pp. 17–21). New York: Raven Press.

Freeman, H. (1993). Moclobemide. *Lancet, 342*, 1528–1532.

Freemont, J., & Craighead, L.W. (1987). Aerobic exercise and cognitive therapy in the treatment of dysphoric moods. *Cognitive Therapy and Research, 2*, 241–251.

Frey-Hewitt, B., Vranivan, K.M., Dreon, D.M., & Wood, P.D. (1990). The effect of weight loss by dieting or exercising on resting metabolic rate in overweight men. *International Journal of Obesity, 14*, 327–334.

Friedman, H. (1968). Magnitude of experimental effect and a taste for its rapid estimation. *Psychological Bulletin, 70*, 245–251.

Frisch, R.E., Wyshak, G., Albright, N.L., Schiff, T.E., & Jones, K.P. (1985). Lower prevalence of breast cancer and cancers of the reproductive system among former college athletes compared to nonathletes. *British Journal of Cancer, 52*, 885–891.

Fry, A.C., Kraemer, W.J., Stone, M.H., Warren, B., Fleck, S.J., Kearney, J.T., & Gordon, S.E. (1994). Endocrine responses to overreaching before and after 1 year of weightlifting. *Canadian Journal of Applied Physiology, 19*, 400–410.

Fry, A.C., Kraemer, W.J., Stone, M.H., Warren, B., Kearney, J.T., Fleck, S.J., & Wesman, C.A. (1993). Endocrine responses to one week of increased volume training and amino acid supplementation in elite junior weightlifters. *International Journal of Sports Nutrition, 3*, 306–322.

Fry, A.C., Kraemer, W.J., Van Borselen, F., Lynch, J.M., Marsit, J.L., Roy, E.P., Triplett, N.T., & Knuttgen, H.G. (1994). Performance decrements with high-intensity resistance exercise overtraining. *Medicine and Science in Sports and Exercise, 26*, 1165–1173.

Fry, A.C., Kraemer, W.J., Van Borselen, F., Lynch, J.M., Triplett, N.T., Koziris, L.P., & Fleck, S.J. (1994). Catecholamine responses to short-term high-intensity resistance exercise overtraining. *Journal of Applied Physiology, 77*, 941–946.

Fry, R.W., Lawrence, S.R., Morton, A.R., Schreiner, A.B., Polglaze, T.D., & Keast, D. (1993). Monitoring training stress in endurance sports using biological parameters. *Clinical Journal of Sport Medicine, 3*, 6–13.

Fry, R.W., Morton, A.R., Garcia-Webb, Crawford, G.P.M., & Keast, D. (1992). Biological responses to overload training in endurance sports. *European Journal of Applied Physiology, 64*, 355–364.

Fry, R.W., Morton, A.R., & Keast, D. (1991). Overtraining in athletes. An update. *Sports Medicine, 12*, 32–65.

Fry, R.W., Morton, A.R., & Keast, D. (1992). Periodisation and the prevention of overtraining. *Canadian Journal of Sport Sciences, 17*, 241–248.

Gaesser, G.A., & Rich, R.G. (1984). Effects of high- and low-intensity exercise training on aerobic capacity and blood lipids. *Medicine and Science in Sports and Exercise, 16*, 269–274.

Gaffney, F.A., Fenton, B.J., Lane, L.D., & Lake, R. (1988). Hemodynamic, ventilatory, and biochemical responses of panic patients and normal controls with sodium lactate infusion and spontaneous panic attacks. *Archives of General Psychiatry, 45*, 53–60.

Galbo, H., Houston, M.D., Christensen, N.J., Holst, J.J., Nielsen, B., Nygaard, E., & Suzuki, J. (1979). The effect of water temperature on the hormonal response to prolonged swimming. *Acta Physiologica Scandinavica, 105*, 326–337.

Garcia, A.W., & King, A.C. (1991). Predicting long-term adherence to aerobic exercise: A comparison of two models. *Journal of Sport and Exercise Psychology, 13*, 394–410.

Gartside, S.E., Cowen, P.J., & Sharp, T. (1992). Evidence that the large neutral amino acid L-valine decreases electrically-evoked release of 5-HT in rat hippocampus in vivo. *Psychopharmacology, 109*, 251–253.

Gauvin, L. (1989). An experimental perspective on the motivational features of exercise and lifestyle. *Canadian Journal of Sport Sciences, 15*, 51–58.

Geller, E.S. (1983). Rewarding safety belt usage at an industrial setting: Tests of treatment generality and response maintenance. *Journal of Applied Behavior Analysis, 16*, 189–202.

Geller, E.S., Mann, M., & Brasted, W. (1977, Aug.). *Trash can design: A determinant of litter-related behavior*. Paper presented at the meeting of the American Psychological Association, San Francisco, CA.

Geracioti, T.D., Jr., Kalogeras, K.T., Pigott, T.A., Demitrack, M.A., Altemus, M., Chrousos, G.P., & Gold, P.W. (1990). In G.D. Burrows, M. Roth, & R. Noyes, Jr. (Eds.), *Handbook of Anxiety: Vol. 3. The neurobiology of anxiety* (pp. 355–364). Amsterdam: Elsevier Science Publishers.

Gerin, C., Becquet, D., & Privat, A. (1995). Direct evidence for the link between monoaminergic pathways and motor activity. I. A study with microdialysis probes implanted in the ventral funiculus of the spinal cord. *Brain Res., 704*, 191–201.

Gerin, C., Legrand, A., & Privat, A. (1994). Study of 5-HT release with a chronically implanted microdialysis probe in the ventral horn of the spinal cord of unrestrained rats during exercise on a treadmill. *Journal of Neuroscience Methods, 52*, 129–141.

Gerra, G., Volpi, R., Delsignore, R., Caccavari, R., Gagiotti, M.T., Montani, G., Maninetti, L., Chiodera, P., & Coiro, V. (1992). ACTH and beta-endorphin responses to physical exercise in adolescent women tested for anxiety and frustration. *Psychiatry Research, 41*, 179–186.

Giraud, O., Cervo, L., Grignaschi, G., & Samanin, R. (1989). Activation of μ opioid receptors in the nucleus raphe dorsalis blocks apomorphine-induced aggression in rats: Serotonin appears not to be involved. *Brain Research, 488*, 174–179.

Gisolfi, C.V., & Christman, J.V. (1980). Thermal effects of injecting norepinephrine into hypothalamus of the rat during rest and exercise. *Journal of Applied Physiology, 49*, 937–941.

Gitlin, M.J., Cochran S.D., & Jamison, K.R. (1989). Maintenance lithium treatment: Side effects and compliance. *Journal of Clinical Psychiatry, 50*, 127–131.

Glämsta, E.-L., Mθrkrid, L., Lantz, I., & Nyberg, F. (1993). Concomitant increase in blood plasma levels of immunoreactive hemorphin-7 and β-endorphin following long distance running. *Regulatory Peptides, 1*, 9–18.

Glass, G.V. (1978). Integrating findings: The meta-analysis of research. *Review of Research in Education, 5*, 351–379.

Glass, G.V., & Kliegl, R. (1983). An apology for research integration in the study of psychotherapy. *Journal of Consulting and Clinical Psychology, 51*, 28–41.

Glasser, W. (1976). *Positive addiction*. New York: Harper & Row.

Glassman, A.H., & Bigger, J.T (1981). Cardiovascular effects of therapeutic doses of tricyclic antidepressants: A review. *Archives of General Psychiatry, 38*, 815–820.

Glazer, A.R., & O'Connor, P.J. (1992). Mood improvements following exercise and quiet rest in bulimic women. *Scandinavian Journal of Medicine and Science in Sports, 3*, 73–79.

Glick, B., & Margolis, R. (1962). A study of the influence of experimental design on clinical outcome in drug research. *American Journal of Psychiatry, 118*, 1087–1096.

Godin, G. (1994). Theories of reasoned action and planned behavior: Usefulness for exercise promotion. *Medicine and Science in Sports and Exercise, 26*, 1391–1394.

Gold, P.W., Goodwin, F.K., & Chrousos, G.P. (1988b). Clinical manifestations of depression, related to the neurobiology of stress [Pt. 2]. *New England Journal of Medicine, 319*, 413–420.

Goldfarb, A.H., Hatfield, B.D., Armstrong, D., & Potts, J. (1990). Plasma beta-endorphin concentration: Response to intensity and duration of exercise. *Medicine and Science in Sports and Exercise, 22*, 241–244.

Goldfarb, A.H., Hatfield, B.D., Potts, J., & Armstrong, D. (1991). Beta-endorphin time course response to intensity of exercise: Effect of training status. *International Journal of Sports and Medicine, 12*, 264–268.

Goodwin, F., & Bunney, W.E. (1971). Depression following reserpine: A re-evaluation. *Seminars in Psychiatry, 3*, 435–448.

Gorman, B.S., Primavera, L.H., & Allison, D.B. (1995). POWPAL: A program for estimating effect sizes, statistical power and sample sizes. *Educational and Psychological Measurement, 55*, 773–776.

Goss, J.D. (1994). Hardiness and mood disturbances in swimmers while overtraining. *Journal of Sport and Exercise Psychology, 16*, 135–149.

Gossard, D., Haskell, W.L., & Taylor, C.B. (1986). Effects of low- and high-intensity home-based exercise training on functional capacity in healthy middle-aged men. *American Journal of Cardiology, 57*, 446–449.

Gøtestam, K.G., & Stiles, T.C. (1990). *Physical exercise and cognitive vulnerability: A longitudinal study*. Paper presented at the Annual Meeting for the Association for the Advancement of Behavior Therapy, San Francisco, CA.

Gray, J.A. (1985). Issues in the neuropsychology of anxiety. In A.H. Tuma & J.D. Masser (Eds.), *Anxiety and the anxiety disorders* (pp. 5–26). Hillsdale, NJ: Lawrence Erlbaum Associates.

Greenberg, R.P., Bornstein, R.F., Zborowski, M.J., Fisher, S., & Greenberg, M.D. (1994). A meta-analysis of fluoxetine outcome in the treatment of depression. *Journal of Nervous and Mental Disease, 182*, 547–555.

Greist, J.H. (1987). Exercise intervention with depressed outpatients. In W.P. Morgan & S.E. Goldston (Eds.), *Exercise and mental health*. Washington, DC: Hemisphere Publishers.

Greist, J.H., Klein, M.H., Eischens, R.R., Faris, J., Gurman, A.S., & Morgan, W.P. (1979). Running as treatment for depression. *Comprehensive Psychiatry, 20*, 41–54.

Grevert, P., Albert, L.H., Inturrisi, C.E., & Goldstein, A. (1983). Effects of eight-hour naloxone infusions on human subjects. *Biological Psychiatry, 18*, 1375–1391.

Griffith, C.R. (1926). *Psychology of coaching*. New York: Charles Scribner.

Griffith, R.O., Dressendorfer, R.H., Fullbright, C.D., & Wade, C.E. (1990). Testicular function during exhaustive endurance training. *The Physician and Sportsmedicine, 18*, 54–64.

Grossman, A., Bouloux, P., Price, P., Drury, P.L., Lam, K.S.L., Turner, T., Thomas, J., Besser, G.M., & Sutton, J. (1984). The role of opioid peptides in the hormonal responses to acture exercise in man. *Clinical Science, 67*, 483–491.

Grosz, H.J., & Farmer B.B. (1969). Blood lactate in the development of anxiety symptoms. *Archives of General Psychiatry, 21*, 611–619.

Gutrie, S.K., Grunhaus, L., & Dantos, E. (1991). Tricyclic antidepressant effects on blood pressure and heart rate following standing and a short walk. *Annals of Clinical Psychiatry, 3*, 153–159.

Guttman, M.C., Pollock, M.L., Foster, C., & Schmidt, D. (1984). Training stress in olympic speed skaters: A psychological perspective. *The Physician and Sportsmedicine, 12*, 45–57.

Hackfort, D., & Schwenkmezger, P. (1989). Measuring anxiety in sport: Perspectives and problems. In D. Hackfort & C.D. Spielberger (Eds.), *Anxiety in sports: An international perspective* (pp. 55–75). New York: Hemisphere.

Hackney, A.C., Pearman, S.N., & Nowacki, J.M. (1990). Physiological profiles of overtrained and stale athletes: A review. *Journal of Applied Sport Psychology, 2*, 21–33.

Handley, S.L., & McBlane, J.W. (1993). 5-HT drugs in animal models of anxiety. *Psychopharmacology, 112*, 13–20.

Hanson, P.G., Vander Ark, C.R., Besozzi, M.C., & Rowe, G.C. (1982). Myocardial infarction in a national class swimmer. *Journal of the American Medical Association, 248*, 2313–2314.

Harter, S. (1983). Developmental perspectives on the self-system. In E.M. Hetherington (Ed.), *Handbook of child psychology: Social and personality development* (Vol. 4. pp. 275–385). New York: John Wiley & Sons.

Harter, S. (1990). Causes, correlates, and the functional role of global self-worth: A life-span perspective. In R.J. Sternberg & J. Kolligian, Jr. (Eds.), *Competence considered* (pp. 67–97). New Haven, CT: Yale University.

Hartley, L.H., Mason, J.W., Hogan, R.P., Jones, L.G., Kotchen, T.A., Mougey, E.H., Wherry, F.E., Pennington, L.L., & Ricketts, P.T. (1972). Multiple hormonal responses to prolonged exercise in relation to physical training. *Journal of Applied Physiology, 33*, 607–610.

Haskell, W.L. (1994a). Dose-response issues from a biological perspective. In C. Bouchard, R.J. Shephard, & T. Stephens (Eds.), *Physical activity, fitness, and health* (pp. 868–882). Champaign, IL: Human Kinetics Publishers.

Haskell, W.L. (1994b). Health consequences of physical activity: Understanding and challenges regarding dose-response. *Medicine and Science in Sports and Exercise, 26*, 649–660.

Hatfield, B.D., Goldfarb, A.H., Sforzo, G.A., & Flynn, M.G. (1987). Serum beta-endorphin and affective responses to graded exercise in young and elderly men. *Journal of Gerontology, 42*, 429–431.

Hatfield, B.D., & Landers, D.M. (1987). Psychophysiology within exercise and sports research: An overview. *Exercise and Sports Sciences Reviews, 15*, 351–387.

Hatfield, B.D., Vaccaro, P., & Benedict, G.J. (1985). Self-concept responses of children to participation in an eight-week jump-rope program. *Perceptual and Motor Skills, 61*, 1275–1279.

Hattie, J. (1992). *Self-concept*. Hillsdale, NJ: Lawrence Erlbaum Associates.

Hedner, T., & Cassuto, J. (1987). Opioids and opioid receptors in peripheral tissues. *Scandinavian Journal of Gastroenterology, 130*(Suppl.), 27–46.

Heidbreder, C., Gewiss, M., Lallemand, S., Roques, B.P., & De Witte, P. (1992). Inhibition of enkephalin metabolism and activation of mu- or delta-opioid receptors elicit opposite effects on reward and motility in the ventral mesencephalon. *Neuropharmacology, 31*, 293–298.

Heinzelmann, F., & Bagley, R.W. (1970). Response to physical activity programs and their effects on health behavior. *Public Health Reports, 86*, 905–911.

Hendrickson, C.D., & Verde, T.J. (1994). Inadequate recovery from vigorous exercise. *The Physician and Sportsmedicine, 22*, 56–64.

Heuser, S.J.E., Wark, H.J., Keul, J., & Holsboer, F. (1991). Hypothalamic-pituitary-adrenal axis function in elderly endurance athletes. *Journal of Clinical Endocrinology and Metabolism, 73*, 485–488.

Heyes, M.P., Garnett, E.S., & Coates, G. (1988). Nigrostriatal dopaminergic activity is increased during exhaustive exercise stress in rats. *Life Sciences, 42*, 1537–1542.

Hill, D.W., Cureton, K.J., & Collins, M.A. (1989). Effect of time of day on perceived exertion at work rates above and below the ventilatory threshold. *Research Quarterly for Exercise and Sport, 60*, 127–133.

Hill, J.O., Davis, J.R., & Tagliaferro, A.R. (1983). Effects of diet and exercise training on thermogenesis in adult female rats. *Physiology and Behavior, 31*, 133–135.

Hirschfeld, R.M.A. (1996). *Advisory panel on depression*. National Depressive and Manic-Depressive Association.

Hirschfeld, R.M.A., & Goodwin, F.K. (1988). Mood disorders. In J.A. Talbott, R.E. Hales, & S.C. Yodofsky (Eds.), *The American Psychiatric Press textbook of psychiatry* (pp. 403–442). Washington, DC: American Psychiatric Press, Inc.

Hoffmann, P., Carlsson, S., Thoren, P. (1990). The effects of μ-, δ-, and κ-opioid receptor antagonists on the pain threshold increase following muscle stimulation in the rat. *Acta Physiol. Scand., 140*, 353–358.

Hoffmann, P., Delle, M., & Thoren, P. (1990). Role of opioid receptors in the long-lasting blood pressure depression after electric muscle stimulation in the hind leg of the rat. *Acta Physiol. Scand., 140*, 191–198.

Hoffmann, P., Elam, M., Thoren, P., & Hjorth, S. (1994). Effects of long-lasting voluntary running on the cerebral levels of dopamine, serotonin and their metabolites in the spontaneously hypertensive rat. *Life Sciences, 54*, 855–861.

Hoffmann, P., Skarphedinsson, J.O., & Thoren, P. (1990). Electric muscle stimulation in the spontaneously hypertensive rat induces a post-stimulatory reduction in activity: Role of different opioid receptors. *Acta Physiologica Scandinavica, 140*, 507–514.

Hoffmann, P., Terenius, L., & Thoren, P. (1990). Cerebrospinal fluid immunoreactive β-endorphin concentration is increased by voluntary exercise in the spontaneously hypertensive rat. *Regulatory Peptides, 28*, 233–239.

Hoffmann, P., Thoren, P., & Ely, D. (1987). Effect of voluntary exercise on open-field behavior and on aggression in the spontaneously hypertensive rat (SHR). *Behavioral and Neural Biology, 47*, 346–355.

Hofstetter, C.R., Hovell, M.F., Macera, C., Sallis, J.F., Spry, V., Barrington, E., & Callender, C. (1991). Illness, injury, and correlates of aerobic exercise and walking: A community study. *Research Quarterly for Exercise and Sport, 62*, 1–9.

Holland, R.L., Sayers, J.A., Keatinge, W.R., Davis, H.M., & Peswami, R. (1985). Effects of raised body temperature on reasoning, memory and mood. *Journal of Applied Physiology, 59*, 1823–1827.

Holloszy, J.O., & Coyle, E.F. (1984). Adaptations of skeletal muscle to endurance exercise and their metabolic consequences. *Journal of Applied Physiology, 56*, 831–840.

Hooper, S.L., Traeger Mackinnon, L., Gordon, R.D., & Bachmann, A.W. (1993). Hormonal responses of elite swimmers to overtraining. *Medicine and Science in Sports and Exercise, 25*, 741–747.

Horne, J.A., & Staff, C.H. (1983). Exercise and sleep: Body heating effects. *Sleep, 6*, 36–46.

Houghten, R.A., Pratt, S.M, Young, E.A., Brown, H., & Spann, D.R. (1986). Effect of chronic exercise on β-endorphin receptor levels in rats. *Monographs of the National Institute of Drug Abuse Research, 75*, 505–508.

Hovell, M.F., Sallis, J.F., Hofstetter, C.R., Spry, V.M., Elder, J.P., Faucher, P., & Caspersen, C.J. (1989). Identifying correlates of walking for exercise: An epidemiologic prerequisite for physical activity promotion. *Preventive Medicine, 18*, 868–866.

Hoyle, R.H. (1993). On the relation between data and theory. *American Psychologist, 48*, 1094–1096.

Huff, D. (1954). *How to lie with statistics.* New York: W.W. Norton & Co. Inc.

Hughes, J.R. (1984). Psychological effects of habitual aerobic exercise: A critical review. *Preventive Medicine, 13*, 66–78.

Humphrey, L.L. (1984). Children's self-control in relation to perceived social environment. *Journal of Personality and Social Psychology, 46*, 178–188.

Isaac, S., & Michael, W.B. (1995). *Handbook in research and evaluation.* San Diego: Educational and Industrial Testing Service.

Jackson, D.N. (1984). *Personality research form manual.* New York: Research Psychologists Press.

Jacobs, B.L., & Fornal, C.A. (1993). 5-HT and motor control: A hypothesis. *Trends in Neurosciences, 16*, 346–352.

Jaffe, J.H., & Martin, W.R. (1985). Opioid analgesics and antagonists. In A. Goodman-Gilman, L.S. Goodman, T.W. Rall, & F. Murad (Eds.), *The pharmacological basis of therapeutics* (pp. 491–531). New York: Macmillan Publishing.

James, W. (1899). Physical training in the educational curriculum. *American Physical Education Review, 4*, 220–221.

Janal, M.N., Colt, E.W.D., Clark, W.C., & Glusman, M. (1984). Pain sensitivity, mood and plasma endocrine levels in man following long-distance running: Effects of naloxone. *Pain, 19*, 13–25.

Janis, L.L., & Mann, L. (1977). *Decision making.* New York: Free Press.

Jaskowski, M.A., Jackson, A.S., Raven, P.B., & Caffrey, J.L. (1989). Enkephalin metabolism: Effect of acute exercise stress and cardiovascular fitness. *Medicine and Science in Sports and Exercise, 21*, 154–160.

Jasnoski, M.L., Holmes, D.S., Solomon, S., & Aguiar, C. (1981). Exercise, changes in aerobic capacity and changes in self-perceptions: An experimental investigation. *Journal of Research in Personality, 15*, 460–466.

Jason, L.A., & Glenwick, D.S. (1980). An overview of behavioral community psychology. In D. Glenwick & L. Jason (Eds.), *Behavioral community psychology: Progress and prospects.* New York: Praeger.

Jefferson, J.W. (1974). Beta-adrenergic receptor blocking drugs in psychiatry. *Archives of General Psychiatry, 31*, 681–691.

Jefferson, J.W. (1975). A review of cardiovascular effects and toxity of tricyclic antidepressants. *Psychosomatic Medicine, 37*, 160–179.

Jefferson, J.W., Greist, J.H., Ackerman, D.L., & Carroll, B.A. (1987). *Lithium encyclopedia for clinical practice* (2nd ed., pp. 292–295). Washington, DC: American Psychiatric Press, Inc.

Jefferson, J.W., Greist, J.H., Clagnaz, P.J., Eischens, R.R., Marten, W.C., & Evenson, M.A. (1982). Effects of strenuous exercise on lithium level in man. *American Journal of Psychiatry, 139*, 1593–1595.

Jennings, G., Nelson, L., Nestel, P., Esler, M., Korner, P., Burton, D., & Bazelmans, J. (1986). The effects of changes in physical activity on major cardiovascular risk factors, hemodynamics, sympathetic function, and glucose utilization in man: A controlled study of four levels of activity. *Circulation, 73*, 30–40.

Jeukendrup, A.E., Hesslink, M.K.C., Snyder, A.C., Kuipers, H., & Keizer, H.A. (1992). Physiological changes in male competitive cyclists after two weeks of intensified training. *International Journal of Sports Medicine, 13*, 534–541.

Ji, L.L., Miller, R.H., Nagle, F.J., Lardy, H.A., & Stratman, F.W. (1987). Amino acid metabolism during exercise in trained rats: The potential role of carnitine in the metabolic fate of branched-chain amino acids. *Metabolism, 36*, 748–752.

Johansson, G., Johnson, J.V., & Hall, E.M. (1991). Smoking and sedentary behavior as related to work organization. *Social Science Medicine, 32*, 837–846.

Johnston-O'Connor, E.J., & Kirschenbaum, D.S. (1986). Something succeeds like success: Positive self-monitoring for unskilled golfers. *Cognitive Therapy and Research, 10*, 123–136.

Judd, L.L., Janowsky, D.S., Segal, D.S., & Huey, L.Y. (1980). Naloxone-induced behavioral and physiological effects in normal and manic subjects. *Archives of General Psychiatry, 37*, 583–586.

Juvent, M., Douchamps, J., Delcourt, E., Kostucki, W., Dulcire, C., d'Hooge, D., & Herchuelz, A. (1990). Lack of cardiovascular side effects of the new tricyclic antidepressant tianeptine. *Clinical Neuropharmacology, 13*, 48–57.

Kalin, N.H., & Dawson, G.W. (1986). Neuroendocrine dysfunction in depression: Hypothalamic-anterior pituitary systems. *Trends in Neurosciences, 9*, 261–266.

Kanfer, F.H., & Karoly, P. (1972). Self-control: A behavioristic excursion into the lion's den. *Behavior Therapy, 3*, 498–516.

Kaplan, R.M., Atkins, C.J., & Reinsch, S. (1984). Specific efficacy expectations mediate exercise compliance in patients with COPD. *Health Psychology, 3*, 223–242.

Karoly, P. (1993). Mechanisms of self-regulation: A systems view. *Annual Review of Psychology, 44*, 23–52.

Karpovich, P.V. (1941). Fatigue and endurance. *Research Quarterly, 12*, 416–422.

Karvonen, M.J., Kentala, J.E., & Mustala, O. (1957). The effects of training on heart rate. *Annales of Medicinae Experimentalis et Biologiae Fenniae, 35*, 308–315.

Katoh, A., Nabeshima, T., & Kameyama, T. (1990). Behavioral changes induced by stressful situations: Effects of enkephalins, dynorphin, and their interactions. *Journal of Pharmacology and Experimental Therapeutics, 253*, 600–607.

Katz, R.J. (1981). Animal models and human depressive disorders. *Neuroscience and Biobehavioral Reviews, 5*, 231–246.

Kavaliers, M., & Innes, D.G.L. (1987). Sex and day-night differences in opiate-induced responses of insular wild deer mice, *Peromyscus maniculatus triangularis. Pharmacology, Biochemistry, and Behavior, 27*, 477–482.

Kavanagh, T., Shephard, R.J., Pandit, V., & Doney, H. (1970). Exercise and hypnotherapy in the rehabilitation of the coronary patient. *Archives of Physical Medicine and Rehabilitation, 51*, 578–587.

Kawakita, K., & Funakoshi, M. (1982). Suppression of the jaw-opening reflex by conditioning A-delta fiber stimulation and electroaccupuncture in the rat. *Experimental Neurology, 78*, 461–465.

Kaye, W.H., Berrettini, W.H., Gwirtsman, H.E., Chretien, M., Gold, P.W., George, D.T., Jimerson, D.C., & Ebert, M.H. (1987). Reduced cerebrospinal fluid levels of immunoreactive pro-opiomelanocortin related peptides (including beta-endorphin) in anorexia nervosa. *Life Sciences, 41*, 2147–2155.

Keir, S., & Lauzon, R. (1980). Physical activity in a healthy lifestyle. In P.O. Davidson & S.M. Davidson (Eds.), *Behavioral medicine: Changing health lifestyles.* New York: Brunner/Mazel, Inc.

Kellerman, J.J., Winter, I., & Kariv, I. (1969). Effect of physical training on neurocirculatory asthenia. *Israel Journal of Medical Science, 5*, 947–949.

Kemper, H. (1994). The natural history of physical activity and aerobic fitness in teenagers. In Dishman, R.K. (Ed.), *Advances in exercise adherence* (pp. 293–318). Champaign, IL: Human Kinetics Publishers.

Kendall, P.C. (1978). Cognitive-behavioral and patient education interventions in cardiac catheterization procedures: The Palo Alto Medical Psychology Project. *Journal of Consulting and Clinical Psychology, 47*, 49–58.

Kennett, G.A., Dickinson, D.L., & Curzon, G. (1985). Enhancement of some 5-HT-dependent behavioural responses following repeated immobilization in rats. *Brain Research, 330*, 253–263.

Kereszty, A. (1971). Overtraining. In L.A. Larson (Ed.), *Encyclopedia of sport sciences and medicine* (pp. 218–222). New York: Macmillan Publishing.

Kerr, J.H., & Svebak, S. (1994). The acute effects of participation in sport on mood: The importance of level of 'antagonistic physical interaction.' *Personality and individual differences, 16*, 159–166.

Kerr, J.H., & Vlaswinkel, E.H. (1990). Effects of exercise on anxiety: A review. *Anxiety Research, 2*, 309–321.

Keverne, E.B., Martensz, N.D., & Tuite, B. (1989). Beta-endorphin concentrations in cerebrospinal fluid of monkeys are influenced by grooming relationships. *Psychoneuroendocrinology, 14*, 155–161.

Khachaturian, H., Lewis, M.E., Schäfer, M.K.H., & Watson, S.J. (1985). Anatomy of the CNS opioid systems. *Trends in Neurosciences, 8*, 111–119.

Kibler, W.B., Chandler, J.T., & Stracener, E.S. (1992). Musculoskeletal adaptations and injuries due to overtraining. In J.O. Holloszy (Ed.), *Exercise and sport sciences reviews* (pp. 99–126). Baltimore: Williams & Wilkins.

King, A.C. (1991). Community intervention for promotion of physical activity and fitness. *Exercise and Sport Sciences Reviews, 19*, 211–260.

King, A.C., Blair, S.N., Bild, D.E., Dishman, R.K., Dubbert, P.M., Marcus, B.H., Oldridge, N.B., Paffenbarger, R.S., Jr., Powell, K.E., & Yeager, K.K. (1992). Determinants of physical activity and interventions in adults. *Medicine and Science in Sports and Exercise, 24*(Suppl.), S221–S236.

King, A.C., Taylor, C.B., Haskell, W.L., & DeBusk, R.F. (1989). Influence of regular aerobic exercise on psychological health: A randomized, controlled trial of healthy middle-aged adults. *Health Psychology, 8*, 305–324.

King, A.L., & Frederiksen, L.W. (1984). Low-cost strategies for increasing exercise behavior: Relapse preparation training and support. *Behavior Modification, 3*, 3–21.

King, C.A., & Kirschenbaum, D.S. (1992). *Helping young children develop social skills*. Pacific Grove, CA: Brooks/Cole Publishing Company.

Kiorman, R., Hilpert, P.L., Michael, R., LaGana, C., & Sveen, O.B. (1980). Effects of coping and mastery modeling on experienced and unexperienced periodontic patients' disruptiveness. *Behavior Therapy 11*, 156–168.

Kirsch, I. (1994). Clinical hypnosis as a nondeceptive placebo: Empirically derived techniques. *American Journal of Clinical Hypnosis, 37*, 95–106.

Kirschenbaum, D.S. (1984). Self-regulation and sport psychology: Nurturing an emerging symbiosis. *Journal of Sport Psychology, 6*, 159–183.

Kirschenbaum, D.S. (1987). Self-regulatory failure: A review with clinical implications. *Clinical Psychology Review, 7*, 77–104.

Kirschenbaum, D.S., & Fitzgibbon, M.L. (1995). Controversy about the treatment of obesity: Criticisms or challenges? *Behavior Therapy, 26*, 43–48.

Kirschenbaum, D.S., & Flanery, R.C. (1984). Toward a psychology of behavioral contracting. *Clinical Psychology Review, 4*, 597–618.

Kirschenbaum, D.S., & Karoly, P. (1977). When self-regulation fails: Tests of some preliminary hypotheses. *Journal of Consulting and Clinical Psychology, 45*, 1116–1125.

Kirschenbaum, D.S., Ordman, A.M., Tomarken, A.J., & Holtzbauer, B. (1982). Effects of differential self-monitoring and level of mastery on sports performance: Brain power bowling. *Cognitive Therapy and Research, 6*, 335–342.

Kirschenbaum, D.S., & Tomarken, A.J. (1982). On facing the generalization problem: The study of self-regulatory failure. In R.C. Kendall (Ed.), *Advances in cognitive-behavior research and therapy: Vol. 1* (pp. 121–200). New York: Academic Press.

Kjaer, M., & Galbo, H. (1988). Effect of physical training on the capacity to secrete epinephrine. *Journal of Applied Physiology, 64*, 11–16.

Kjaer, M., Secher, N.H., Bach, F.W., Sheikh, S., & Galbo, H. (1989). Hormonal and metabolic responses to exercise in humans: Effect of sensory nervous blockade. *American Journal of Physiology, 257*, E95-E101.

Klein, M.H., Greist, J.H., Gurman, A.S., Neimeyer, R.A., Lesser, D.P., Bushnell, N.J., & Smith, R.E. (1985). A comparative outcome study of group psychotherapy vs. exercise treatments for depression. *International Journal of Mental Health, 13*, 148–177.

Knapp, D.N. (1988). Behavioral management techniques and exercise promotion. In R.K. Dishman (Ed.), *Exercise adherence: its impact on public health* (pp. 203–236). Champaign, IL: Human Kinetics Publishers.

Kniffki, K.D., Mense, S., & Schmidt, R.F. (1981). Muscle receptors with fine afferent fibers which may evoke circulatory reflexes. *Circulation Research, 48*(Suppl. 1.), I-25–I-31.

Koltyn, K.F., & Morgan, W.P. (1990). Psychological and physiological alterations following whole-body cooling and vigorous exercise. *Medicine and Science in Sports and Exercise, 22*, 78.

Koltyn, K.F., & Morgan, W.P. (1992a). Influence of underwater exercise on anxiety and body temperature. *Scandinavian Journal of Medicine and Science in Sports, 2*, 249–253.

Koltyn, K.F., & Morgan, W.P. (1992b). Efficacy of perceptual vs. heart rate monitoring in the development of endurance. *British Journal of Sports Medicine, 26*, 132–134.

Koltyn, K.F., & Morgan, W.P. (1993). The influence of wearing a wetsuit on core temperature and anxiety responses during underwater exercise. *Medicine and Science in Sports and Exercise, 25*, S45.

Koltyn, K.F., Raglin, J.S., O'Connor, P.J., & Morgan, W.P. (1995). Influence of weight training on state anxiety, body awareness and blood pressure. *International Journal of Sports Medicine, 16*, 266–269.

Koltyn, K.F., Robins, H.I., Schmitt, C.L., Cohen, J.D., & Morgan, W.P. (1992). Changes in mood state following whole-body hyperthermia. *International Journal of Hyperthermia, 8*, 305–307.

Koltyn, K.F., Shake, C.L., & Morgan, W.P. (1993). Interaction of exercise, water temperature and protective apparel on body awareness and anxiety. *International Journal of Sport Psychology, 24*, 297–305.

Koob, G.F. (1989). Anhedonia as an animal model of depression. In G.F. Koob, C.L. Ehlers, & D.J. Kupfer (Eds.), *Animal models of depression* (pp. 162–183). Boston: Birkhauser Boston, Inc.

Korol, B., Land, W.J., & Brown, M.J. (1965). Effects of chronic chlorpromazine administration on systemic arterial blood pressure in schizophrenic patients: Relationship of body position to blood pressure. *Clinical Pharmacology and Therapeutics, 6*, 587–591.

Kottke, T.E. (1992). Cardiac rehabilitation 1992. *Keio Journal of Medicine, 41*, 123–127.

Koutedakis, Y., Frischknecht, R., Budgett, R., Vrbova, G., & Sharp, R. (1993). Impaired voluntary force production of quadriceps in overtrained subjects. *Journal of Physiology, 459*, 151.

Kraemer, R.R., Dzewaltowski, D.A., Blair, M.S., Rinehardt, K.F., & Castracane, V.D. (1990). Mood alteration from treadmill running and its relationship to beta-endorphin, corticotropin, and growth hormone. *Journal of Sports Medicine and Physical Fitness, 31*, 241–246.

Kraemer, W.J., Armstrong, L.E., Marchitelli, L.J., Hubbard, R.W., & Leva, N. (1987). Plasma opioid peptide responses during heat acclimation in humans. *Peptides, 8*, 715–719.

Kuczmarski, R.J., Flegal, K.M., Campbell, S.M., & Johnson, C.L. (1994). Increasing prevalence of overweight among U.S. adults: The National Health and Nutrition Examination Surveys, 1960–1991. *Journal of the American Medical Association, 272*, 205–212.

Kugler, J., Dimsdale, J., Hartley, L.H., & Sherwood, J. (1990). Hospital supervised vs. home exercise in cardiac rehabilitation. *Archives of Physical Medicine and Rehabilitation, 71*, 322–325.

Kugler, J., Seelbach, H., & Kruskemper, G.M. (1994). Effects of rehabilitation exercise programmes on anxiety and depression in coronary patients: A meta-analysis. *British Journal of Clinical Psychology, 33*, 401–410.

Kuhn, D.M., Wolf, W.A., & Youdim, M.B.H. (1986). Serotonin neurochemistry revisited: A new look at some old axioms. *Neurochemistry International, 8*, 141–154.

Kuipers, H., & Keizer, H.A. (1988). Overtraining in elite athletes. Review and directions for the future. *Sports Medicine, 6*, 79–92.

Kurosawa, M., Okada, K., Sato, A., & Uchida, S. (1993). Extracellular release of acetylcholine, noradrenaline and serotonin increases in the cerebral cortex during walking in conscious rats. *Neuroscience Letters, 161*, 73–76.

Kuusinen, J., & Heinonen, M. (1972). Immediate aftereffects of the Finnish sauna on psychomotor performance and mood. *Journal of Applied Physiology, 56*, 336–340.

Lacey, J.I. (1967). Somatic patterning and stress: Some revisions of the activation theory. In M.H. Appley & R. Trumbell (Eds.), *Psychological stress* (pp. 14–37). New York: Appleton-Century-Crofts.

Lader, M. (1985). Benzodiazepines, anxiety and catecholamines: A commentary. In A.H. Tuna & J. Maser (Eds.), *Anxiety and the anxiety disorders*, (pp. 77–83). Hillsdale NJ: Lawrence Erlbaum Associates.

Langenfeld, M.E., Hart, L.S., & Kao, P.C. (1987). Plasma β-endorphin responses to one-hour bicycling and running at 60% VO_2max. *Journal of Sports Medicine and Physical Fitness, 19*, 83–86.

Langley, J.N. (1901). Observations on the physiological action of extracts of the suprarenal bodies. *Journal of Physiology (Cambridge), 27*, 237–256.

Laurent, J.P., Mangold, M., Humbel, U., & Haefely, W. (1983). Reduction by two benzodiazepines and pentobarbitone of the multiunit activity in substantia nigra, hippocampus, nucleus locus coeruleus, and nucleus raphe dorsalis of encephale isole rats. *Neuropharmacology, 22*, 501–511.

Layman, E. (1960). Physical activity as a psychiatric adjunct. In W.R. Johnson (Ed.), *Science and medicine of exercise and sports* (pp. 703–725). New York: Harper and Brothers.

Lee, I.M., & Paffenbarger, R.S., Jr. (1992a). Physical activity and risk of prostatic cancer among college alumni. *American Journal of Epidemiology, 135*, 169–179.

Lee, I.M., & Paffenbarger, R.S., Jr. (1992b). Quetelet's index and risk of colon cancer in college alumni. *Journal of the National Cancer Institute, 84,* 1326–1331.

Lehmann, M., Baumgartl, P., Wiesenck, C., Seidel, A., Baumann, H., Fischer, S., Spori, U., Gendrisch, G., Kaminski, R., & Keul, J. (1992). Training-overtraining: Influence of a defined increase in training volume vs training intensity on performance, catecholamines, and some metabolic parameters in experienced middle- and long-distance runners. *European Journal of Applied Physiology, 64,* 169–177.

Lehmann, M., Dickhuth, H.H., Gendrisch, G., Lazar, W., Thum, M., Kaminiski, R., Aramendi, J.F., Peterke, E., Wieland, W., & Kuel, J. (1991). Training-overtraining: A prospective, experimental study with experienced middle- and long-distance runners. *International Journal of Sports Medicine, 12,* 444–452.

Lehmann, M., Foster, C., & Keul, J. (1993). Overtraining in endurance athletes: A brief review. *Medicine and Science in Sports and Exercise, 25,* 854–862.

Lehmann, M., Schnee, W., Scheu, R., Stockhausen, W., & Bachl, N. (1992). Decreased nocturnal catecholamine excretion: Parameter for an overtraining syndrome in athletes? *International Journal of Sports Medicine, 13,* 236–242.

Leon, A.S., Connett, J., Jacobs, D.R., & Rauramaa, R. (1987). Leisure-time physical activity levels and risk of coronary heart disease and death: The multiple risk factor intervention trial. *Journal of the American Medical Association, 258,* 2388–2395.

Leventhal, M., Zimmerman, R., & Gutmann, M. (1984). Compliance: A self-regulatory perspective. In D. Gentry (Ed.), *Handbook of behavioral medicine.* New York: Guilford Publications.

Levin, S. (1991). Overtraining causes olympic-sized problems. *The Physician and Sportsmedicine, 19,* 112–118.

Levitt, E.E. (1971). Research on psychotherapy with children. In A.E. Bergin & S.L. Garfield (Eds.), *Handbook of psychotherapy and behavior change: an empirical analysis* (pp. 474–494). New York: John Wiley & Sons.

Levitt, E.E. (1980). The experimental measurement of anxiety. *The psychology of anxiety* (pp. 47–71). Hillsdale, NJ: Lawrence Erlbaum Associates.

Levy, L.H. (1967). Awareness, learning, and the beneficent subject as expert witness. *Journal of Personality and Social Psychology, 6,* 365–370.

Leysen, J.E. (1989). Use of 5-HT receptor agonists and antagonists for the characterization of their respective receptor sites. In A.B. Boulton, G.B. Baker, & A.V. Juorio (Eds.), *Neuromethods: Vol. 12. Drugs as tools in neurotransmitter research* (pp. 299–349). Clifton, NJ: The Humana Press.

Lichtman, S., & E.G. Poser (1983). The effects of exercise on mood and cognitive functioning. *Journal of Psychosomatic Research, 27,* 43–52.

Liederback, M., Glein, G.W., & Nicholas, J.A. (1992). Monitoring training status in professional ballet dancers. *Journal of Sports Medicine and Physical Fitness, 32,* 187–195.

Lobstein, D.D., & Rasmussen, C.L. (1991). Decreases in resting plasma beta-endorphin and depression scores after endurance training. *Journal of Sports Medicine and Physical Fitness, 31,* 543–551.

Lockette, W., McCurdy, R., Smith, S., & Carretero, O. (1987). Endurance training and $\alpha2$-adrenergic receptors on platelets. *Medicine and Science in Sports and Exercise, 19,* 7–10.

Long, B.C. (1984). Aerobic conditioning and stress inoculation: A comparison of stress-management interventions. *Cognitive Therapy and Research, 8,* 517–542.

Long, B.J., Calfas, Sallis, J.F., Patrick, K., Darmstadter, B., & Campbell, J. (1994). Evaluation of patient physical activity after counseling by primary care providers. [Abstract] *Medicine and Science in Sports and Exercise, 26(Suppl.),* S4.

Lubin, B. (1967). *Manual for depression adjective checklist.* San Diego, CA: Educational and Industrial Testing Service.

Luchins, D.J. (1983). Review of clinical and animal studies comparing the cardiovascular effects of doxepin and other tricyclic antidepressants. *American Journal of Psychiatry, 140,* 1006–1009.

Luger, A., Deuster, P.A., Kyle, S.B., et al. (1987). Acute hypothalamic-pituitary-adrenal responses to the stress of treadmill exercise: Physiological adaptations to physical training. *New England Journal of Medicine, 316,* 1309–1315.

Lundborg, P., Åstrøm, H., Bengtsson, C., Fellenius, E., von Schenck, H., Svensson, L., & Smith, U. (1981). Effect of beta-adrenoreceptor blocade on exercise performance and metabolism. *Clinical Science, 61*, 299–305.

Luoto, K. (1964). Personality and placebo effects upon timing behavior. *Journal of Abnormal and Social Psychology, 68*, 54–61.

Lyon, L.J., & Antony, J. (1982). Reversal of alcoholic coma by naloxone. *Annals of Internal Medicine, 96*, 464–465.

Maas, J.W. (1979). Neurotransmitters and depression: Too much, too little, or unstable? *Trends in the Neurosciences, 2*, 306–308.

Maas, J.W., & Leckman, J.F. (1983). Relationships between central nervous system noradrenergic function and plasma and urinary MHPG and other norephrinephrine metabolites. *MHPG: Basic mechanisms and psychopathology* (pp. 33–43). New York: Academic Press.

Macera, C.A., Jackson, K.L., Hagenmaier, G.W., Kronenfeld, J.J., Kohl, H.W., & Blair, S.N. (1989). Age, physical activity, physical fitness, body composition, and incidence of orthopedic problems. *Research Quarterly for Exercise and Sport, 60*, 225–233.

Macera, C.A., Pate, R.R., Powell, K.E., Jackson, K.L., Kendrick, J.S., & Craven, T.E. (1989). Predicting lower-extremity injuries among habitual runners. *Archives of Internal Medicine, 149*, 2565–2568.

Mahmarian, J.J., Verani, M.S., & Pratt, C.M. (1990). Hemodynamic effects of intravenous and oral sotalol. *American Journal of Cardiology*, 65, 28A-34A.

Mahoney, M.J., & Thoresen, C.E. (1974). *Self-control: Power to the person.* Monterey, CA: Brooks/Cole.

Maki,T., Kontula, K., & Harkonen, M. (1990). The beta-adrenergic system in man: Physiological and pathophysiological response. *Scandinavian Journal of Clinical Laboratory Investigation, 50* (Suppl. 201), 25–43.

Malmborg, R., Isaacson, S., Kallivroussis, G. (1974). The effect of beta-blocade and/or physical training in patients with angina pectoris. *Current Therapeutic Research Clinical and Experimental, 16*, 171–183.

Mansour, A., Khachaturian, H., Lewis, M.E., Akil, H., & Watson, S.J. (1988). Anatomy of CNS opioid receptors. *Trends in Neurosciences, 11*, 308–314.

Manuck, S.B., Olsson, G., Hjemdahl, P., et al. (1992). Does cardiovascular reactivity to mental stress have prognostic value in postinfarction patients? A pilot study. *Psychosomatic Medicine, 54*, 1992.

Marcus, B.H., Banspach, S.W., Lefebvre, R.C., Rossi, J.S., Carleton, R.A., & Abrams, D.B. (1992). Using the stages of change model to increase the adoption of physical activity among community participants. *American Journal of Health Promotion, 6*, 424–429.

Marcus, B.H., Eaton, C.A., Rossi, J.S., & Harlow, L.L. (1994). Self-efficacy, decision making, and stages of change: An integrated model of physical exercise. *Journal of Applied Social Psychology, 24*, 489–508.

Marcus, B.H., & Owen, N. (1992). Motivational readiness, self-efficacy, and decision-making for exercise. *Journal of Applied Social Psychology, 22*, 3–16.

Marcus, B.H., Rakowski, W., & Rossi, J.S. (1992). Assessing motivational readiness and decision-making for exercise. *Health Psychology, 11*, 257–261.

Marcus, B.H., Rossi, J.S., Selby, V.C., Niaura, R.S., & Abrams, D.B. (1992). The stages and processes of exercise adoption and maintenance in a workshop sample. *Health Psychology, 11*, 386–395.

Marcus, B.H., & Simkin, L.R. (1993). The stages of exercise behavior. *Journal of Sports Medicine and Physical Fitness, 33*, 83–88.

Marlatt, G.A., & Gordon, J.R. (Eds.). (1985) *Relapse prevention.* New York: Guilford Publications.

Marsden, C.A., Conti, J., Strope, E., Curzon, G., & Adams, R.N. (1979). Monitoring 5hydroxytryptamine release in the brain of the freely moving unanesthetized rat using in vivo voltammetry. *Brain Research, 171*, 85–99.

Marsh, H.W. (1990). A multidimensional self-concept: A social psychological perspective. *Annual Review of Psychology, 38*, 299–337.

Marsh, H.W. (1993). Relations between global and specific domains of self: The importance of individual importance, certainty, and ideals. *Journal of Personality and Social Psychology, 65,* 975–992.

Marsh, H.W., & Redmayne, R.S. (1994). A multidimensional physical self-concept and its relation to multiple components of physical fitness. *Journal of Sport and Exercise Psychology, 16,* 45–55.

Marsh, H.W., Richards, G.E., & Barnes, J. (1986a). Multidimensional self-concepts: The effect of participation in an Outward Bound program. *Journal of Personality and Social Psychology, 50,* 195–204.

Marsh, H.W., Richards, G.E., & Barnes, J. (1986b). Multidimensional self-concepts: A long-term follow-up of the effect of participation in Outward Bound program. *Personality and Social Psychology, 12,* 475–492.

Marsh, H.W., Richards, G.E., Johnson, S., Roche, L., & Tremayne, P. (1994). Physical self-description questionnaire: Psychometric properties and a multi-trait-multi-method analysis of relationships to existing instruments. *Journal of Sport and Exercise Psychology, 16,* 270–305.

Marsh, H.W., & Sonstroem, R.J. (1995). Importance ratings and specific components of physical self-concept: Relevance to predicting global self-concept and exercise. *Journal of Sport and Exercise Psychology, 17,* 84–104.

Martel, F.L., Nevison, C.M., Rayment, F.D., Simpson, M., & Keverne, E.B. (1993). Opioid receptor blockade reduces maternal affect and social grooming in rhesus monkeys. *Psychoneuroendocrinology, 18,* 307–321.

Martin, J.E. (1981). Exercise management: Shaping and maintaining physical fitness. *Behavioral Medicine Advances, 4,* B-5.

Martin, J.E., & Dubbert, P.M. (1982a). Exercise applications and promotion in behavioral medicine: Current status and future directions. *Journal of Consulting and Clinical Psychology, 50,* 1004–1017.

Martin, J.E., & Dubbert, P.M. (1982b). Exercise and health: The adherence problem. *Behavioral Medicine Update, 4,* 17–24.

Martin, J.E., Dubbert, P.M., Katell, A.D., Thompson, J.K., Raczynski, J.R., Lake, M., Smith, P.O., Webster, J.S., Sikova, T., & Cohen, R.E. (1984). The behavioral control of exercise in sedentary adults: Studies 1–6. *Journal of Consulting and Clinical Psychology, 52,* 795–811.

Martinsen, E.W. (1987a). The role of aerobic exercise in the treatment of depression. *Stress Medicine, 3,* 93–100.

Martinsen, E.W. (1987b). Exercise and medication in the psychiatric patient. In W.P. Morgan & S.E. Goldston (Eds.), *Exercise and mental health* (pp. 85–95). Washington, DC: Hemisphere.

Martinsen, E.W. (1990). Benefits of exercise for the treatment of depression. *Sports Medicine, 9,* 380–389.

Martinsen, E.W. (1994). Physical activity and depression: Clinical experience. *Acta Psychiatrica Scandinavica Supplement, 377,* 23–27.

Martinsen, E.W., Hoffart, A., & Solberg, Ø. (1989a). Comparing aerobic and nonaerobic exercise in the treatment of clinical depression: A randomized trial. *Comprehensive Psychiatry, 30,* 324–331.

Martinsen, E.W., Hoffart, A., & Solberg, Ø. (1989b). Aerobic and non-aerobic forms of exercise in the treatment of anxiety disorders. *Stress Medicine, 5,* 115–120.

Martinsen, E.W., & Medhus, A. (1989). Exercise adherence and patients' evaluation of exercise in a comprehensive treatment programme for depression. *Nordic Journal of Psychiatry, 43,* 521–529.

Martinsen, E.W., Medhus, A., & Sandvik, L. (1985). Effects of aerobic exercise on depression: A controlled study. *British Medical Journal, 291,* 109.

Martinsen, E.W., Sandvik, L., & Kolbjomsrüd, O.B. (1989). Aerobic exercise in the treatment of nonpsychotic mental disorders. *Nordic Journal of Psychiatry, 43,* 411–415.

Martinsen, E.W., Strand, J., Paulsson, G., & Kaggestad, J. (1989). Physical fitness in patients with anxiety and depressive disorders. *International Journal of Sports Medicine, 10,* 58–61.

Matthews, K.A., Weiss, S.M., Detre, T., Dembroski, T.M., Falkner, B., Manuck, S.B., & Williams, R.B. (1986). *Handbook of stress, reactivity & cardiovascular disease.* New York: John Wiley & Sons.

Maynert, E.W., & Levi, R. (1964). Stress-induced release of brain norepinephrine and its inhibition by drugs. *Journal of Pharmacology and Experimental Therapy, 143*, 90–95.

Mazzeo, R.S. (1991). Catecholamine responses to acute and chronic exercise. *Medicine and Science in Sports and Exercise, 23*, 839–845.

McCann, I.L., & Holmes, D.S. (1984). Influence of aerobic exercise on depression. *Journal of Personality and Social Psychology, 46*, 1142–1147.

McCubbin, J.A., Cheung, R., Montgomery, T.B., Bulbulian, R., & Wilson, J.F. (1992). Aerobic fitness and opioidergic inhibition of cardiovascular stress reactivity. *Psychophysiology, 29*, 687–697.

McCulloch, T.L., & J.S. Bruner (1939). The effect of electric shock upon subsequent learning in the rat. *Journal of Psychology, 7*, 333–336.

McDonald, D.G., & Hodgdon, J.A. (1991). *The psychological effects of aerobic fitness training: Research and theory.* New York: Springer-Verlag.

McGowan, R.W., Pierce, E.F., Eastman, N., Tripathi, H.L., Dewey, T., & Olson, K. (1993). Beta-endorphins and mood states during resistance exercise. *Perceptual and Motor Skills, 76*, 376–378.

McGowan, R.W., Pierce, E.G., & Jordan, D. (1991). Mood alterations with a single bout of physical activity. *Perceptual and Motor Skills, 72*, 1203–1209.

McMenamy, R.H. (1965). Binding of indole analogues to human serum albumin. Effects of fatty acids. *Journal of Biological Chemistry, 24*, 4235–4243.

McMurray, R.G., Sheps, D.S., & Guinan, D.M. (1984). Effects of naloxone on maximal stress testing in females. *Journal of Applied Physiology, 56*, 436–440.

McNair, D.M., Lorr, M., & Droppleman, L.F. (1971). *Profile of mood state manual.* San Diego: Educational and Industrial Testing Service.

McNair, D.M., Lorr, M., & Droppleman, L.F. (1981). *Profile of mood state manual.* San Diego: Educational and Industrial Testing Service.

McNair, D.M., Lorr, M., & Droppleman, L.F. (1992). *Profile of mood state manual.* San Diego: Educational and Industrial Testing Service.

McPhillips, J.B., Pellettera, K.M., Barrett-Connor, E., Wingard, D.L., & Criqui, M.H. (1989). Exercise patterns in a population of older adults. *American Journal of Preventive Medicine, 5*, 65–72.

Meeusen, R., Thoren, K., Chaouloff, F., Sarre, S., DeMerleir, K., Ebinger, G., & Michotte, Y. (1996, in press). Effects of trytophan and/or acute running on extracellular 5-HT and 5-HIAA levels in the hippocampus of food-deprived rats. *Brain Research.*

Meichenbaum, D., & Turk, D.C. (1987). *Facilitating a treatment adherence: A practitioner's handbook.* New York: Plenum Publishing Corp.

Melamed, B.G., & Siegel, L.J. (1975). Reduction of anxiety in children facing hospitalization and surgery by use of filmed modeling. *Journal of Consulting and Clinical Psychology, 43*, 511–521.

Mellergard, P., & Nordstrom, C.H. (1990). Epidural temperature and possible intracerebral temperature gradients in man. *British Journal of Neurosurgery, 4*, 31–39.

Mellerowicz, H., & Barron, D.K. (1971). Overtraining. In L.A. Larson (Ed.), *Encyclopedia of sport sciences and medicine* (pp. 1310–1312). New York: Macmillan.

Menzaghi, F., Heinrichs, S.C., Pich, E.M., Weiss, F., & Koob, G.F. (1993). The role of limbic and hypothalamic corticotropin-releasing factor in behavioral responses to stress. *Annals of the New York Academy of Sciences, 82*, 142–154.

Messer, B., & Harter, S.V. (1986). *Manual for the adult self-perception profile.* Denver: University of Denver Press.

Messick, S. (1989). Validity. In R.L. Linn (Ed.), *Educational measurement* (3rd ed., pp. 13–104). New York: Macmillan.

Metzger, J.M., & Stein, E.A. (1984). β-endorphin and sprint training. *Life Sciences, 34*, 1541–1547.

Meyer, A.J., Nash, J.D., McAlister, A.L., Maccoby, N., & Farquhar, J.W. (1980). Skills training in a cardiovascular health education campaign. *Journal of Consulting and Clinical Psychology, 48,* 129–142.

Michael-Titus, A., Dourmap, N., Caline, H., Costentin, J., & Schwartz, J.C. (1989). Role of endogenous enkephalins in locomotion and nociception studied with peptidase inhibitors in two inbred strains of mice (C57BL/6J and DBA/2J). *Neuropharmacology, 28,* 117–122.

Michael, E.R. (1961). Overtraining in athletics. *Journal of Sports Medicine and Physical Fitness, 1,* 99.

Michaels, R.R., Huber, M.J., & McCann, D.S. (1976). Evaluation of transcendental meditation as a method of reducing stress. *Science, 192,* 1242–1244.

Middleton, H.C., Maisley, D.N., & Mills, I.H. (1987). Do antidepressants cause postural hypotension by blocking cardiovascular reflexes? *European Journal of Clinical Pharmacology, 31,* 647–653.

Miller, E.B., Pain, R.W., & Skripal, P.J. (1978). Sweat lithium in manic-depression. *British Journal of Psychiatry, 133,* 477–478.

Mills, J.L. (1993). Data torturing. *New England Journal of Medicine, 329,* 1196–1199.

Mills, P.J., & Dimsdale, J.E. (1991). Cardiovascular reactivity to psychosocial stressors: A review of the effects of beta-blockade. *Psychosomatics, 32,* 209–220.

Mitchell, J.H., & Schmidt, R.F. (1983). Cardiovascular reflex control by afferent fibers from skeletal muscle receptors. In J.T. Shepherd & F.M. Abboud (Eds.), *Handbook of physiology, The cardiovascular system* (pp. 623–658). Washington, DC: American Physiological Society.

Mizutani, M., Hashimoto, R., Ohta, T., Nakazawa, K., & Nagatsu, T. (1994). The effect of exercise on plasma biopterin levels. *Neuropsychobiology, 29,* 53–56.

Mogenson, G.J., Brudzynski, S.M., Wu, M., Yang, C.R., & Yim, C.C.Y. (1993). From motivation to action: A review of dopaminergic regulation of limbic→nucleus accumbens→ventral pallidum→pedunculopontine nucleus circuitries involved in limbic-motor integration. In P.W. Kalivas & C.D. Barnes (Eds.), *Limbic motor circuits and neuropsychiatry.* Boca Raton, FL: CRC Press.

Mole, P.A., Stern, J.S., Schultz, C.L., Bernauer, E.M., & Holcomb, B.J. (1989). Exercise reverses depressed metabolic rate produced by severe caloric restriction. *Medicine and Science in Sports and Exercise, 21,* 29–33.

Molnar, G.W., & Read, R.C. (1974). Studies during open-heart surgery on the special characteristics of rectal temperature. *Journal of Applied Physiology, 36,* 333–336.

Mondin, G.W., Morgan, W.P., Piering, P.N., Stegner, A.J., Stotesbery, C.L., Trine, M.R., & Wu. M.-Y. (1996). Psychological consequences of exercise deprivation in habitual exercisors. *Medicine and Science in Sports and Exercise, 28.*

Montgomery, S.A., & Åsberg, M. (1979). A new depression scale designed to be sensitive to change. *British Journal of Psychiatry, 134,* 382–389.

Moore, J. (1984). On behaviorism, knowledge, and causal explanation. *Psychological Record, 34,* 73–97.

Morgan, W.P. (1968a). Selected physiological and psychomotor correlates of depression in psychiatric patients. *Research Quarterly, 39,* 1037–1043.

Morgan, W.P. (1968b). Hyperponetic states and psychopathology: A review. *American Corrective Therapy Journal, 22,* 165–167.

Morgan, W.P. (1969a). Physical fitness and emotional health: A review. *American Corrective Therapy Journal, 23,* 124–127.

Morgan, W.P. (1969b). A pilot investigation of physical working capacity in depressed and non-depressed psychiatric males. *Research Quarterly, 40,* 859–861.

Morgan, W.P. (1970a). Physical fitness correlates of psychiatric hospitalization. In G.S. Kenyon (Ed.), *Contemporary psychology of sport.* Chicago: Athletic Institute.

Morgan, W.P. (1970b). Physical working capacity in depressed and non-depressed psychiatric females: A preliminary study. *American Corrective Therapy Journal, 24,* 14–16.

Morgan, W.P. (1972). Basic considerations. In W.P. Morgan (Ed.), *Ergogenic aids in muscular performance* (pp. 3–31). New York: Academic Press.

Morgan, W.P. (1973a). Psychological factors influencing perceived exertion. *Medicine and Science in Sports and Exercise, 5,* 97–103.

Morgan, W.P. (1973b). Efficacy of psychobiologic inquiry in the exercise and sport sciences. *Quest, 20,* 39–47.

Morgan, W.P. (1973c, January). Influence of acute physical activity on state anxiety. *Proceedings of the National College Physical Education Meetings,* 113–121.

Morgan, W.P. (1974). Exercise and mental disorders. In A.J. Ryan & F.L. Allman, Jr. (Eds.), *Sports medicine* (pp. 671–674). New York: Academic Press.

Morgan, W.P. (1977, January). Involvement in vigorous physical activity with special reference to adherence. *Proceedings, of the National College Physical Education Association,* 235–246.

Morgan, W.P. (1978). Sport personology: The credulous-skeptical argument in perspective. In W.F. Straub (Ed.), *Sport psychology: An analysis of athlete behavior.* Ithaca, NY: Mouvement Publications.

Morgan, W.P. (1979a). Negative addiction in runners. *The Physician and Sportsmedicine, 7,* 57–70.

Morgan, W.P. (1979b). Anxiety reduction following acute physical activity. *Psychiatric Annals, 9,* 36–45.

Morgan, W.P. (1981). Psychological benefits of physical activity. In F.J. Nagle & H.J. Montoye (Eds.), *Exercise, health, and disease* (pp. 299–314). Springfield, IL: Charles C Thomas.

Morgan, W.P. (1982). Psychological effects of exercise. *Behavioral Medicine Update, 4,* 25–30.

Morgan, W.P. (1984). Physical activity and mental health. In H. Eckert & H.J. Montoye (Eds.), *The Academy papers* (pp. 132–145). Champaign, IL: Human Kinetics Publishers.

Morgan, W.P. (1985a). Affective beneficence of vigorous physical activity. *Medicine and Science in Sports and Exercise, 17,* 94–100.

Morgan, W.P. (1985b). Selected psychological factors limiting performance: A mental health model. In D.H. Clarke & H.M. Eckert (Eds.), *Limits of human performance* (pp. 70–80). Champaign, IL: Human Kinetics Publishers.

Morgan, W.P. (1987). Reduction of state anxiety following acute physical activity. In W.P. Morgan & S.E. Goldston (Eds.), *Exercise and mental health* (pp. 105–109). New York: Hemisphere Publishing, Inc.

Morgan, W.P. (1991). Monitoring and prevention of the staleness syndrome. *Proceedings of the Second IOC World Congress on Sport Sciences* (pp. 19–23). Barcelona: Plaza & Janés Editores, S.A.

Morgan, W.P. (1994a). Psychological components of effort sense. *Medicine and Science in Sports and Exercise, 26,* 1071–1077.

Morgan, W.P. (1994b). Physical activity, fitness and depression. In C. Bouchard, R.J. Shephard, & T. Stephens (Eds.), *Physical activity, fitness and health* (pp. 851–867). Champaign, IL: Human Kinetics Publishers.

Morgan, W.P. (1995). Anxiety and panic in recreational scuba divers. *Sports Medicine, 20,* 398–421.

Morgan, W.P., & Borg, G. (1976). Perception of effort in the prescription of physical activity. In T. Craig (Ed.), *The humanistic and mental health aspects of sports, exercise, and recreation.* Chicago: American Medical Association.

Morgan, W.P., Brown, D.R., Raglin, J.S., O'Connor, P.J., & Ellickson, K.A. (1987). Psychological monitoring of overtraining and staleness. *British Journal of Sports Medicine, 21,* 107–114.

Morgan, W.P., & Costill, D.L. (1996). Selected psychological characteristics and health behaviors of aging marathon runners: A longitudinal study. *International Journal of Sports Medicine, 17,* 305–312.

Morgan, W.P., Costill, D.L., Flynn, M.G., Raglin, J.S., & O'Connor, P.J. (1988). Mood disturbance following increased training in swimmers. *Medicine and Science in Sports and Exercise, 20,* 408–414.

Morgan, W.P., & Ellickson, K.A. (1989). Health, anxiety and physical exercise. In C.D. Spielberger & D. Hackbart (Eds.), *Anxiety in sports: An international perspective.* Washington, DC: Hemisphere.

Morgan, W.P., & Goldston, S.E. (Eds.) (1987). *Exercise and Mental Health.* Washington, DC: Hemisphere.

Morgan, W.P., & Hammer, W.M. (1974). Influence of competitive wrestling upon state anxiety. *Medicine and Science in Sports, 6*, 58–61.

Morgan, W.P., & Horstman, D.H. (1978). Psychometric correlates of pain perception. *Perceptual and Motor Skills, 47*, 27–39.

Morgan, W.P., & Horstman, D.H., Cymerman, A., & Stokes, J. (1980). Exercise as a relaxation technique. *Primary Cardiology, 6*, 48–57.

Morgan, W.P., & O'Connor, P.J. (1988). Exercise and mental health. In R.K. Dishman (Ed.), *Exercise adherence: Its impact on public health* (pp. 91–121). Champaign, IL: Human Kinetics Publishers.

Morgan, W.P., & O'Connor, R.J. (1989). Psychological effects of exercise and sports. In A.J. Ryan & F. Allman (Eds.), *Sports medicine* (pp. 671–689). Orlando, FL: Academic Press.

Morgan, W.P., O'Connor, P.J., Ellickson, K.A., & Bradley, P.W. (1988). Personality structure, mood states, and performance in elite male distance runners. *International Journal of Sport Psychology, 19*, 247–263.

Morgan, W.P., O'Connor, P.J., & Koltyn, K.F. (1990). Psychological benefits of physical activity through the life span: Methodological issues. In R. Telama (Ed.), *Physical education and lifelong physical activity* (pp. 65–72). Jyvaskyla, Finland: Reports of Physical Culture and Health.

Morgan, W.P., O'Connor, P.J., Sparling, P.B., & Pate, R.R. (1987). Psychological characterization of the elite female distance runner. *International Journal of Sports Medicine, 8*(Suppl. 2), 124–131.

Morgan, W.P., Olson, E.B., Jr., & Pedersen, N.P. (1982). A rat model of psychopathology for use in exercise science. *Medicine and Science in Sports and Exercise, 14*, 91–100.

Morgan, W.P., & Pollock, M.L. (1978). Physical activity and cardiovascular health: Psychological aspects. In F. Landry & W. Orban (Eds.), *Physical activity and human well-being* (pp. 163–181). Miami: Symposia Specialists.

Morgan, W.P., & Raven, W.P. (1985). Prediction of distress for individuals wearing industrial respirators. *American Industrial Hygiene Association Journal, 46*, 363–368.

Morgan, W.P., Roberts, J.A., Brand, F.R., & Feinerman, A.D. (1970). Psychological effect of chronic physical activity. *Medicine and Science in Sports, 2*, 213–217.

Morgan, W.P., Roberts, J.A., & Feinerman, A.D. (1971). Psychologic effect of acute physical activity. *Archives of Physical Medicine and Rehabilitation, 52*, 422–425.

Morris, J.N., Clayton, D.G., Everitt, M.G., Semmence, A.M., & Burgess, E.H. (1990). Exercise in leisure time: Coronary attach and death rates. *British Heart Journal, 63*, 325–334.

Morrison, J.K. (1980). The public's current beliefs about mental illness: Serious obstacles to effective community psychology. *American Journal of Community Psychology, 8*, 697–707.

Moses, J., Steptoe, A., Mathews, A., & Edwards, S. (1989). The effects of exercise training on mental well-being in the normal population: A controlled trial. *Journal of Psychosomatic Research, 33*, 47–61.

Mougin, C., Baulayy, A., Henriet, M.T., Haton, D., Jacquier, M.C., Turnill, D., Berthelay, S., & Gallard, R.C. (1987). Assessment of plasma opioid peptides, β-endorphin and met-enkephalin, at the end of an international nordic ski race. *European Journal of Applied Physiology, 56*, 281–286.

Mougin, C., Henriet, M.T., Baulay, A., Haton, D., Berthelay, S., & Gaillard, R.C. (1988). Plasma levels of beta-endorphin, prolactin and gonadotropins in male athletes after an international nordic ski race. *European Journal of Applied Physiology, 57*, 425–429.

Muñoz, R.F., Holon, S.D., McGrath, E., Rehm, L.P., & VandenBos, G.R. (1994). On the AHCPR *Depression in Primary Care* guidelines: Further considerations for practitioners. *American Psychologist, 49*, 42–61.

Murphy, S.M., Fleck, S.T., Dudley, G., & Callister, R. (1990). Psychological and performance concomitants of increased training volume in elite athletes. *Journal of Applied Sport Psychology, 2*, 34–50.

Mutrie, N. (1988). Exercise as a treatment for moderate depression in the UK health service. In *Sport, health, psychology and exercise*. Symposium conducted at the Bisham Abbey National Sports Centre, Buckinghamshire, England.

Nabeshima, T., Kamei, H., & Kameyama, T. (1988). Opioid κ receptors correlate with the development of conditioned suppression of motility in mice. *European Journal of Applied Physiology, 152*, 129–133.

Nadel, E.R., & Horvath, S.M. (1970). Comparison of tympanic membrane and deep body temperatures in man. *Life Science, 9*, 869–875.

National Institute of Mental Health. (1995). *Statistical Reports* (Publication OM-00–4000). Rockville, MD: Author.

Nelson, T.F., & Morgan, W.P. (1994). Acute effects of exercise on mood in depressed female students. *Medicine and Science in Sports and Exercise, 26*(Suppl.), 156.

Newsholme, E.A., Blomstrand, E., McAndrew, N., & Parry-Billings, M. (1992). Biochemical causes of fatigue and overtraining. In R.J. Shephard & P.O. Astrand (Eds.), *Endurance in sport* (pp. 351–364). London: Blackwell Scientific Publications, Inc.

Newton, L.E., Hunter, G., Bammon, M., & Roney, R. (1993). Changes in psychological state and self-reported diet during various phases of training in competitive bodybuilders. *Journal of Strength and Conditioning Research, 7*, 153–158.

Nicoloff, G., & Schwenk, T.L. (1995). Using exercise to ward off depression. *The Physician and Sportsmedicine, 23*, 44–57.

Nielsen, B., & Jessen, C. (1992). Evidence against brain-stem cooling by face fanning in severely hyperthermic humans. *Pflugers Archives, 422*, 168–172.

Nolen-Hoeksema, S., & Morrow, J. (1993). Effects of rumination and distraction on naturally occurring depressed mood. *Cognition and Emotion, 7*, 561–570.

Norman, R.M.G. (1986). The nature and correlates of health behavior. *Health promotion studies: Series No. 2*. Ottawa, Canada: Health and welfare.

Norman, T.C., Mathews, W., & Yohe C.D. (1987). A case study on the effects of strenous exercise on serum lithium levels. *Nebraska Medical Journal, 72*, 224–225.

Norris, R., Carroll, D., & Cochrane, R. (1992). The effects of physical activity and exercise training on psychological stress and well-being in an adolescent population. *Journal of Psychsomatic Medicine, 36*, 55–65.

North, T.C., McCullagh, P., & Tran, Z.V. (1990). Effects of exercise on depression. *Exercise and Sport Sciences Reviews, 18*, 379–415.

Nouri, S., & Beer, J. (1989). Relations of moderate physical exercise to scores on hostility, aggression, and trait-anxiety. *Perceptual and Motor Skills, 68*, 1191–1194.

O'Connor, P.J., Bryant, C.X., Veltri, J.P., & Gebhardt, S.M. (1993). State anxiety and ambulatory blood pressure following resistance exercise in females. *Medicine and Science in Sports and Exercise, 25*, 516–521.

O'Connor, P.J., Carda, R.D., & Graf, B.K. (1991). Anxiety and intense running exercise in the presence and absence of interpersonal competition. *International Journal of Sports Medicine, 12*, 423–426.

O'Connor, P.J., & Davis, J.C. (1992). Psychobiologic responses to exercise at different times of the day. *Medicine and Science in Sports and Exercise, 24*, 714–719.

O'Connor, P.J., Morgan, W.P., & Raglin, J.S. (1991). Psychobiologic effects of 3 days of increased training in female and male swimmers. *Medicine and Science in Sports and Exercise, 23*, 1055–1061.

O'Connor, P.J., Morgan, W.P., Raglin, J.S., Barksdale, C.M., & Kalin, N.H. (1989). Mood state and salivary cortisol levels following overtraining in female swimmers. *Psychoneuroendocrinology, 14*, 303–310.

O'Connor, P.J., Petruzzelo, S.J., Kubitz, K.A., & Robinson, T.L. (1995). Anxiety responses to maximal exercise testing. *British Journal of Sports Medicine, 29*, 97–102.

O'Connor, P.J., & Youngstedt, S.D. (1995). Influence of exercise on human sleep. In J.O. Holloszy (Ed.), *Exercise and sport sciences reviews* (Vol. 23, pp. 105–134). Baltimore: Williams & Wilkins.

Ojanen, M. (1994). Can the true effects of exercise on psychological variables be separated from placebo effects? *International Journal of Sport Psychology, 25*, 63–80.

Oldridge, N.G. (1982). Compliance and exercise in primary and secondary prevention of coronary heart disease: A review. *Preventive Medicine, 11*, 56–70.

Oldridge, N.G., Donner, A., Buck, C.W., Jones, N.L., Anderson, G.A., Parker, J.O, Cunningham, D.A., Kavanagh, T., Rechnitzer, P.A., & Sutton, J.R. (1983). Predictive indices for dropout: The Ontario Exercise Heart Collaborative Study experience. *American Journal of Cardiology, 51*, 70–74.

O'Leary, K.D., & Borkovec T.D. (1978). Conceptual, methodological, and ethical problems of placebo groups in psychotherapy research. *American Psychologist, 33*, 821–830.

Olehansky, M.A., Zoltick, J.M., Herman, R.H., Mougey, E.H., & Meyerhoff, J.L. (1990). The influence of fitness on neuroendocrine responses to exhaustive treadmill exercise. *European Journal of Pharmacology, 59*, 405–410.

Olson, E.B., Jr., & Morgan, W.P. (1982). Rat brain monoamine levels related to behavioral assessment. *Life Sciences, 30*, 2095–2100.

Olson, G.A., Olson, R.D., Kastin, A.J., & Coy, D.H. (1982). Endogenous opiates: 1981. *Peptides, 3*, 1039–1072.

Oltras, C.M., Mora, F., & Vives, F. (1987). Beta-endorphin and ACTH in plasma: Effects of physical and psychological stress. *Life Sciences, 40*, 1683–1686.

Orne, M.T. (1962). On the social psychology of the psychological experiment: With particular reference to demand characteristics and their implications. *American Psychologist, 17*, 776–783.

Ossip-Klein, D.J., Doyne, E.J., Bowman, E.D., Osborn, K.M., McDougall-Wilson, I.B., & Neimeyer, R.A. (1989). Effects of running or weight lifting on self-concept in clinically depressed women. *Journal of Consulting and Clinical Psychology, 57*, 158–161.

Owen, N., Lee, C., Naccarrella, L., & Haag, K. (1987). Exercise by mail: A mediated behavior-change program for aerobic exercise. *Journal of Sport Psychology, 9*, 346–357.

Paffenbarger, R.S., Hyde, R.T., Wing, A.L., & Hsieh, C. (1986). Physical activity, all-cause mortality, and longevity of college alumni. *New England Journal of Medicine, 314*, 605–613.

Paffenbarger, R.S., Jr., Hyde, R.T., Wing, A.L., & Steinmetz, C.H. (1984). A natural history of athleticism and cardiovascular health. *Journal of the American Medical Association, 252*, 491–495.

Paffenbarger, R.S., Jr., Lee, I-M., & Leung, R. (1994). Physical activity and personal characteristics associated with depression and suicide in American college men. *Acta Psychiatrica Scandinavia, (Suppl 377)*, 16–22.

Panksepp, J. (1990). The psychoneurology of fear: Evolutionary perspectives and the role of animal models in understanding human anxiety. In G.D. Burrows, M. Roth, & R. Noyes, Jr. (Eds.), *Handbook of anxiety* (Vol. 3, pp. 3–58). Amsterdam: Elsevier Science Publishing Co., Inc.

Parmenter, D.C. (1923). Some medical aspects of the training of college athletes. *Boston Medical and Surgical Journal, 189*, 45–50.

Parry-Billings, M., Budgett, R., Koutedakis, Y., Blomstrand, E., Brooks, S., Williams, C., Calder, P.C., Pilling, S., Baigrie, R., & Newsholme, E.A. (1992). Plasma amino acid concentrations in the overtraining syndrome: Possible effects on the immune system. *Medicine and Science in Sports and Exercise, 24*, 1353–1358.

Pate, R.R., Pratt, M., Blair, S.N., Haskell, W.L., Macera, C.A., & Bouchard, C. (1995). Physical activity and public health: A recommendation from the Centers for Disease Control and the American College of Sports Medicine. *Journal of the American Medical Association, 273*, 402–407.

Paterson, S.J., Robson, L.E., & Kosterlitz, H.W. (1983). Classification of opioid receptors. *British Medical Bulletin, 39*, 31–36.

Patten, S. (1990). Propanolol and depression: Evidence from antihypertension trials. *Canadian Journal of Psychiatry, 35*, 257–259.

Paulhus, D.L. (1991). Measurement and control of response bias. In J.P. Robinson, P.R. Shaver, & L. Wrightsman (Eds.), *Measures of personality and social-psychological attitudes* (pp. 17–59). San Diego: Academic Press.

Pender, N.J., Sallis, J.F., Long, B.J., & Calfas, K.J. (1994). Health care provider counseling to promote physical activity. In R.K. Dishman (Ed.), *Advances in exercise adherence* (pp. 213–235). Champaign, IL: Human Kinetics Publishers.

Peronnet, F., Cleroux, J., Perrault, H., Cousineau, D., De Champlain, J., & Nadeau, R. (1981). Plasma norepinephrine response to exercise before and after training in humans. *Journal of Applied Physiology, 51*, 812–815.

Peronnet, F., & Szabo, A. (1993). Sympathetic response to acute psychosocial stressors in humans: Linkage to physical exercise and training. In P. Seraganian (Ed.), *Exercise psychology: The influence of physical exercise on psychological processes* (pp. 172–217). New York: John Wiley & Sons, Inc.

Persson, S., Jonsdottir, I., Thoren, P., Post, C., Nyberg, F., & Hoffmann, P. (1993). Cerebrospinal fluid dynorphin-converting enzyme activity is increased by voluntary exercise in the spontaneously hypertensive rat. *Life Sciences, 53*, 643–652.

Peters, E.M., & Bateman, E.D. (1983). Ultramarathon running and upper respiratory tract infections. *South African Journal of Medicine, 64*, 582–584.

Peterson, L., & Ridley-Johnson, R. (1980). Pediatric hospital response to survey on prehospital preparation for children. *Journal of Pediatric Psychology, 5*, 1–7.

Peterson, L., & Shigetomi, C. (1981). The use of coping techniques to minimize anxiety in hospitalized children. *Behavior Therapy, 12*, 1–14.

Petruzello, S.J., & Landers, D.M. (1994). State anxiety reduction and exercise: Does hemispheric activation reflect such changes? *Medicine and Science in Sports and Exercise, 26*, 1028–1035.

Petruzello, S.J., Landers, D.M., Hatfield, B.D., Kubitz, K.A., & Salazar, W. (1991). A meta-analysis on the anxiety reducing effects of acute and chronic exercise: Outcomes and mechanisms. *Sports Medicine, 11*, 142–182.

Petruzello, S.J., Landers, D.M., & Salazar, W. (1993). Exercise and anxiety reduction: Examination of temperature as an explanation for affective change. *Journal of Sport and Exercise Psychology, 15*, 63–76.

Peyrin, L. (1990). Urinary MHPG sulfate as a marker of central norepinephrine metabolism: A commentary. *Journal of Neural Transmitters, 80*, 51–65.

Piepoli, M., & Coats, A.J.S. (1994). Effects of exercise on the autonomic control of the heart: Training or overtraining? *Cardiovascular Research, 28*, 141–142.

Pitts, F.N., & McClure, J.N. (1967). Lactate metabolism in anxiety neurosis. *New England Journal of Medicine, 277*, 1329–1336.

Plante, T.G., & Rodin, J. (1990). Physical fitness and enhanced psychological health. *Current Psychology: Research & Reviews, 9*, 3–24.

Plotsky, P.M., Cunningham, E.T., Jr., & Widmaier, E.P. (1989). Catecholaminergic modulation of corticotropin-releasing factor and adrenocorticotropin secretion. *Endocrine Reviews, 10*, 437–458.

Plummer, O.K., & Koh, Y.O. (1987). Effect of "aerobics" on self-concepts of college women. *Perceptual and Motor Skills, 65*, 271–275.

Plutchik, R., Platarnan, S.R., & Fieve, R.R. (1969). Three alternatives to the double-blind. *Archives of General Psychiatry, 20*, 428–432.

Polivy, J. (1994). Physical activity, fitness, and compulsive behaviors. In C. Bouchard, R.J. Shephard, & T. Stephens (Eds.), *Physical activity, fitness, and health* (pp. 868–882). Champaign, IL: Human Kinetics Publishers.

Pollock, M.L. (1988). Prescribing exercise for fitness and health. In R.K. Dishman (Ed.), *Exercise adherence: Its impact on public health* (pp. 259–277). Champaign, IL: Human Kinetics Publishers.

Pollock, M.L., Carroll. J.F., Graves, J.E., Leggett, S.H., Braith, R.W., Limacher, M., & Hagberg, J.M. (1991). Injuries and adherence to walk/jog and resistance programs in the elderly. *Medicine and Science in Sports and Exercise, 23*, 1194–1200.

Pollock, M.L., Gettman, L.R., Milesis, C.A., Bah, M.D., Durstine, L., & Johnson, R.B. (1977). Effects of frequency and duration of training on attrition and incidence of injury. *Medicine and Science in Sports, 9*, 31–36.

Porsolt, R.D., LePichon, M., & Jalfre, M. (1977). Depression: A new animal model sensitive to antidepressant treatments. *Nature, 226*, 730–732.

Post, R.M., Kotin, J., Goodwin, F.K., & Gordon, E.K. (1973). Psychomotor activity and cerebrospinal fluid amine metabolites in affective illness. *American Journal of Psychiatry, 130*, 67–72.

Powell, K.E., & Blair, S.N. (1994). The public health burdens of sedentary living habits. Theoretical but realistic estimates. *Medicine and Science in Sports and Exercise, 26,* 851–856.

Powell, K.E., & Paffenbarger, R.S., Jr. (1985). Workshop on epidemiologic and public health aspects of physical activity and exercise: A summary. *Public Health Reports, 100,* 118–126.

Powell, K.E., Spain, K.G., Christenson, G.M., & Mollenkamp, M.P. (1986). The status of the 1990 objectives for physical fitness and exercise. *Public Health Reports, 10,* 15–21.

Powell, K.E., Thompson, P.D., Caspersen, C.J., & Kendrick, J.S. (1987). Physical activity and the incidence of coronary heart disease. *Annual Review of Public Health, 8,* 353.

Powles, A.C.P. (1981). The effects of drugs on the cardiovascular response to exercise. *Medicine and Science in Sports and Exercise, 13,* 252–258.

Prange, A.J. (1964). The pharmacology and biochemistry of depression. *Diseases of the Nervous System, 25,* 217–221.

Prochaska, J.O., & DiClemente, C.C. (1983). The stages and processes of self-change in smoking: Towards an integrative model of change. *Journal of Consulting in Clinical Psychology, 51,* 390–395.

Prochaska, J.O., & Marcus, B.H. (1994). The transtheoretical model: The applications to exercise. In R.K. Dishman (Ed.), *Advances in exercise adherence* (pp. 161–180). Champaign, IL: Human Kinetics Publishers.

Prochaska, J.O., Velicer, W.F., DiClemente, C.C., & Fava, J. (1988). Measuring processes of change: Applications to the cessation of smoking. *Journal of Consulting and Clinical Psychology, 56,* 520–528.

Purvis, J.W., & Morgan, W.P. (1978). Influence of repeated maximal testing on anxiety and work capacity in college women. *Research Quarterly, 49,* 512–519.

Radosevich, P.M., Nash, J.A., Lacy, D.B., O'Donovan, C., Williams, P.E., & Abumrad, N.N. (1989). Effects of low- and high-intensity exercise on plasma and cerebrospinal fluid levels of ir-β-endorphin, ACTH, cortisol, norepinephrine and glucose in the conscious dog. *Brain Research, 498,* 89–98.

Raglin, J.S. (1990). Exercise and mental health: Beneficial and detrimental effects. *Sports Medicine, 9,* 323–329.

Raglin, J.S. (1992). Anxiety and sport performance. In J.O. Holloszy (Ed.), *Exercise and sport sciences reviews* (pp. 243–274). Baltimore: Williams & Wilkins.

Raglin, J.S. (1993). Overtraining and staleness: Psychometric monitoring of endurance athletes. In R.B. Singer, M. Murphey, & L.K. Tennent (Eds.), *Handbook of research on sport psychology* (pp. 840–850). New York: Macmillan.

Raglin, J.S., Eksten, F, & Garl, T. (1995). Mood state responses to a pre-season conditioning program in male collegiate basketball players. *International Journal of Sport Psychology, 26,* 214–225.

Raglin, J.S., & Morgan, W.P. (1985). Influence of vigorous exercise on mood states. *Behavior Therapist, 8,* 179–183.

Raglin, J.S., & Morgan, W.P. (1987). Influence of exercise and quiet rest on state anxiety and blood pressure. *Medicine and Science in Sports and Exercise, 19,* 456–463.

Raglin, J.S., & Morgan, W.P. (1994). Development of a scale for use in monitoring training-induced distress in athletes. *International Journal of Sports Medicine, 15,* 84–88.

Raglin, J.S., Morgan, W.P., & Luchsinger, A.E. (1990). Mood and self-motivation in female rowers. *Medicine and Science in Sports and Exercise, 22,* 849–853.

Raglin, J.S., Morgan, W.P., & O'Connor, P.J. (1991) Changes in mood state during training in female and male college swimmers. *International Journal of Sports Medicine, 12,* 585–589.

Raglin, J.S., Stager, J.M., Koceja, D.M., & Harms, C.A. (1996). Changes in mood state, neuromuscular function, and performance during a season of training in female collegiate swimmers. *Medicine and Science in Sports and Exercise, 28,* 372–377.

Raglin, J.S., Turner, P.E., & Eksten, F. (1993). State anxiety and blood pressure following 30 min of leg ergometry or weight training. *Medicine and Science in Sports and Exercise, 25,* 1044–1048.

Raglin, J.S., & Wilson. M. (1996). State anxiety following 20-min of leg ergometry at differing intensities. *International Journal of Sports Medicine, 17,* 467–471.

Rainey, D., & Wigtil, J. (1985). Aerobic running as a counseling technique for undergraduates with low self-esteem. *Journal of College Student Personnel, 16*, 53–57.

Randall, W.C., Rawson, R.O., McCook, R.C., & Peiss, C.N. (1963). Central and peripheral factors in dynamic thermo-regulation. *Journal of Applied Physiology, 18*, 61–64.

Ransford, C.P. (1982). A role for amines in the antidepressant effect of exercise: A review. *Medicine and Science in Sports and Exercise, 14*, 1–10.

Rappaport, J. (1977). *Community psychology: Values, research, and action.* New York: Holt, Rinehart & Winston.

Rawson, R.O., & Hammell, H.T. (1963). Hypothalamic and tympanic membrane temperature in rhesus monkey. *Federation Proceedings, 22*, 283.

Redmond, D.E. (1985). Neurochemical basis for anxiety and anxiety disorders: Evidence from drugs which decrease human fear or anxiety. In A.H. Tuma & J.D. Maser (Eds.), *Anxiety and the anxiety disorders* (pp. 533–555). Hillsdale, NJ: Lawrence Erlbaum Associates.

Reeves, D.L., Levison, D.M., Justesen, D.R., & Lubin, B. (1985). Endogenous hyperthermia in normal human subjects: Experimental study of emotional states (II). *International Journal of Psychosomatics, 32*, 18–23.

Regier, D.A., Boyd, J.H., Burke, J.D., Rae, D.S., Myers, J.K., Kramer, M., Robins, L.N., George, L.K., Karno, M., & Locke, B.Z. (1988). One-month prevalence of mental disorders in the United States. *Archives of General Psychiatry, 45*, 977–986.

Rejeski, W.J., Hardy, C.J., & Shaw, J. (1991). Psychometric confounds of assessing state anxiety in conjunction with bouts of vigorous exercise. *Journal of Sport and Exercise Psychology, 13*, 65–74.

Rezvani, A.H., Gordon, C.J., & Heath, J.E. (1982). Action of preoptic injections of Bendorphin on temperature regulation in rabbits. *American Journal of Physiology, 243*: R104–R111.

Roberts, A.H., Kewman, D.G., Mercier, L., & Hovell, M. (1993). The power of nonspecific effects in healing: Implications for psychosocial and biological treatments. *Clinical Psychology Review, 13*, 375–391.

Roberts, A.C., McClure, R.D., Weiner, R.I., & Brooks, G.A. (1993). Overtraining affects male reproductive status. *Fertility and Sterility, 60*, 686–692.

Roberts, J.A., & Morgan, W.P. (1971). Effect of type and frequency of participation in physical activity upon physical working capacity. *American Corrective Therapy Journal, 25*, 99–104.

Robins, H.I., Dennis, W.H., Neville, A.J., Hvgander, A., Shecterle, L.M., Martin, P.A., Grossman, J., Gillis, W., Steeves, R.A., & Davis, T.E. (1985). Whole body hyperthermia clinical trials. *Proceedings of the Seventh Annual Conference of the IEEE Engineering in Medicine and Biology Society*, Chicago: IEEE.

Robins, H.I., Kalin, N.H., Shelton, S.E., Martin, P.A., Schecterle, L.M., Barksdale, C.M., Neville, A.J., & Marshall, J. (1987). Rise in plasma beta-endorphin, ACTH and cortisol in cancer patients undergoing whole-body hyperthermia. *Hormonal and Metabolic Research, 19*, 441–443.

Robins, H.I., Kalin, N.H., Shelton, S.E., Schecterle, L.M., Barksdale, C.M., Martin, P.A., & Marshall, J. (1987). Neuro-endocrine changes in patients undergoing whole-body hyperthermia. *International Journal of Hyperthermia, 3*, 99–105.

Roethlisberger, F.J., & Dickson, W.J. (1939). *Management and the worker.* Cambridge, MA: Harvard University Press.

Rohles, F.H., Nevins, R.G., & Springer, W.E. (1967). Temporal characteristics of body temperature during high thermal stress. *Journal of Aerospace Medicine, 38*, 286–290.

Romanowski, W., & Grabiec, S. (1974). The role of serotonin in the mechanism of central fatigue. *Acta Physiologica Polonica, 25*, 127–134.

Rose, G. (1969). Physical activity and coronary heart disease. *Proceedings of the Royal Society of Medicine, 62*, 1183.

Rosen, G. (1958). *A history of public health.* New York: MD Publications.

Rosenberg, M. (1979). *Conceiving the self.* New York: Basic Books.

Rosenthal, R. (1966). *Experimenter effects in behavioral research.* New York: Meredith Publishing.

Rosenthal, R. (1991). *Meta-analytic procedures for social research.* Beverly Hills, CA: Sage Publications.

Rosenthal, R., & Rosnow, R.L. (1969). *Artifact in behavioral research.* New York: Academic Press.

Rosenthal, R., & Rosnow, R.L. (1975). *The volunteer subject.* New York: John Wiley & Sons, Inc.

Roth, D.L. (1989). Acute emotional and psychological effects of aerobic exercise. *Psychophysiology, 26*, 593–602.

Rowland, T.W. (1986). Exercise fatigue in adolescents: Diagnosis of athlete burnout. *The Physician and Sportsmedicine, 14*, 69–77.

Rueter, M., Mutrie, N., & Harris, D. (1982). *Running as an adjunct to counseling in the treatment of depression.* Master's thesis. State College, PA: The Pennsylvania State University.

Rusko, H.K., Härkönen, M., & Pakarinen, A. (1994). Overtraining effects on hormonal and autonomic regulation in young cross-country skiers. *Medicine and Science in Sports and Exercise, 26*, S64.

Ryan, A.J. (1983). Overtraining of athletes: A round table. *The Physician and Sportsmedicine, 11*, 93–110.

Sable, D.L., Brammell, H.L., Sheehan, M.W., Nies, A.S., Gerber, J., & Horwitz, L.D. (1982). Attenuation of exercise conditioning by beta-adrenergic blocade. *Circulation, 65*, 679–684.

Sachar, E.J. (1985). Disorders of feeling: Affective diseases. In E.R. Kandel & J.H. Schwartz (Eds.), *Principles of neural science* (2nd ed., pp. 717–725). New York: Elsevier.

Sallis, J.F., Haskell, W.L., Fortmann, S.P., Vranizan, K.M., Taylor, C.B., & Solomon, D.S. (1986). Predictors of adoption and maintenance of physical activity in a community sample. *Preventive Medicine, 15*, 331–341.

Sallis, J.F., & Hovell, M.F. (1990). Determinants of exercise behavior. *Exercise and Sport Sciences Reviews, 18*, 307–330.

Sallis, J.F., Hovell, M.F., & Hofstetter, C.R. (1992). Predictors of adoption and maintenance of vigorous physical activity in men and women. *Preventive Medicine, 21*, 237–251.

Sallis, J.F., Hovell, M.F., Hofstetter, C.R., Elder, J.P., Faucher, P., Spry, V.M., Barrington, E., & Hackley, M. (1990). Lifetime history of relapse from exercise. *Addictive Behaviors, 15*, 573–579.

Sallis, J.F., Hovell, M.F., Hofstetter, C.R., Faucher, P., Elder, J.P., Blanchard, J., Caspersen, C.J., Powell, K.E., & Christenson, G.M. (1989). A multivariate study of determinants of vigorous exercise in a community sample. *Preventive Medicine, 18*, 20–34.

Sallis, J.F., Hovell, M.F., Hofstetter, C.R., Elder, J.P., Hackley, M., Caspersen, C.J., & Powell, K.E. (1990). Distance between homes and exercise facilities related to frequency of exercise among San Diego residents. *Public Health Reports, 105*, 179–185.

Sallis, J.F., Simons-Marton, B.J., Stone, E.J., Corbin, C.B., Epstein, L.H., Faucette, N., Iannoti, R.J., Killen, J.D., Klesges, R.C., Petray, C.K., Rowland, T.W., & Taylor, W.C. (1992). Determinants of physical activity and interventions in youth. *Medicine and Science in Sports and Exercise, 24*, 5248–5257.

Sanghera, M.K., & German, D.C. (1983). The effects of benzodiazepine anxiolytics on locus coeruleus unit activity. *Journal of Neural Transmitters, 57*, 267–275.

Sapolsky, R.M., Krey, L.C., & McEwen, B.S. (1984). Stress down-regulates corticosterone receptors in a site-specific manner in the brain. *Endocrinology, 114*, 287–292.

Sarbin, T.R., & Mancuso, J.C. (1970). Failure of a moral enterprise: Attitudes of the public toward mental illness. *Journal of Consulting and Clinical Psychology, 35*, 159–173.

Schildkraut, J.J. (1975). Catecholamine metabolism and affective disorders: studies of MHPG excretion. In E. Usdin & S. Snyder (Eds.), *Frontiers in catecholamine research* (pp. 1165–1171). New York: Pergamon Press.

Schildkraut, J.J., Orsulak, P.J., Schatzberg, A.F., & Rosenbaum, A.H. (1983). Relationship between psychiatric diagnostic groups of depressive disorders and MHPG. In J.W Maas (Ed.), *MHPG basic mechanisms and psychopathology* (pp. 129–144). New York: Academic Press.

Schlicht, W. (1994). Does physical exercise reduce anxious emotions? A meta-analysis. *Anxiety, Stress, and Coping, 6*, 275–288.

Schwarz, L., & Kindermann, W. (1990). 13-endorphin, adrenocorticotropic hormone, cortisol and catecholamines during aerobic and anaerobic exercise. *European Journal of Applied Physiology, 61*, 165–171.

Seals, D.R. (1991). Sympathetic neural adjustments to stress in physically training and untrained humans. *Hypertension, 17*, 36–43.

Segura, R., & Ventura, J.L. (1988). Effect of L-tryptophan supplementation on exercise performance. *International Journal of Sports Medicine, 9*, 301–305.

Seraganian, P. (1993). *Exercise psychology*. London: Wiley-Interscience.

Sexton, H., Mære, Å., & Dahl, N.H. (1989). Exercise intensity and reduction of neurotic symptoms: A controlled follow-up study. *Acta Psychiatrica Scandinavia, 80*, 231–235.

Sforzo, G.A., Seeger, T.F., Pert, C.B., Pert, A., & Dotson, C.O. (1986). In vivo opioid receptor occupation in the rat brain following exercise. *Medicine and Science in Sports and Exercise, 18*, 380–384.

Shaikh, M.B., Lu, C.L., & Siegel, A. (1991). An enkephalinergic mechanism involved in amygdaloid suppression of affective defence behavior elicited from the midbrain periaqueductal gray in the cat. *Brain Research, 559*, 109–117.

Sharkey, B.J. (1970). Intensity and duration of training and the development of cardiorespiratory endurance. *Medicine and Science in Sports and Exercise, 2*, 197–202.

Sharkey, B.J., & Holleman, J.P. (1967). Cardiorespiratory adaptations to training at specified intensities. *The Research Quarterly, 38*, 698–704.

Sharp, N.C.C., & Koutedakis, Y. (1992). Sport and the overtraining syndrome: Immunological aspects. *British Medical Bulletin, 48*, 518–533.

Shephard, R.J. (1968). Intensity, duration, and frequency of exercise as determinants of the response to a training regime. *International Z Angew Physiology einschl Arbeitsphysiology, 26*, 272–278.

Shephard, R.J. (1990). Cost and benefits of an exercising versus a non-exercising society. In C. Bouchard, R.J. Shephard, T. Stephens, J.R. Sutton, & B.D. McPherson (Eds.), *Exercise, fitness, and health: A consensus of current knowledge* (pp. 49–60). Champaign, IL: Human Kinetics Publishers.

Sherman, W.M., & Maglischo, E.W. (1991). Minimizing chronic athletic fatigue among swimmers: Special emphasis on nutrition. *Gatorade Sports Science Institute's Sports Science Exchange, 4*, 1–5.

Sherman, A.D., & Petty, F. (1982). Additivity of neurochemical changes in learned helplessness. *Behavior and Neural Biology, 35*, 344–353.

Sherman, A.D., Sacwuitne, J.L., & Petty, F. (1982). Selectivity of the learned helplessness model of depression. *Pharmacology and Biochemistry Behavior, 16*, 449–454.

Shimomitsu, T. (1993). The relation between plasma changes in B-endorphin level and mood states after ultraendurance exercise. *Journal of the Tokyo Medical College, 51*, 116–124.

Shippenberg, T.S., Bals-Kubik, R., & Herz, A. (1987). Motivational properties of opioids: Evidence that an activation of δ-receptors mediates reinforcement processes. *Brain Research, 436*, 234–239.

Shopsin, B., Gershon, S., Goldstein, M., Friedman, E., & Wilk, S. (1975). Use of synthesis inhibitors in defining a role for biogenic amines during imipramine treatment in depressed patients. *Psychopharmacology, 1*, 239–249.

Shyu, B.C., Andersson, S.A., & Thoren, P. (1982). Endorphin mediated increase in pain threshold induced by long-lasting exercise in rats. *Life Sciences, 30*, 833–840.

Shyu, B.C., & Thoren, P. (1986). Circulatory events following spontaneous muscle exercise in normotensive and hypertensive rats. *Acta Physiolgica Scandinavica, 128*, 515–524.

Siever, L.J., & Davis, K.L. (1985). Overview toward a dysregulation hypothesis of depression. *American Journal of Psychiatry, 142*, 1017–1031.

Silva, J.M. (1990). An analysis of the training stress syndrome in competitive athletics. *Journal of Applied Sport Psychology, 2*, 5–20.

Sime, W.E. (1977). A comparison of exercise and mediation in reducing physiological response to stress. *Medicine and Science in Sports and Exercise, Suppl. 9*, 55.

Sime, W.E. (1977). A comparison of exercise and meditation in reducing physiological response to stress. *Medicine and Science in Sports and Exercise, Suppl. 9*, 55.

Sime, W.E. (1987). Exercise in the treatment and prevention of depression. In W.P. Morgan & S.E. Goldston (Eds.)., *Exercise and mental health* (pp. 145–152). Washington, DC.

Simons, C.W., & Birkimer, J.C. (1988). An exploration of factors predicting the effects of aerobic conditioning on mood state. *Journal of Psychosomatic Research, 32*, 63–75.

Simons, A.D., McGowan, C.R., Epstein, L.H., Kupfer, D.J., & Robertson, R.J. (1985). Exercise as a treatment for depression: An update. *Chemical Psychology Review, 5,* 553–568.

Singh, N.P., Despars, J.A., Stansbury, D.W., Avalos, K., & Light, R.W. (1993). Effects of buspirone on anxiety levels and exercise tolerance in patients with chronic airflow obstruction and mild anxiety. *Chest, 103,* 800–804.

Skinner, J.S., Baldini, F.D., & Gardner, A.W. (1990). Assessment of fitness. In C. Bouchard, R.J. Shephard, T. Stephens, J.R. Sutton, & B.D. McPherson (Eds.), *Exercise, fitness and health: A consensus of current knowledge* (pp. 63–70). Champaign, IL: Human Kinetics Publishers.

Smith, M.L., Hudson, D.L., Graitzer, H.M., & Raven, P.B. (1989). Exercise training bradycardia: The role of autonomic balance. *Medicine and Science in Sports and Exercise, 21,* 40–44.

Smith, R.E. (1993). A positive approach to enhancing sport performance: Principles of positive reinforcement and performance feedback. In J.M. Williams (Ed.), *Applied sport psychology: Personal growth to peak performance* (pp. 25–35). Mountain View, CA: Mayfield Publishing.

Smith, D.F. (1973). The effect of exercise on renal clearance of lithium, sodium, potassum and creatinine in the rat. *International Pharmacopsychiatry, 8,* 217–220.

Smoak, B., Deuster, P., Rabin, D., & Chrousos, G. (1991). Corticotropin-releasing horrnone is not the sole factor mediating exercise-induced adrenocorticotropin release in humans. *Journal of Clinical Endocrinology and Metabolism, 73,* 302–306.

Snodgrass, J.G., Levy-Berger, G., & Haydon, M. (1985). *Human experimental psychology.* New York: Oxford University Press.

Snow-Harter, C., & Marcus, R. (1991). Exercise bone mineral density, and osteoporosis. *Exercise and Sport Sciences Reviews, 19,* 351–388.

Snyder, A.C., Jeukendrup, A.E., Hesselink, M.K.C., Kuipers, H., & Foster, C. (1993). A physiological/psychological indicator of over-reaching during intensive training. *International Journal of Sports Medicine, 14,* 29–32.

Somers, V.K., Leo, K.C., Shields, R., Clary, M., & Mark, A.L. (1992). Forearm endurance training attenuates sympathetic nerve response to isometric handgrip in normal humans. *Journal of Applied Physiology, 72,* 1039–1043.

Sonstroem, R.J. (1976). The validity of self-perceptions regarding physical and athletic ability. *Medicine and Science in Sports and Exercise, 8,* 126–132.

Sonstroem, R, J. (1978). Physical estimation and attraction scales: Rationale and research. *Medicine and Science in Sports, 10,* 97–102.

Sonstroem, R.J. (1984). Exercise and self-esteem. *Exercise and Sport Sciences Reviews, 12,* 23–155.

Sonstroem, R.J. (1988). Psychological models. In R.K. Dishman (Ed.), *Exercise adherence: Its impact on public health* (pp. 125–154). Champaign, IL: Human Kinetics Publishers.

Sonstroem, R.J. (1995). Improving compliance with exercise programs. In J.S. Torg & R.J. Shephard (Eds.), *Current therapy in sports medicine* (3rd ed., pp. 608–611). St. Louis: Mosby-Year Book, Inc.

Sonstroem, R.J., Harlow, L.L., Gemma, L.M., & Osborne, S. (1991). Test of structural relationships within a proposed exercise and self-esteem model. *Journal of Personality Assessment, 56,* 348–364.

Sonstroem, R.J., Harlow, L.L., & Josephs, L. (1994). Exercise and self-esteem: Validity of model expansion and exercise associations. *Journal of Sport and Exercise Psychology, 16,* 29–42.

Sonstroem, R.J., Harlow, L.L., & Salisbury, K.A. (1993). Path analysis of a self-esteem model across a competitive swim season. *Research Ouarterly for Exercise and Sport, 64,* 335–342.

Sonstroem, R.J., & Kampper, K.P. (1980). Prediction of athletic participation in middle school males. *Research Quarterly for Exercise and Sport, 51,* 685–694.

Sonstroem, R.J., & Morgan, W.P. (1989). Exercise and self-esteem: Rationale and model. *Medicine and Science in Sports and Exercise, 21,* 329–337.

Sonstroem, R.J., Speliotis, E.D., & Fava, J.L. (1992). Perceived physical competence in adults: An examination of the Physical Self-Perception Profile. *Journal of Sport and Exercise Psychology, 14,* 207–221.

Sothmann, M.S. (1991). Catecholamines, behavioral stress, and exercise: Introduction to the symposium. *Medicine and Science in Sports and Exercise, 23*, 836–838.

Sothmann, M.S., Blaney, J., & Woulfe, T. (1990). Plasma free and sulfoconjugated catecholamines during sustained exercise. *Journal of Applied Physiology, 68*, 452–456.

Sothmann, M.S., & Ismail, A.H. (1985). Factor analytic derivation of the MHPG/NM ratio. Implications for studying the link between physical fitness and depression. *Biology and Psychiatry, 20*, 570–583.

Spanagel, R., Herz, A., Bals-Kubik, R., & Shippenberg, T.S. (1991). β-endorphhin-induced locomotor stimulation and reinforcement are associated with an increase in dopamine release in the nucleus accumbens. *Psychopharmacology, 104*, 51–56.

Spielberger, C.D. (1972). Anxiety as an emotional state. In C.D. Spielberger (Ed.), *Anxiety: Current trends in theory and research* (Vol. 1., pp. 23–49). New York: Academic Press.

Spielberger, C.D. (1983). *Manual for the State-Trait Anxiety Inventory (form Y)*. Palo Alto, CA: Consulting Psychologists Press, Inc.

Spielberger, C.D. (1989). Stress and anxiety in sports. In D. Hackfort & C.D. Spielberger (Eds.), *Anxiety in sports: An international perspective* (pp. 3–17). New York: Hemisphere Publishers, Inc.

Spitzer, R.L., Endicott, J., & Robins, E. (1978). Research diagnostic criteria. *Archives of General Psychiatry, 35*, 773–782.

Stachenfeld, N.S., Gleim, G.W., & Nicholas, J.A. (1992). Endurance training. How much is too much? *The Physician and Sportsmedicine, 20*, 129–132.

Stalonas, P.M., Jr., Johnson, W.G., & Christ, M. (1978). Behavior modification for obsesity: The evaluation of exercise, contingency management, and program adherence. *Journal of Consulting and Clinical Psychology, 46*, 463–469.

Stein, J.M., Papp, L.A., Klein, D.F., Cohen, S., Simon, J., Ross, D., Martinez, J., & Gorman, J.M. (1992). Exercise tolerance in panic disorder patients. *Biological Psychiatry, 32*, 281–287.

Stein, P.N., & Motta, R.W. (1992). Effects of aerobic and nonaerobic exercise on depression and self-concept. *Perceptual and Motor Skills, 74*, 79–89.

Steinhardt, M.A., & Young, D.R. (1992). Psychological attributes of participants and non-participants in a worksite health and fitness center. *Behavioral Medicine, 18*, 40–46.

Stemmler, G. (1989). The autonomic differentiation of emotions revisted: Convergent and discriminant validation. *Psychophysiology, 26*, 617–632.

Stephens, T. (1988). Physical activity and mental health in the United States and Canada: Evidence from four population surveys. *Preventive Medicine, 17*, 35–47.

Stephens, T., & Craig, C.L. (1990). *The well-being of Canadians: Highlights of the 1988 Campbell's survey*. Ottawa: Canadian Fitness and Lifestyle Research Institute.

Steptoe, A., & Bolton, J. (1988). The short-term influence of high and low intensity physical exercise on mood. *Psychology and Health, 2*, 91–106.

Steptoe, A., & Cox, S. (1988). Acute effects of aerobic exercise on mood. *Health Psychology, 7*, 329–340.

Steptoe, A., Edwards, S., Moses, J., & Mathews, A. (1989). The effects of exercise training on mood and perceived coping ability in anxious adults from the general population. *Journal of Psychosomatic Research, 33*, 537–547.

Stern, M.J., & Cleary, P. (1981). Psychosocial changes observed during a low-level exercise program. *Archives of Internal Medicine, 141*, 1463–1467.

Stern, M.J., & Cleary, P. (1982). The national exercise and heart disease project: Long-term psychosocial outcome. *Archives of Internal Medicine, 142*, 1093–1097.

Stewart, A.L., King, A.C., & Haskell, W.L. (1993). Endurance exercise and health-related quality of life in 50–65-year-old adults. *The Gerentologist*, 782–789.

Stone, E.A., & Platt, J.E. (1982). Brain noradrenergic receptors and resistance to stress. *Brain Research, 237*, 405–414.

Stone, E.A. (1973). Accumulation and metabolism of NE in rat hypothalamus after exhautive stress. *Journal of Neurochemistry, 21*, 589–601.

Stone, M.H., Keith, R.E., Kearney, J.T., Fleck, S.H., Wilson, G.D., & Triplett, N.T. (1991). Overtraining: A review of the signs, symptoms and possible causes. *Journal of Applied Sport Science Research, 5*, 35–50.

Stotesbery, C.L., Stegner, A.J., Morgan, W.P. (1996). Influence of physical activity performed in a naturalistic setting on anxiety and depression. *Medicine and Science in Sports and Exercise*, Suppl. *26*, 29.

Stratton, J.R., & Halter, J.B. (1985). Effect of a benzodiazepine (Alprazolam) on plasma epinephrine and norepinephrine levels during exercise stress. *Cardiovascular Pharmacology, 56*, 136–139.

Strom-Olsen, R., & Weil-Malherbe, H. (1958). Humoral changes in manic-depressive psychosis with particular reference to the excretion of catecholamines in urine. *Journal of Mental Science, 104*, 696–704.

Sulser, F., Ventulani, J., & Mobley, P. (1978). Mode of action of antidepressant drugs. *Biochemistry and Pharmacology, 27*, 257–261.

Svedenhag, J., Wallin, B.G., Sundlof, G., & Henriksson, J. (1984). Skeletal muscle sympathetic activity at rest in trained and untrained subjects. *Acta Physiologica Scandinavica, 120*, 499–504.

Tanabe, K., & Takauri, S. (1964). Effects of cooling and warming the common carotid arteries on the brain and tympanic temperatures in the rabbit. *Japanese Journal of Pharmacology, 14*, 67–79.

Taylor, C.B., King, R., Ehlers, A., Margraf, J., Clark, D., Hayward, C., Roth, W.T., & Agras, S. (1987). Treadmill exercise test and ambulatory measures in panic attacks. *American Journal of Cardiology, 60*, 48J-52J.

Taylor, C.B., Sallis, J.F., & Needle, R. (1985). The relation of physical activity and exercise to mental health. *Public Health Reports, 100*, 195–202.

Tendzegolskis, Z., Viru, A., & Orlova, E. (1991). Exercise-induced changes of endorphin contents in hypothalamus, hypophysis, adrenals and blood plasma. *International Journal of Sports Medicine, 12*, 495–497.

Tharp, G.D., & Barnes, M.W. (1990). Reduction of saliva immunoglobulin levels by swim training. *European Journal of Applied Physiology, 60*, 61–64.

Tharp, G.D., & Carson, W.H. (1975). Emotionality changes in rats following chronic exercise. *Medicine and Science in Sports, 7*, 123–126.

Thayer, R.E. (1967). Towards a theory of multidimensional activation (arousal). *Motivation and Emotion, 2*, 1–34.

Thomas, L. (1977). On the science and technology of medicine. In J.H. Knowles (Ed.), *Doing better and feeling worse: Health in the United States*. New York: W.W. Norton & Co.

Thompson, C.D., & Martin, J.E. (1984). Exercise in health modification: Assessment and training guidelines. *The Behavior Therapist, 7*, 5–8.

Thoreau, H.D. (1978). In R. Epstein & S. Phillips (Eds.) *The natural man: A Thoreau Anthology*. Wheaton, IL: The Theosophical Publishing House.

Thoren, P., Floras, J.S., Hoffmann, P., & Seals, D.R. (1990). Endorphins and exercise: Physiological mechanisms and clinical implications. *Medicine and Science in Sports and Exercise, 22*, 417–428.

Thorndike, E.L. (1920). A constant error in psychological ratings. *Journal of Applied Psychology, 4*, 25–29.

Trine, M.R., & Morgan, W.P. (1995). Influence of time of day on psychological responses to exercise: A review. *Sports Medicine, 20*, 328–337.

Trine, M.R., & Morgan, W.P. (1996, in press). Influence of time of day on the anpiolytic effects of exercise. *International Journal of Sports Medicine*.

Tuomisto, J., & Mannisto, P. (1985). Neurotransmitter regulation of anterior pituitary hormones. *Pharmacology Review, 37*, 249–332.

Turk, D.C., Rudy, T.E., & Salovey, P. (1984). Health protection: Attitudes and behaviors of LPNs, teachers, and college students. *Health Psychology, 3*, 189–210.

Udenfriend, S. (1958). Metabolism of 5-hydroxytryptamine. In G.P. Lewis (Ed.), *5-Hydroxytryptamine: Proceedings of a Symposium Held in London on 1st-2nd April 1957* (pp. 43–49). New York: Pergamon Press.

Udenfriend, S., & Dairman, W. (1971). Regulation of norepinephrine synthesis. In G. Weber (Ed.), *Advances in enzyme regulation* (Vol. 9, pp. 145–165). Oxford: Pergamon Press.

Ungerstedt, U. (1971). Stereotaxic mapping of the monoamine pathway in the rat brain. *Acta Physiologica Scandinavica, 367*, 1–48.

U.S. Department of Health and Human Services & Public Health Service. (1990). *Healthy people 2000: National health promotion and disease prevention objectives.* Washington, DC: U.S. Government Printing Office.

Uusitupa, M., Aro, A., & Pietkainen, M (1980). Severe hypoglycaemia caused by physical strain and pindolol therapy. *Annals of Clinical Research, 12*, 25–27.

Vailas, A.C., Morgan, W.P., & Vailas, J.C. (1990). Physiologic and cellular basis of overtraining. In W.B. Leadbetter, J.A. Buckwalter, & S.L. Gordon (Eds.), *Inflammation and healing of sports induced soft tissue injury* (pp. 677–686). American Orthopaedic Society.

Valenstein, E.S. (1986). *Great and desperate cures.* New York: Basic Books.

Valentino, R.J. (1988). Corticotropin-releasing factor (CRF) and physiological stressors alter activity of rat noradrenergic locus coeruleus (LC) neurons in a similar manner. *Journal of Cell Biochemistry, (Suppl. 12D)*, 317.

Van Dale, D., Saris, W.H.M., & Ten Hoor, F. (1990). Weight maintenance and resting metabolic rate, 18–40 months after a diet/exercise treatment. *International Journal of Obesity, 14*, 347–359.

Vanhees, L., Fagard, R., Amery, A. (1982). Influence of beta adrenergic blocade of effects of physical training in patients with ischemic heart disease. *British Heart Journal, 48*, 33–38.

Veale, D.M.W. (1991). Psychological aspects of staleness and dependence on exercise. *International Journal of Sports Medicine, 12*(Suppl. 1.), S19-S22.

Veith, R.C., Raskind, M.A., Caldwell, J.H., Barnes, R.F., Gumbrecht, G., & Rithie, J.L. (1982). Cardiovascular effects of tricyclic antidepressants in depressed patients with chronic heart disease. *New England Journal of Medicine, 306*, 954–959.

Velicer, W.F., DiClemente, C.C., Prochaska, J.O., & Brandenburg, N. (1989). A decisional balance measure for assessing and predicting smoking status. *Journal of Personality and Social Psychology, 48*, 1279–1289.

Verde, T., Thomas, S., & Shephard, R.J. (1992). Potential markers of heavy training in highly trained distance runners. *British Journal of Sports Medicine, 26*, 167–175.

Viegener, B.J., Perri, M.G., Nezu, A.M., Renjilian, D.A., McKelvey, W.F., & Schein, R.L. (1990). Effects of an intermittent, low-fat, low-calorie diet in the behavioral treatment of obesity. *Behavior Therapy, 21*, 499–509.

Viti, A., Lupo, C., Lodi, L., Bonifazi, M., & Martelli, G. (1989). Hormonal changes after supine posture, immersion and swimming. *International Journal of Sports Medicine, 10*, 402–405.

Vogel, G.R., Neill, D., Hagler, M., & Kors, D. (1990). A new animal model of endogenous depression: A summary of present finding. *Neuroscience and Biobehavioral Reviews, 14*, 85–91.

Vogt, M. (1954). The concentration of sympathin in different parts of the central nervous system under normal conditions and after administration of drugs. *Journal of Physiology (Cambridge), 154*, 52–67.

Vohra, J., Burrows, J.D., & Sloma, J. (1975). Assessment of cardiovascular side effects of therapeutic doses of tricyclic antidepressant drugs. *Australian and New Zealand Journal of Medicine, 5*, 7–11.

Volterra, A., Brunello, N., Cagiano, R., Cuomo, V., & Racagni, G. (1984). Behavioural and biochemical effects in C57BL/6J mice after a prolonged treatment with the δ-opiate antagonist ICI 154129. *Journal of Pharmacy and Pharmacology, 36*, 849–851.

von Euler, C., & Soderberg, V. (1957). The influence of hypothalamic thermoreceptive structures on the electro-encephalogram and gamma motor activity. *Electroencephalography and Clinical Neurophysiology, 9*, 391–408.

Vranic, M., & Wasserman, D. (1990). Exercise, fitness, and diabetes. In C. Bouchard, R.J. Shephard, T. Stephens, J. Sutton, & B. McPherson (Eds.), *Exercise, fitness and health: A consensus of current knowledge* (pp. 467–490). Champaign, IL: Human Kinetics Publishers.

Walker, J.M., Berntson, G.G., Paulucci, T.S., & Champney, T.C. (1981). Blockade of endogenous opiates reduces activity in the rat. *Pharmacology, Biochemistry and Behavior, 14*, 113–116.

Wang, Y., & Morgan, W.P. (1992). The effect of imagery perspectives on the psychophysiological responses to imagined exercise. *Behavioral Brain Research, 52*, 167–174.

Wankel, L.M., Yardley, J.K., & Graham, J. (1985). The effects of motivational interventions upon the exercise adherence of high and low self-motivated adults. *Canadian Journal of Applied Sport Sciences, 10,* 147–155.

Ward, A., & Morgan, W.P. (1984). Adherence patterns of healthy men and women enrolled in an adult exercise program. *Journal of Cardiac Rehabilitation, 4,* 143–152.

Watson, S.J., Khachaturian, H., Lewis, M.E., & Akil, H. (1986). Chemical neuroanatomy as a basis for biological psychiatry. In P.A. Berger & H.K.H. Brodie (Eds.), *Biological psychiatry* (pp. 4–33). New York: Basic Books.

Watson, G.S., Zador, P.L., & Wilks, A. (1980). The repeal of helmet use laws and increased motorcyclist mortality in the United States, 1975–1978. *American Journal of Public Health, 70,* 579–585.

Weisner, J.B., & Moss, R.L. (1986). Suppression of receptive and proceptive behavior in ovariectomized, estrogen-progesterone-primed rats by intraventricular beta-endorphin: Studies of behavioral specificity. *Neuroendocrinology, 43,* 57–62.

Weiss, J.M., Goodman, P.A., Losito, B.G., Corrigan, S., Charry, J.M., & Bailey, W.H. (1981). Behavioral depression produced by an uncontrollable stressor: Relationship to norepinephrine, dopamine, and serotonin levels in various regions of rat brain. *Brain Research, 3,* 167–205.

Weiss, J.M., & Simson, P.G. (1989). Electrophysiology of the locus coeruleus: Implications for stress-induced depression. In G.F. Koob, C.L. Ehlers, & D.J. Kupfer (Eds.), *Animal models of depression* (pp. 111–134). Boston: Birkhauser Boston, Inc.

Weiss, J.M., Simson, P.G., Hoffman, L.J., Ambrose, M.J., Cooper, S., & Webster, A. (1986). Infusion of adrenergic receptor agonists and antagonists into locus coeruleus and ventricular system of the brain: Effects on swim-motivated and spontaneous motor activity. *Neuropharmacology, 25,* 367–384.

Wells, L.E., & Marvell, G. (1976). *Self-esteem: Its conceptualization and measurement.* Newberry Park, CA: Sage Publications.

Wertz, A.L., Koltyn, K.F., & Morgan, W.P. (1992). The effects of acute exercise and relaxation on state anxiety, body awareness, and blood lactate. *Medicine and Science in Sports and Exercise, Vol. 24* (Suppl.), S149.

Wertz-Garvin, A., Trine, M.R., & Morgan, W.P. (1996). Affective and metabolic responses to autogenic relaxation and quiet rest in the seated and supine positions. *Medicine and Science in Sports and Exercise,* Suppl. *28,* 30.

Westhall, C. (1863). *The modern method of training for running, walking, rowing, & boxing. Including hints on exercise, diet, clothing and advice to trainers* (7th ed.). London: Ward, Lock and Taylor.

Whatmore, G.B., & Ellis, P.M. (1959). Some neurophysiologic aspects of depressed states: An electromyographic study. *Archives of General Psychiatry, 6,* 243–253.

Whitby, J.D., & Dunkin, L.J. (1971). Cerebral, esophageal and naso-pharyngeal temperatures. *British Journal of Anaesthesiology, 43,* 673–675.

White, J. (1994). Hoyfield's fatigue linked to his heart. *The Physician and Sportsmedicine, 14,* 69–77.

White, C.C., Powell, K.E., Hogelin, G.C., Gentry, E.M., & Forman, M.R. (1987). Behavioral risk factor surveys: IV. The descriptive epidemiology of exercise. *American Journal of Preventive Medicine, 3,* 304–310.

White, J.E., Dishman, R.K., Bunnell, B.N., Warren, G.L., Mougey, E.H., & Meyerhoff, J.L. (1993). Chronic treadmill training moderates plasma ACTH responses to homotypic and heterotypic stress. *Medicine and Science in Sports and Exercise, 25*(Suppl.), S91.

White, R.W. (1959). Motivation reconsidered: The concept of competence. *Psychological Review, 66,* 297–333.

White-Welkley, J.E., Bunnell, B., Mougey, E.H., Meyerhoff, J.L., & Dishman, R.K. (1995). Treadmill training and estradiol differentially modulate hypothalamic-pituitary-adrenal cortical responses to acute running and immobilization. *Physiology and Behavior, 57,* 533–540.

White-Welkley, Warren, G.L., Bunnell, B.N., Mougey, E.H., Meyerhoff, J.L., & Dishman, R.K. (1996). Treadmill exercise training and estradiol increase plasma ACTH and prolactin after novel footshock. *Journal of Applied Physiology, 80,* 931–939.

Whybrow, P.C., Akiskal, H.S., & McKinney, W.T., Jr. (1984). *Mood disorders: Toward a new psychobiology.* New York: Plenum Press.

Wildmann, J., Krüger, A., Schmole, M., Niemann, J., & Matthaei, H. (1986). Increase of circulating beta-endorphin-like immunoreactivity correlates with the change in feeling of pleasantness after running. *Life Sciences, 38*, 997–1003.

Wilfley, D., & Kunce, J. (1986). Differential physical and psychological effects of exercise. *Journal of Consulting Psychology, 33*, 337–342.

Williams, R.S., Eden, R.S., Moll, M.E., Lester, R.M., & Wallace, A.G. (1981). Autonomic mechanisms of training bradycardia:β-adrenergic receptors in humans. *Journal of Applied Physiology, 51*, 1232–1237.

Wilson, A., & Krane, R. (1980). Change in self-esteem and its effects on depression. *Cognitive Therapy and Research, 4*, 419–421.

Wilson, W.M., & Marsden, C.A. (1996). In vivo measurement of extracellular serotonin in the ventral hippocampus during treadmill running. *Behav. Pharmacol., 7*, 101–104.

Winder, W.W., Hagberg, J.M., Hickson, R.C., Ehsani, A.A., & McLane, J.A. (1978). Time course of sympathoadrenal adaptation to endurance exercise training in man. *Journal of Applied Physiology, 45*, 370–374.

Winder, W.W., Hickson, R.C., Hagberg, J.M., Ehsani, A.A., & McLane, J.A. (1979). Training-induced changes in hormonal and metabolic responses to submaximal exercise. *Journal of Applied Physiology, 46*, 766–771.

Wittig, A.F., Houmard, J.A., & Costill, D.L. (1989). Psychological effects during reduced training in distance runners. *International Journal of Sports Medicine, 10*, 97–100.

Wolf, J.G. (1971). Staleness. In L.A. Larson (Ed.), *Encyclopedia of sport sciences and medicine* (pp. 1048–1051). New York: MacMillan Publishing Company.

Wong, C.K., Lau, C.P., Leung, W.H., & Cheng, C.H. (1990). Usefulness of labetolol in chronic atrial fibrillation. *American Journal of Cardiology, 66*, 1212–1215.

Wood, P.D., Stefanick, M.L., Williams, P.T., & Haskell, W. (1991). The effects on plasma lipoproteins of a prudent weight-reducing diet with or without exercise in overweight men and women. *New England Journal of Medicine, 325*, 461–466.

Workman, E.A., & Short, D.D. (1993). Atypical antidepressants versus imipramine in the treatment of major depression: A meta-analysis. *Journal of Clinical Psychiatry, 54*, 5–12.

Wylie, R.C. (1979). *The self-concept: Theory and research in selected topics* (Vol. 2., Rev. ed.). Lincoln, NB: University of Nebraska Press.

Yao, T., Andersson, S., & Thoren, P. (1982a). Long-lasting cardiovascular depression induced by acupunture-like stimulation of the sciatic nerve in unanaesthetized spontaneously hypertensive rats. *Brain Research, 240*, 77–85.

Yao, T., Andersson, S., & Thoren, P. (1982b). Long-lasting cardiovascular depressor response following sciatic stimulation in spontaneously hypertensive rats: Evidence for the involvement of central endorphin and serotonin systems. *Brain Research, 244*, 295–303.

Yehuda, S., & Kastin, A.J. (1980). Peptides and thermoregulation. *Neuroscience Biobehavioral Review, 4*, 459–471.

Young, D.R., Haskell, W.L., Taylor, C.B., & Fortmann, S.P. (1996). Effect of community health education on physical activity knowledge, attitudes and behavior: the Stanford 5-city project. *American Journal of Epidemiology, 145*, 610–620.

Youngstedt, S.D., Dishman, R.K., Cureton, K.J., & Peacock, L.J. (1993). Does body temperature mediate anxiolytic effect of acute exercise? *Journal of Applied Physiology, 74*, 825–831.

Yusef, S., Wittes, J., & Friedman, L. (1988). Overview of results of randomized clinical trials in heart disease. Part I: Treatments following myocardial infarction. *Journal of the American Medical Association, 260*, 2088–2093.

Zarcharko, R.M., & Anisman, H. (1989). Pharmacological, biochemical, and behavioral analyses of depression. In G.F. Koob, C.L. Ehlers, & D.J. Kupfer (Eds.), *Animal models of depression* (pp. 204–238). Boston: Birkhauser.

Zastowny, T.R., Kirschenbaum, D.S., & Meng, I. (1986). Effects of stress inoculation training on children before, during, and after hospitalization for surgery. *Journal of Consulting and Clinical Psychology, 5*, 231–247.

Zifa, E., & Fillion, G. (1992). 5-hydroxytryptamine receptors. *Pharmacological Reviews, 44*, 401–458.

Zung, W.W.K. (1965). Self-Rating Depression Scale. *Archives of General Psychiatry, 12*, 63–70.

Zwiren, L.D., Freedson, P.S., Ward, A., Wilke, S., & Rippe, J.M. (1991). Estimation of VO_2max: A comparitive analysis of five exercise tests. *Research Quarterly for Exercise and Sport, 62*, 73–78.

Index

Printed in Great Britain
by Amazon

23145906R00170